T5-CVL-714

MEDICAL RADIOLOGY
Diagnostic Imaging

Editors:
A.L. Baert, Leuven
K. Sartor, Heidelberg
J.E. Youker, Milwaukee

Springer
Berlin
Heidelberg
New York
Barcelona
Hong Kong
London
Milan
Paris
Singapore
Tokyo

P. Rogalla · J. Terwisscha van Scheltinga
B. Hamm (Eds.)

Virtual Endoscopy and Related 3D Techniques

With Contributions by

A. J. Aschoff · C. I. Bartram · T. R. Fleiter · S. Gottschalk · R. Klingebiel · N. Meiri
E. M. Merkle · P. Rogalla · J. Terwisscha van Scheltinga · T. H. Wiese · C. Wisianowsky

Series Editor's Foreword by
A. L. Baert

With 189 Figures in 581 Separate Illustrations, 82 in Color

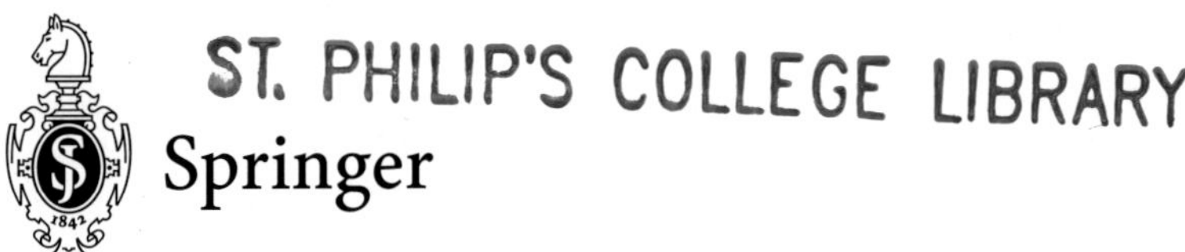

Springer

Patrik Rogalla, MD
Department of Radiology, Charité Hospital
Humboldt-Universität zu Berlin
Schumannstrasse 20/21
10117 Berlin
Germany

Jeroen Terwisscha van Scheltinga, MSc
Philips Medical Systems, Easy Vision Modules
P.O. Box 10000
5680 DA Best
The Netherlands

Bernd Hamm, MD
Professor, Department of Radiology, Charité Hospital
Humboldt-Universität zu Berlin
Schumannstrasse 20/21
10117 Berlin
Germany

Medical Radiology · Diagnostic Imaging and Radiation Oncology
Continuation of
Handbuch der medizinischen Radiologie
Encyclopedia of Medical Radiology

ISBN 3-540-65157-8 Springer-Verlag Berlin Heidelberg New York

Library of Congress Cataloging-in-Publication Data

Virtual endoscopy and related 3D techniques / P. Rogalla, J. Terwisscha van Scheltinga, B. Hamm (Eds.) ; with contributions by A. J. Aschoff ... [et al.].
p. ; cm. -- (Medical radiology)
Includes bibliographical references and index.
ISBN 3540651578 (alk. paper)
1. Endoscopic surgery. 2. Three-dimensional imaging in medicine. 3. Image processing--Computer programs. I. Rogalla, P. (Patrik) II. Terwisscha van Scheltinga, J. (Jeroen), 1966- III. Hamm, Bernd, Prof. Dr. IV. Series.
[DNLM: 1. Surgical Procedures, Endoscopic--methods. 2. Image Processing, Computer-Assisted--methods. 3. Tomography, X-Ray Computed--methods. WO 505 V819 2000]
RD33.53 . V57 2000
616.07'57--dc21 99-051749

Springer-Verlag Berlin Heidelberg New York
a member of BertelsmannSpringer Science+Business Media GmbH

Printed in Germany

Cover-Design and Typesetting: Verlagsservice Teichmann, 69256 Mauer

SPIN: 106 972 31 21/3130 – 5 4 3 2 1 0 – Printed on acid-free paper

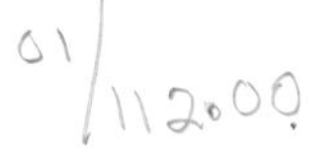

Foreword

The role and impact of computer technology on the clinical practice of radiology is becoming more important every day. Whereas more basic and theoretic research in this area is within the realm of computer engineers and physicists, an intense collaboration between these scientists and radiologists is necessary in order to develop the results evolving from basic research into tools that can be tested and implemented in the field of clinical imaging.

The exact place of three-dimensional reconstruction techniques within the spectrum of modern imaging methods remains to be determined.

The editors and contributing authors are outstanding specialists in the field of 3D imaging.

They have been able to provide radiologists in this volume with the latest information and should enable them to acquire a deeper insight about limits and possibilities of these new imaging methods.

I do hope that radiologists, internal medicine specialists and surgeons will find this volume a useful reference and a source to enlarge their knowledge and skills in 3D imaging.

I would appreciate every constructive criticism that might be offered.

Leuven ALBERT L. BAERT

Preface

Three-dimensional reconstruction techniques were introduced into diagnostic radiology more than 10 years ago, but were handicapped by strong artifacts and limited spatial resolution. At that time, the imaging modalities – mainly computed tomography with incremental scanning technology – were unable to acquire continuous, complete data, leading to pronounced stairstepping artifacts in the three-dimensional reconstructions, for instance of the bones. Furthermore, because the studies took a long time to perform, homogeneous contrasting of the vasculature was impossible without the administration of enormous amounts of contrast material.

Modalities providing continuous and complete data information have now become available: spiral computed tomography (spiral CT), electron beam tomography (EBT), and magnetic resonance imaging (MRI) with breathhold sequences. Using the source data from these modalities, high resolution, three dimensional volumetric reconstructions can be produced.

The difficulty in segmenting the structures to be visualised posed the primary problem in establishing a role for 3D images. As virtual endoscopy was introduced in the mid-1990s, it was also characterised by relatively poor image quality. With rapid technological improvements, mainly due to advanced software solutions, i.e. volume rendering techniques, the source of the data (CT, EBT, MRI) has decreased in importance. The key to diagnostic 3D reconstruction and virtual endoscopy lies in the contrast between various tissues, whichever imaging modality is used. As an example, superb 3D reconstructions and virtual endoscopy of the abdominal aorta can be calculated from CT or from MRI data with no noticeable difference in the resulting spatial 3D resolution and diagnostic yield.

The fact that all the diagnostic information is contained in the originally acquired cross sectional images has justifiably given rise to the question of whether or not 3D imaging and virtual endoscopy are, despite the very impressive views, superfluous in terms of the diagnostic information they supply. However, the production of a 3D image helps the radiologist and the clinician to put the numerous individual pieces together into a single picture. In this respect, 3D reconstruction and virtual endoscopy function as a data compressor, allowing the reader to focus on specific organs and findings, free from the mental task of reconstructing 2D into t3D images.

In many fields, radiologists are challenged by the necessity of continuing professional education and are required to adapt to a different approach to diagnostics. For example, how many radiologists have educational and practical experience with fibreoptic endoscopy of the colon? Often interpreted as a potential competitor or threat to true endoscopy, it should be remembered that virtual endoscopy is not intended to imitate and replace true endoscopy, but rather to complement it by providing additional supportive information. For example, virtual endoscopy allows visualization of the neighbouring structures outside the viewed organ, which assists in the localisation of pathology. Other methodological advantages are the ability to bypass an occluded or stenotic area and continue with the virtual visualization, viewing in a forward or reverse direction, and, finally, to provide an endoscopic picture of areas, such as the majority of the small intestine, that cannot be reached by true endoscopy.

As with all imaging modalities, it is important to also recognise the limitations of the technique in order to supply accurate patient assessments. Of particular importance is information regarding imaging and rendering artifacts – an issue that is still inadequately investigated and documented. At the present stage of development, virtual endoscopy portrays a static picture, it cannot supply information on the dynamic changes of organs. However, as the speed of the source modalities increases, the future could offer the possibility of including dynamic information in a virtual reconstruction – thus leading to true virtual reality.

As virtual endoscopy becomes more widely used and accepted in university as well as other hospitals, its value for visual demonstration of findings to clinical colleagues, and its great potential for enhancing education when creatively adopted as a teaching device for students and residents – even for clinicians will become irrefutable.

The main applications of virtual endoscopy are currently in the respiratory system, the intestinal tract – mainly the colon – and the vascular system, although its clinical and diagnostic roles in the latter are as yet unclear. Applications in the remaining areas of the body, such as the nose and paranasal sinuses, the urinary tract and the neurological system, are more or less experimental, but in the near future, likely to become routine. Alongside the improvements in the imaging modalities delivering the source data, rapid improvements in the software for three dimensional postprocessing appear to play a crucial part in the further maturation of virtual endoscopy. It can be expected that with increased hardware power, real-time navigation with excellent spatial resolution and true 3D visualization on dedicated screens will be an inevitable progression in the time to come.

The authors hope that this book will be an informative source for radiologists and other professionals and students in the field of medicine willing and able to approach innovation with an open mind. Although often a target of criticism, this fascinating field has drawn much interest from clinicians, researchers and technicians alike, who have worked together and continue to do so, allowing rapid development and progress. We hope we have succeeded in conveying this fascination and that this book will inspire our readers to continue broadening the horizons of this breathtaking new technique.

Berlin, Best

Patrik Rogalla
Jeroen Terwisscha van Scheltinga
Bernd Hamm

Contents

1 Technical Background

J. Terwisscha van Scheltinga

CONTENTS

J. Terwisscha van Scheltinga, MSc
Philips Medical Systems, Easy Vision Modules, P.O. Box 10000, 5680 DA Best, The Netherlands

1.1 Introduction

In recent years the computerized postprocessing of image data from cross-sectional imaging modalities has received progressively increasing recognition in the field of medicine. This development has various reasons. Firstly, the technical developments of examination modalities such as CT and MRI, as well as SPECT, PET, and ultrasound, have swiftly improved along with continuously increasing spatial resolution, which means not only a growing memory capacity for the computer, but also that additional image information is included in each slice. For any given volume, more slices can be produced in an ever-decreasing amount of time. Secondly, rapidly growing computer performance has created the opportunity to display complex relations, be it anatomical structures or functional information, in a simplified and comprehensible manner. For example, the new multislice CT scanners allow examination protocols of the chest which produce more than 500 slices per examination; in comparison, a chest CT 10 years ago with 10 mm slice thickness consisted of about 25 slices. The explanation for this impressive difference is the current capacity of the multislice CT scanner to produce a 1 mm slice thickness along with overlapping reconstruction intervals of 0.5 mm. In addition, modern modalities produce data sets which, when obtained in a single breathhold (in other words, without any pause or movement artifacts), represent the examined volume relatively well. Such data sets are therefore referred to as "volume data sets."

For years now, various postprocessing techniques have been available and are evaluated not only in terms of their ability to display anatomy and pathology, but also with respect to their ability to make the volume "viewable" to the viewer or radiologist in the shortest possible amount of time. In this case, "viewable" indicates not only that the interpretation of the image data must proceed within an economically effective time, but, moreover, that the viewer is enabled to recognize a pathological condition as a deviation from a normal variant. To refer back to the example of the thorax with 500 images: if each image were to be viewed before one could proceed to the next image, the viewer would require an enormous amount of time in order to sift through all the slices. An additional consideration is that since the expected variations from one image to the next are minimal, the danger arises that changes would not be recognized as such at all. Being able to appreciate all images in a movie-mode, as permitted by most workstations, represents only one of the numerous possibilities of overcoming this problem and allowing effective evaluation of volume data sets.

Virtual endoscopy is one of the most recent innovations in the spectrum of postprocessing techniques. The predominant motive here is, similarly, to present the image data included in the original slices in such a fashion that the viewer or radiologist is able to differentiate between that which is healthy and that which is pathological. In this state of rapidly progressing technical developments in computers and software, it is difficult to provide an up-to-date report on the technical background of virtual endoscopy. Furthermore, the terminology has become so extensive that a normal human being is hardly capable of understanding the slew of jargon without an accompanying dictionary. It is therefore a goal of the first chapter of this book to provide a basic understanding of the technical background and terminology of virtual endoscopy. A further aim is to put professionals who are interested in the technical details in a position to become better informed about problems, artifacts and possible improvements in volume visualization technology.

1.2 At a Glance...

Volume visualization is a term that embodies the ability to visualize volumetric data sets produced by modern CT and MR scanners. Volume visualization projects a given volumetric data set as a whole, resulting in a single image of the projected volume data. To produce images with a realistic appearance, the surfaces present in the volume data are commonly illuminated using a surface shading algorithm.

In conventional computer graphics, surfaces are represented by geometric "primitives." It is also possible to use this surface rendering for volume visualization by extracting a surface representation from the volume data. The first widely used volume visualization method is the cuberille surface model (Herman and Liu 1979). Based on an intensity threshold, volume elements are segmented. The cuberille model consists of the rectilinear voxel faces of these segmented voxels. The marching cubes algorithm (Lorensen and Cline 1987) generates a more precise surface model by locating the iso surface within the voxels. Dividing cubes (Cline et al. 1988) generates a cloud of points instead of a surface representation.

Volume rendering is able to display the volume data directly. With ray casting (Tuy and Tuy 1984), for each image pixel a ray is cast into the volume, along which the first visible voxel is shown. Levoy (1988) enhanced this method by resampling the volume data at evenly spaced sample locations. These samples are translucent, which requires compositing of the samples to form a single image pixel. Direct volume rendering by Drebin et al. (1988) also uses translucency with compositing, but the view projection is performed by transforming the volume data instead of using ray casting. Splatting (Westover 1990) transforms each voxel of the volume data to the screen space, after which it is composited with previously projected voxels.

Surface shading is an essential part of volume visualization. Depth shading (Herman and Udupa 1981) only uses the distance to the observer to vary the surface color. Depth gradient shading (Gordon et al. 1985) uses the local variation in distances to the observer to perform shading. Gray-level gradient shading (Höhne and Bernstein 1986) calculates an approximation of the surface orientation, used for shading, from the volume data itself.

Surface rendering first extracts a surface representation from the volume data. This intermediate description of the surface is rendered using conventional computer graphics methods, often supported by graphics hardware. Volume rendering is capable of directly rendering the volume data itself, without the necessity of a conversion to another representation.

Virtual endoscopy, the technique of interest here, visualizes inner structures using a perspective projection. For easy navigation, or to generate animations, a path through the inner structure is needed. Because manually tracking such a path may be difficult, or at least time consuming, computer assistance known as path tracking is required. The above listed procedures are clarified more extensively in the following pages.

1.3 Volume Data

Modern CT and MRI scanners produce a set of contiguous cross sectional images. When these individual slices are combined a gray level volumetric data set of voxels is formed. Voxels (volume elements) are the basic elements of volumetric data, similar to picture elements, which are called pixels. Volume visualization techniques visualize such a volumetric data set as a whole, producing a single projected image of the volume data.

The volume data can be regarded as a discrete sampling of a continuous intensity field, which can be reconstructed by an interpolation function. By selecting only one specific intensity value it is possible to define an iso surface in this continuous field. This is the basic method that is used to select the visible data from the volume data. In certain instances an iso surface selection may not be sufficient, for example, when certain structures are blocking the view. In this situation, the iso surface selection can be restricted solely to the structures of interest, thereby making the structures that originally obstructed the view invisible. This is handled via a segmentation process.

1.3.1 Interpolation

The voxels in the volume data are positioned on a grid. When intermediate intensity values are needed, the surrounding voxels are used to calculate this intensity value. This interpolation reconstructs a continuous function from discrete sample points. A very simple interpolation technique is replication, where simply the intensity of the closest voxel is taken. However because this technique results in obstructing artifacts, it is not widely used. In comparison, trilinear interpolation produces better results. It uses the eight surrounding voxels to calculate the sample intensity, based on the distance to the sample location. Higher order interpolation techniques, e.g., cubic splines, give even better results, but are computationally very expensive as the number of operations increases rapidly for 3D interpolation.

1.3.2 Volume Gradient

An important factor in volume visualization is the volume gradient. The volume gradient is used to provide the surface normal (the vector perpendicular to the local surface orientation) in surface shading. It is also an indication of the presence of a surface (via the magnitude of the gradient vector).

The central difference method described by Höhne and Bernstein (1986) computes the volume gradient at a voxel location. To calculate the gradient component for each (x, y, z) direction, both neighboring voxels of a voxel in each component direction are subtracted. This is illustrated in Fig. 1.1a for the x-direction. This produces a gradient component at the voxel location. Interpolation of these gradient components can provide the gradient at an arbitrary sample location.

Another method to calculate the volume gradient is the intermediate difference method (Terwisscha van Scheltinga et al. 1996). Here, two neighboring voxels are subtracted to give a gradient component halfway to these voxels (Fig. 1.1b). This results in three new grids (one for each component) which are shifted half a voxel in each corresponding component direction. An interpolation for each component is used to calculate the gradient at the sample location.

Note that on the voxel grid locations the two methods give the same results. The advantage of the intermediate difference method is that the gradient is calculated using a one-voxel distance instead of two for the central difference method. This results in a better image quality, especially in regions with higher frequencies.

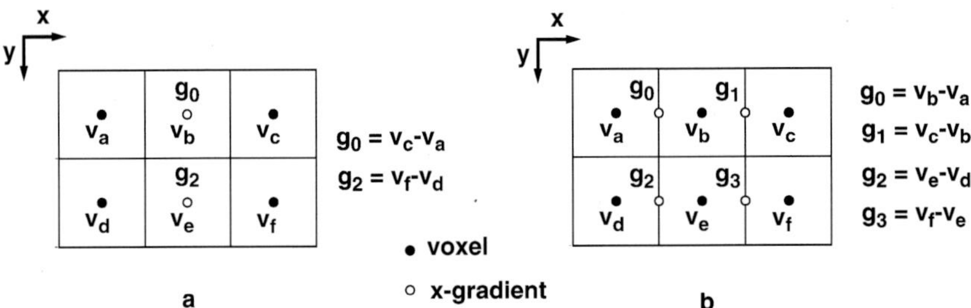

Fig. 1.1. Volume gradient calculated using the central (**a**) and intermediate (**b**) difference

1.3.3 Segmentation

To display specific structures present in the volume data, they first need to be identified. The intensity value is often a good indicator for the presence of a structure. Thus a basic selection method is thresholding: the voxels or points with intensity values within an intensity range are selected. Sometimes this thresholding is part of the rendering method itself, so that no explicit segmentation step is required. When only a threshold is used, an iso surface image is generated.

Thresholding is often just the basis for further segmentation based on this initial selection. Well-known techniques are (de)selecting connected regions via a seed point. Or regions can be expanded (via a dilation operation) or shrunken (via an erosion operation). Other postprocessing operations include or exclude regions based on properties like size, shape, location or other characteristics, or by manual editing.

Segmentation methods often label individual voxels as belonging to a certain region or not. These binary segmentation methods approach difficulties at the borders of regions (Fig. 1.2). Because only a fraction of each voxel at the border is occupied (the partial volume effect), the intensity of such a border voxel quickly falls outside the selected threshold range. As a result such a border voxel is not included in the selection. This may translate into a false appearance of holes in thin structures.

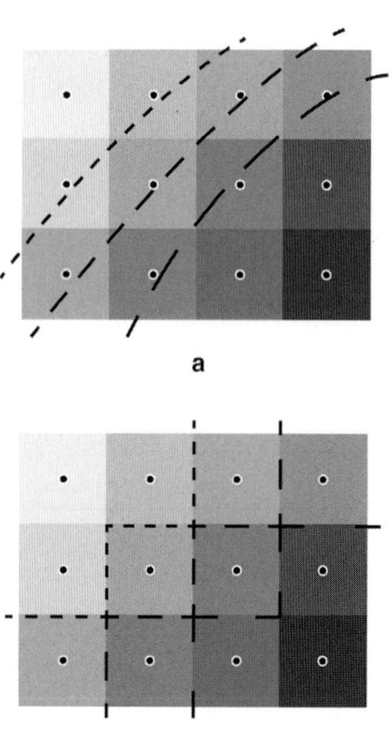

Fig. 1.2. Iso surface (**a**) compared to binary segmentation (**b**) for several threshold values

Advanced segmentation methods not only include or exclude voxels, but are also able to label individual voxels as partly occupied by a certain region. This probabilistic segmentation is often used in volume rendering methods, which are described later.

1.4 View Projections

Since the volume data are three-dimensional, they cannot be viewed directly. In order to visualize the volume data in a single (2D) image, a projection of the volume data onto a projection plane is needed. This projection plane is similar to a film in a camera. The following text represents only an introduction to the technique of projecting volume data onto a plane, and therefore readers who are interested in an extensive explanation, including a mathematical description, are referred, for example, to Foley et al. (1990).

In this procedure, every point of the volume data is transformed to a point on the projection plane. This transformation is defined by a straight projection ray (projector) which starts at a center of projection and passes through the volume point that is projected. The intersection point of this projector, or ray, with the projection plane is the projected position. Under certain circumstances parts of the volume data may not be visible; this occurs when the projector does not intersect with the projection plane. Normally the center of projection, or viewpoint, is positioned at a certain distance on a line perpendicular to the projection plane and through its center. So the viewpoint, together with the position, orientation and size of the projection plane, define the view. This is illustrated in Fig. 1.3.

Note that all points on the projection ray map back to the same position on the projection plane. Normally only the point closest to the viewpoint is visible. But when this point is translucent, the next closest point appears to shine through this first translucent point.

View projections can be divided into two basic classes: parallel projection, where the viewpoint is positioned at an infinite distance, and perspective projection. When separate view projections for both eyes are used, this is called stereoscopic projection. It gives one the illusion of being able to perceive differences in depth, as in real life. With stereoscopic projection two actual projections (for the left and right eye) are needed.

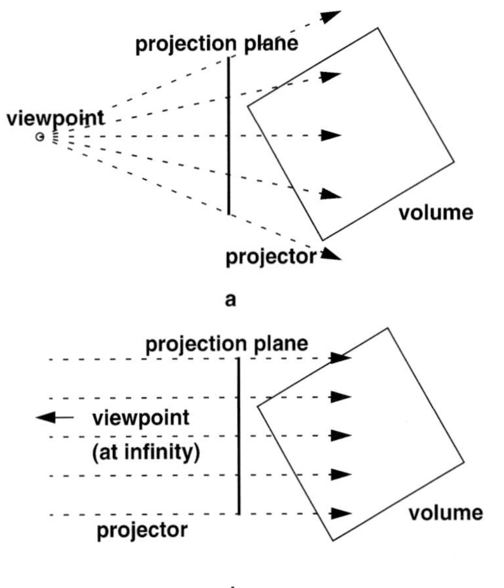

Fig. 1.3. Perspective (**a**) and parallel (**b**) view projection

1.4.1
Parallel Projection

When the viewpoint is positioned at an infinite distance, the projection rays are parallel to each other. This parallel projection is illustrated in Fig. 1.3b. Parallel projection has certain characteristics. The projection is generally faster than perspective projection, as it is simpler to perform. Furthermore, the relative sizes and angles of objects are preserved in the final image. For example, parallel lines remain parallel in the projected image. This absence of distortion in the produced images is an advantage of parallel projection because it allows measurements to be performed on the projection plane.

1.4.2
Perspective Projection

With perspective projection, objects are projected towards a single point behind the projection plane. This is referred to as the center of projection or the viewpoint. Figure 1.3a shows this perspective projection. Perspective projection causes a distortion of object shapes. The reason for the distortion is that objects that are located closer to the viewpoint appear larger in the projected image than objects that are located further away. In this respect, perspective projection is similar to viewing in real life. It results in realistic images and can provide essential depth cues. However, the perspective distortion precludes accurate, direct measurements of objects in the projected plane.

1.4.3
Stereoscopic Projection

Stereoscopic projection is not an additional projection method, but rather, a combination of two normal perspectives instead of one. In the human visual system, the eyes view a scene from slightly different positions. Figure 1.4 shows how the two projection planes mainly overlap each other, but are shifted partially to the left and right. Because the viewpoints are positioned at slightly different locations, the objects are seen from somewhat different angles. These left and right images are fused in the brain, thereby giving the perception of depth.

Several techniques exist to view such a pair of stereoscopic images. A well-known technique is to use glasses with polarizing filters. While the left (right) image is displayed on a standard monitor, the vision of the right (left) eye is blocked by the filter. Because the images are swapped very fast, both eyes continuously see only their designated image. Another technique is using a screen where the image seen is dependent on the angle from which it is viewed.

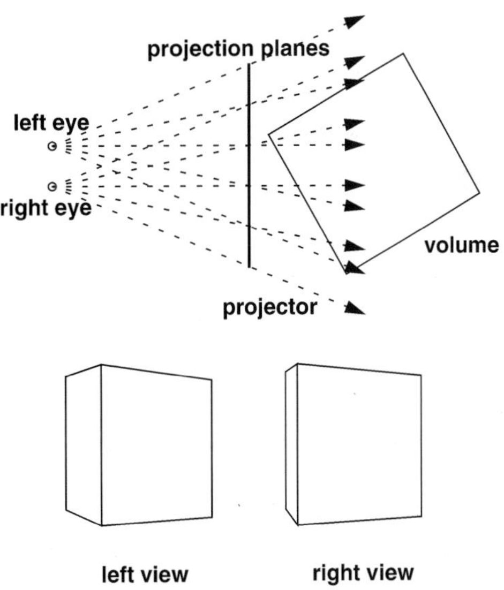

Fig. 1.4. Stereoscopic projection

1.5 Surface Shading

The intensity and color visible at a specific surface location is determined by the surface shading model. This process of surface shading adds realism to an image, so it is a very important aspect of volume visualization. The absence of surface shading makes it very difficult to guess the surface orientation, or relative positions of surfaces.

1.5.1 Depth Cueing

A simple but effective means to enhance the notion of depth is called depth cueing. In fact, in the early days of volume visualization, this was the only method available for surface shading (HERMAN and UDUPA 1981). With depth cueing, points closer to the viewer appear brighter than points farther away. This simulates the effect of atmospheric attenuation.

This effect is often limited to a specific depth range which means only objects within this range are optically distinguished through a varying intensity. Closer objects have a normal (bright) intensity, whereas objects behind this range have the darkest intensity.

It is also possible to simulate fog by extending this model with an atmospheric color. With distant objects, this atmospheric color is nearly all that is visible, at which point the object itself becomes very vague.

As it is very complicated to signify small intensity changes, visualization of small depth differences is poor. However, depth cueing is a useful technique to view or enhance visualization of the global surface structure. Visualization of local surface curvature is much better with surface illumination, which is discussed next.

1.5.2 Phong Illumination Model

Surface illumination imitates the interaction of light with a surface. A very popular surface illumination model is the Phong model (PHONG 1975). This model consists of three components: ambient, diffuse and specular reflection. Although the various existing derivatives of the Phong model (BLINN 1977; SCHLICK 1994) give similar results, they allow for a more efficient implementation than that which is possible in the original model.

As opposed to indirect light, which represents light reflected from other surfaces, direct light arrives uninterrupted from the light source and is the most important illumination parameter. The direct source is largely dependent on the surface orientation. This surface orientation is described by the surface normal, which is perpendicular to the local surface. The surface normal is used to calculate the direct lighting components.

The surface normal can be estimated by using the depth buffer. This is a depth gradient method (GORDON and REYNOLDS 1985) that uses differences in depth values of neighboring pixels in order to calculate a surface normal. Another method is to use the volume gradient direction as the surface normal. This is the preferred method as it gives a much more realistic and detailed presentation (HÖHNE and BERNSTEIN 1986).

1.5.2.1 Ambient Light

The ambient component models indirect light, reflected from other surfaces in the environment. It is independent of the surface orientation, as the light is arriving from all directions. The ambient light component for a surface point is defined by: $I_{ambient} = I_a k_a$. The intensity of the incoming ambient light is given by I_a. The ambient reflection coefficient k_a ranges from 0 to 1 and determines the amount of ambient light which is reflected by the surface. Because the ambient light is assumed uniform in the environment, the ambient component is modeled as a constant value.

1.5.2.2 Diffuse Reflection

The diffuse component models the direct light, which is scattered on the surface into all directions. It is dependent on the angle θ between the surface normal *N* and the direction to the light source *L* (Fig. 1.5). The intensity is highest at those surface points where the incoming light is perpendicular to the surface and drops to zero where the incoming light is parallel to the surface. When θ exceeds 90°, the surface is not lit up, otherwise it can be shown that the amount of incoming light is proportional to $\cos\theta$. Thus the diffuse light component is defined by: $I_{diffuse} = I_p k_d \cos\theta$. The intensity of the point light source is given by I_p. The diffuse reflection coefficient k_d ranges from 0 to 1 and indicates how much of the incoming light is reflected for a particular surface.

The reflected diffuse light color depends on the surface color and the incoming light color. Normally the incoming light is white, which means that the reflected diffuse light would then have the surface col-

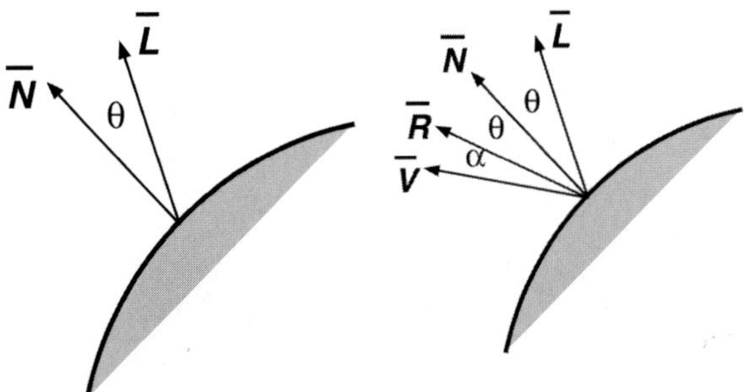

Fig. 1.5. Diffuse reflection

Fig. 1.6. Specular reflection

or. As the intensity depends on the orientation of the surface towards the light source, it provides vital clues about the surface orientation.

1.5.2.3 Specular Reflection

Another direct lighting component is specular reflection. It models the mirror-like reflection of light on a surface. On a perfect mirror, incoming light is reflected in a single direction. This direction of reflection *R* is the light vector *L* mirrored about the surface normal *N*. But usually a shiny surface is not a perfect mirror, and the light is not reflected in this reflection direction only, but also in other directions with a lower intensity. The angle a between the reflection vector and the vector to the viewpoint *V* specifies the intensity of the reflection (Fig. 1.6). When this angle a increases, the reflected light rapidly decreases in intensity. This fall-off speed is controlled by the specular exponent *n*. The specular light component is defined as: $I_{specular} = I_p k_s \cos^n \alpha$. The specular reflection coefficient k_s ranges from 0 to 1 and indicates the intensity of the specular reflected light for a particular type of surface.

Because the specular reflection is only visible from a certain direction, it is dependent on the viewer's position. Especially with motion, this gives important hints about the surface orientation. The color of the reflected light has the same color as the incoming light, as it is simply reflected.

1.5.2.4 Surface Illumination

The total illumination of a surface point is given by the addition of the ambient, diffuse and specular components. The effect of the individual components is illustrated in Fig. 1.7. Figure 1.7a shows a scene shaded with depth cueing and the ambient component only. Figure 1.7b shows the same scene with the diffuse component added, which results in a much better image. Finally, in Fig. 1.7c and 1.7d the specular component with a low (c) and high (d) specular exponent is added, which adds realism to the image.

1.5.3 Material Properties

The material properties define the appearance of a surface. A logical parameter is, of course, the surface color. It can, for example, be used to distinguish (segmented) surfaces from each other. Another property is whether the surface looks dull (for example, chalk) or shiny (for example, polished metal). This is defined by the Phong parameters.

The ambient component of the Phong model can be regarded as the brightness parameter of a material, the diffuse component as the contrast parameter, while the specular component is a shininess parameter. The specular exponent controls the extent of the highlighting, in which case higher values result in a weaker highlighting.

1.6 3D Rendering

For interpreting volume data two classes of rendering techniques are applicable. Surface rendering requires a surface description, which is extracted from the volume data. Volume rendering directly renders the volume data, without the need for such an intermediate description.

1.6.1 Surface Rendering

Surface rendering is a conventional computer graphics technique that is widely supported by specialized graphics hardware. It uses a surface description to model the object surface. This description normally consists of a mesh of polygons. To visualize this surface, individual polygons are projected and combined with previously projected polygons, resulting in the final image which depicts the surface.

To visualize volume data, a surface description needs to be extracted. This triangulation process could be based on a segmentation performed earlier or on an iso value segmentation.

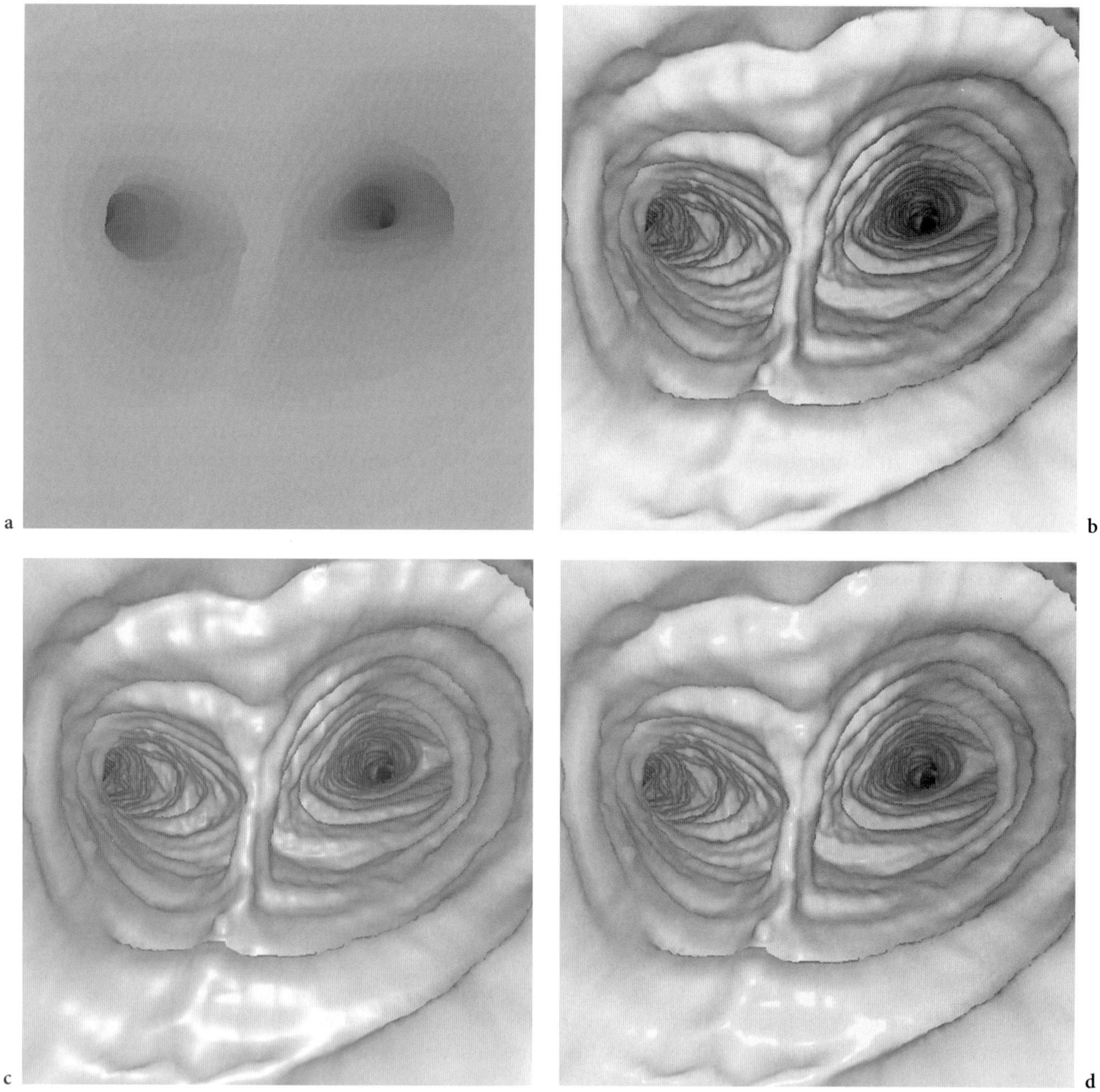

Fig. 1.7. Scene shaded with depth cueing and the ambient component (**a**), addition of the diffuse component (**b**), addition of the specular component with low specular exponent (**c**), and high specular exponent (**d**)

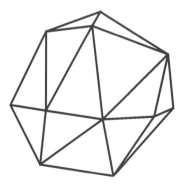

Fig. 1.8. Triangle mesh

1.6.1.1
Surface Description

The most common surface description is a set of connected planar polygons, or a polygon mesh. As a polygon is flat, the points forming the boundary of a polygon (called vertices) must lie in one plane. To avoid a violation of this requirement, triangles are often used, as the three vertices of a triangle always form a plane. Figure 1.8 shows an example of a triangle mesh.

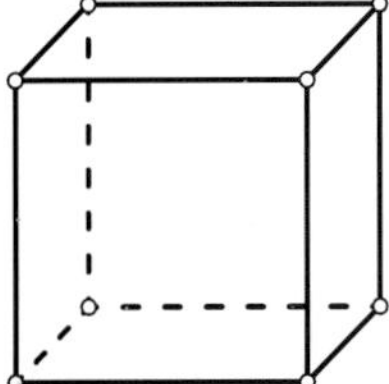

Fig. 1.9. Voxel cube bounded by eight voxels

A representation of a curved surface is possible by approximating it with small flat surfaces. Normally a polygon mesh is closed; this means it is not possible to move from one side of the surface to the other without crossing the surface.

1.6.1.2 Surface Extraction

A widely used surface extraction method algorithm is the marching cubes algorithm (LORENSEN and CLINE 1987). Considering the production of a set of triangles this process is called triangulation. The marching cubes algorithm creates triangle meshes by examining basic cells (cubes bounded by eight voxels) in the volume data. A threshold value selects an iso surface for which a description is generated. Once the surface description is obtained, the original volume data is no longer needed. However, if the threshold value is changed, a complete new surface description must be regenerated.

A cube is defined by the inclusion of eight contiguous voxels from two adjacent slices (Fig. 1.9). Each vertex of this cube is classified as inside or outside the surface by comparing its intensity value with the iso surface value. From these eight classifications, an eight-bit index is built by combining the boolean values. This index is used to select an edge list. This edge list is then used to define the triangles present in the cube by describing which three of the 12 cube edges delimit a triangle. The position of the intersection along the edge is found by an interpolation of the vertex intensities. Up to four triangles may be needed to describe the iso surface in the cube. Finally surface normals for each triangle vertex are calculated by interpolating the volume gradients at the cube vertices. Using the symmetry of the cube, the 256 possible cases of iso surface intersection can be reduced to 14. These cases are shown in Fig. 1.10.

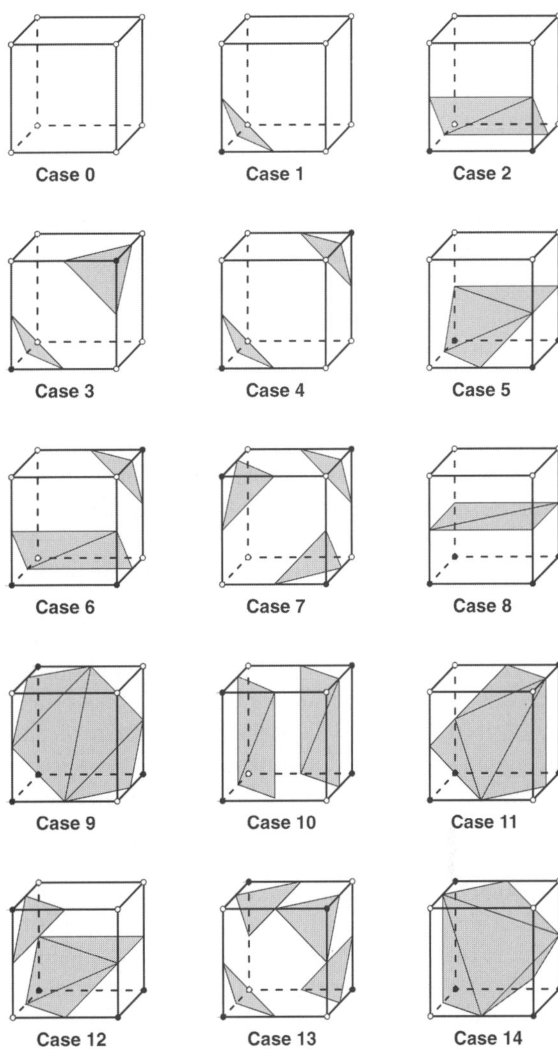

Fig. 1.10. Marching cubes iso surface intersection cases

Sometimes the original algorithm generates triangle sets containing holes, the reason being that ambiguous cases exist where the triangles of adjacent cubes are not connected correctly. Many authors have proposed solutions, for example the marching tetrahedra algorithm by SHIRLEY and TUCHMAN (1990).

The triangulation process can easily result in millions of (very small) triangles. Thus the hardware memory requirements are large and the rendering speed is rather slow. These drawbacks have necessitated a simplification of the triangle meshes, in order to reduce the number of triangles. Nevertheless, this decimation of triangle meshes (SCHROEDER et al. 1992) should maintain a good approximation of the original mesh. The algorithm examines triangles containing a certain vertex. If the decimation criterion is satisfied, the vertex and associated triangles are removed, and the resulting hole is filled with new triangles. This is repeated for other vertices until no further decimation is possible. The originally generated triangles are already a planar approximation of the iso surface, so this decimated triangle mesh results in a further loss of detail.

1.6.1.3 Rendering the Surface Description

Each vertex of a polygon is projected onto the projection plane. Shading is often performed only at these vertices using the provided surface normal. With flat shading, the polygon adapts a single color from one of its vertices. With smooth shading, the vertex colors are interpolated to the interior pixels of the polygon. This results in shading errors, which are especially visible at highlighted locations. When, alternatively, the surface normal is interpolated over the polygon, and the shading is performed for every pixel, accurate results can be achieved.

The polygon mesh surface description can be rendered using a standard software library interface, for example, OpenGL (Woo et al. 1997).

Multiple polygons can overlap each other in the image. But only the (parts of) polygons in front of others are visible. Therefore the visibility of a (part of the) polygon needs to be determined before it is actually stored in the image. This is called hidden-surface removal. A possibility is to sort the polygons before projecting them. Sorting is, however, not always possible as the polygons may intersect each other, or overlap cyclically. A simple but effective solution is to use the depth value of each projected pixel to determine whether it is visible or hidden behind another surface, a technique that is described in the next section.

1.6.1.4 Depth Buffer

To determine whether a newly projected pixel is visible compared to previously rendered pixels, a depth buffer is used. This depth buffer (or *z*-buffer) has the same size as the image, and contains a depth value for each image pixel. The depth of every new surface pixel is compared to the corresponding depth value stored in the depth buffer. Only when the pixel is in front of a previously rendered pixel, is the pixel stored in the image, and the depth buffer is adjusted accordingly.

With a depth buffer, the polygons can be projected in an arbitrary order. Furthermore, potential intersections of polygons are irrelevant. If a rough front-to-back depth sorting of polygons is performed, then most of the hidden surfaces will require no expensive shading. The depth buffer is useful not only during the rendering stage itself, but also for merging other objects or images afterwards.

1.6.2 Volume Rendering

With volume rendering, the volume data itself is directly interpreted, without an explicit surface representation. A classification function defines the visible and invisible parts of a volume, based on the intensity values in the volume. Many variants of volume rendering exist, so there is not a single true volume rendering method. Although volume rendering is often associated with translucent images, it is also capable of creating surface shaded images.

1.6.2.1 Classification

The classification function defines the visibility of materials present in the data set. It is commonly assumed that different materials map to different intensity levels; therefore, the classification function maps intensity levels to opacity values. A low opacity value results in a translucent or even invisible object, while a high opacity value results in a clearly visible object. When the classification is restricted to segmented regions, only these regions are visualized.

When a simple threshold is used to select an iso surface, the classification maps all intensity values below the threshold to a low or zero opacity, and all intensities above this threshold to a high opacity (Fig. 1.11a). The classification function is often smoothed as in Fig. 1.11b, which generates a fuzzy classification.

The basic classification function assigns an opacity value to each intensity level. Levoy (1988) proposed that the opacity be scaled by the local gradient magnitude (the gradient vector size). The gradient magnitude is a good indicator for the presence of a surface. Consequently, this scaling suppresses the opacity forming the interior of tissues, while enhancing the opacity at surfaces. The resulting images show semi-transparent surfaces. An example of such a tissue transition projection (TTP) image is given in Fig. 1.12.

1.6.2.2 Splatting

An object order volume rendering method projects the volume data in voxel order onto the projection plane. With splatting (Westover 1990), each voxel is projected onto the projection plane. A voxel contributes to multiple image pixels, which is defined by a footprint. The contribution of the voxel to an image pixel is highest at the center of the footprint. The

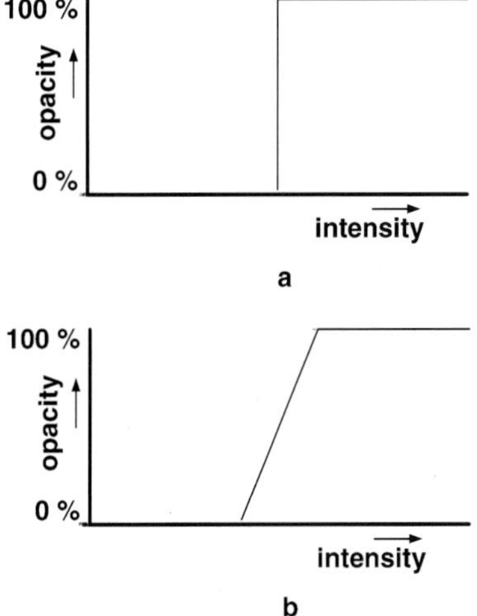

Fig. 1.11. A threshold classification function (**a**) and a smoothed classification function (**b**)

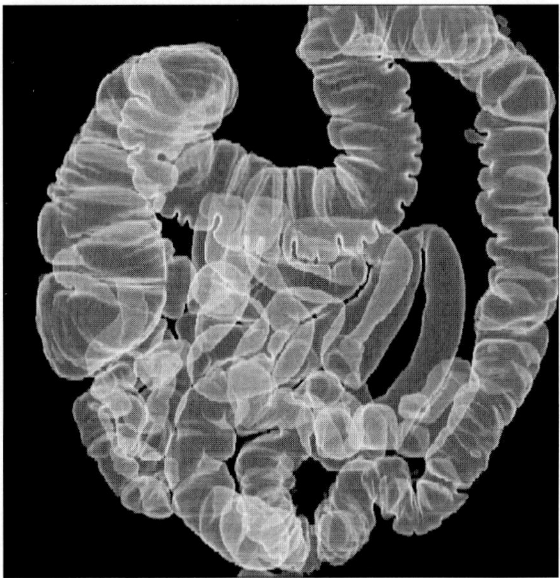

Fig. 1.12. A TTP image of the colon

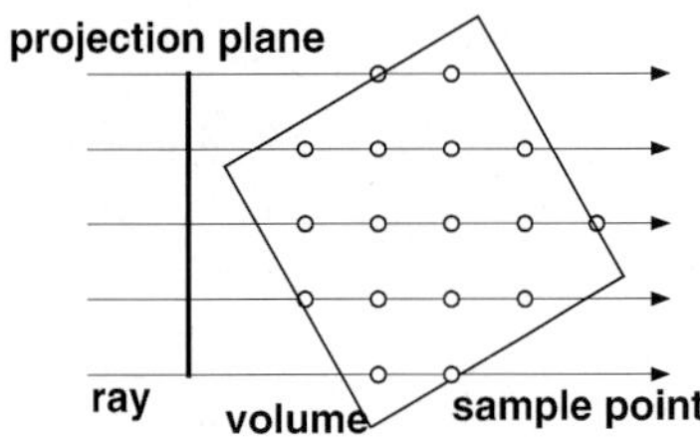

Fig. 1.13. Ray casting

footprints of adjacent voxels overlap each other; hence, an individual image pixel is normally the result of an accumulation of several projected voxels.

Because the resolution of splatting is restricted to the voxel size, and because the footprint causes blurring of the image, splatting is of limited use.

1.6.2.3 Ray Casting

A commonly used volume rendering method to project the volume data is ray casting (Levoy 1988). With ray casting the volume data is processed in image (pixel) order. A ray is cast through the volume data for each pixel of the output image. Along this ray, opacity and color values are calculated at evenly spaced sample positions. This is illustrated in Fig. 1.13. When all sample points of the ray are composited, the result is a single image pixel.

The samples along a ray are composited using alpha blending. The process of alpha blending is illustrated in Fig. 1.14, where two adjacent samples are consolidated to form a composited sample. The front sample with opacity a_f and color contribution C_f is composited with the back sample with opacity α_b and color contribution C_b. The color contribution C is defined as the alpha blended contribution of the sample color c: $C = c\alpha$. The composited color C_c is given by: $C_c = C_f+(1-\alpha_f)\ C_b$. The composited opacity is given by: $\alpha_c = \alpha_f+(1-\alpha_f)\ \alpha_b$. As expected, a front opacity of 1 results in no contribution from the back sample.

In Levoy's algorithm, the classification and shading is performed at voxel locations. Interpolation is used to calculate the opacity and color at the sample locations. Image quality is improved when the classification and shading is performed at sample loca-

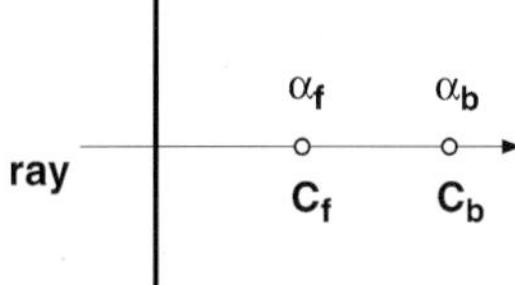

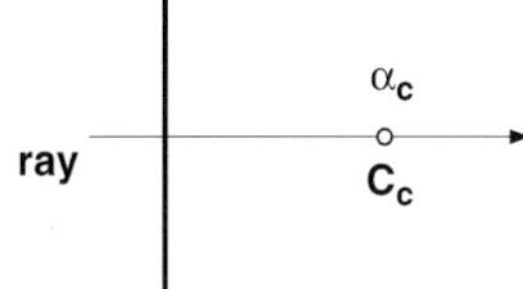

Fig. 1.14. Compositing

tions (Terwisscha et al. 1996). Therefore, the intensity level and volume gradient are calculated at the sample location via interpolation.

To optimize ray casting, Levoy (1990) skips empty (invisible) cells. In other words, a hierarchical spatial enumeration is used to quickly identify (groups of) cells containing only voxels with zero opacity. Such cells are completely invisible and need no processing. When a group of cells is visible, the test is performed on the cells at a lower level. Another optimization is labeled adaptive ray termination. When the composed opacity along the ray reaches a certain level, further processing is abandoned, as the contribution to the pixel is negligible.

When the classification function is simply a threshold, it offers the opportunity to locate the iso surface exactly by using iso surface volume rendering (Bosma et al. 1998; Parker et al. 1998). Instead of taking samples along each ray, the first intersection of a ray with the iso surface is detected. Shading is then performed at this intersection point.

To detect the ray-surface intersection, the ray traverses voxel cells in the volume data. If the cell contains intensity values both above and below the iso value, the cell contains the iso surface. If a cell contains the iso surface, an analytic computation locates the intersection points. Multiple intersections are possible because the iso surface generally is curved. It is also possible that no intersection point exists, in which case the ray misses the iso surface present in the cell. The closest intersection point (the first) is used as the iso surface location.

Instead of generating an explicit polygonal surface representation as in marching cubes, the intersection of a ray with the iso surface is calculated directly from the volume data. Therefore changing the iso value is possible without the need for an expensive surface extraction step.

Traversing cells is the most expensive part of this method. Thus to optimize iso surface volume rendering, a multi-level spatial hierarchy similar to Levoy's hierarchical spatial enumeration is useful. Accordingly, cells are hierarchically grouped into larger cells. When minimum and maximum values for such cell groups are available, these cell groups can be skipped if the minimum value is above the iso value, or the maximum value is below this iso value.

1.7 Rendering Artifacts

Several artifacts may occur when rendering volume data. Examples are staircasing, aliasing, rippling, slicing and highlight flashing. These artifacts are mainly caused by interpolation errors. The avoidance of these artifacts is often a trade-off between image quality and speed.

1.7.1 Staircasing

When the slice distance is large compared to the pixel size, a staircasing effect may occur. Normally interpolation of the volume data results in a smooth iso surface, but with a large slice distance this is a problem, as illustrated in Fig. 1.15. To prevent this staircasing effect the slice distance of the volume data should be similar to the slice pixel size. Another possibility is to use a specialized interpolation technique aimed at reducing this effect.

1.7.2 Aliasing

Aliasing occurs as a result of interference between the resample grid and the voxel grid. When the resample grid resolution with ray casting is too small with respect to the voxel grid, ringing artifacts can occur. Enlarging the resolution of the image can prevent this. With virtual endoscopy aliasing is not a problem, as the images are normally zoomed and thus have a high resolution compared to the volume data.

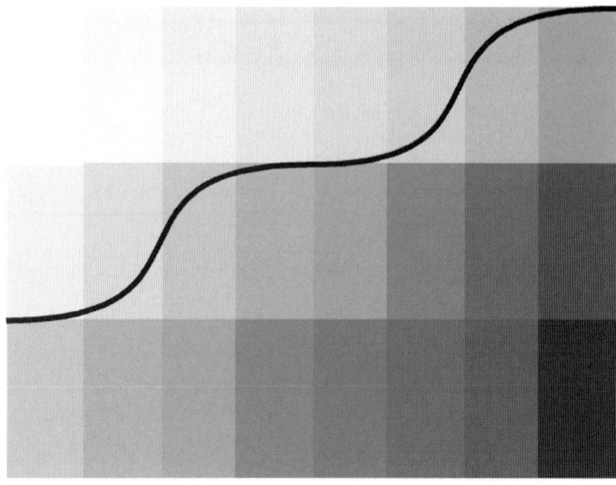

Fig. 1.15. The staircase effect

1.7.3 Rippling

With volume rendering individual voxels are sometimes visible via rippling artifacts when an image is zoomed-in. These artifacts are caused by an incorrect order of operations. When classification and shading is performed at voxel locations and these results are interpolated to sample locations, the voxels show up in the image. But this rippling disappears when first the volume data is interpolated to the sample location, and then classification and shading is performed. An example showing the rippling effect is shown in Fig. 1.16.

1.7.4 Slicing

When with ray casting the sampling distance along a ray is too large, slices may appear in the image (see Fig. 1.17). The discrete depth locations at which samples are taken then become visible as slices. This effect occurs when the sample rate is not adjusted while zooming-in on the image. It is solved by increasing the sample rate at higher zoom rates, but this results in a slower rendering speed as more samples are taken along each ray.

1.7.5 Highlight Flashing

With surface rendering, the specular highlights may suddenly flash on or off during interaction. Because shading is only performed at vertices, specular shading is not always correct for the other pixels of the polygon. Instead of interpolating colors over the polygon, the surface normal should be interpolated. But this also requires shading for every polygon pixel, a costly affair.

1.8 Virtual Endoscopy

Virtual endoscopy visualizes the inner surfaces of structures present in volumetric data in 3D images. To simulate true endoscopy, surface shaded images are generated using a perspective projection. As navigating through the inner structures quickly becomes a complicated procedure, often a (possibly branched) path through the structure is used. This path can be used to interactively investigate the inner structure or to generate an animation along the path.

1.8.1 Visualization Settings

To visualize the interior surface of tubular structures, the visible surface needs to be selected. Normally a simple threshold is sufficient, resulting in an iso surface display. A segmentation step may sometimes be necessary, however, to remove blocking structures.

For virtual endoscopy, the parallel projection is not very useful. The explanation is that only a small part of

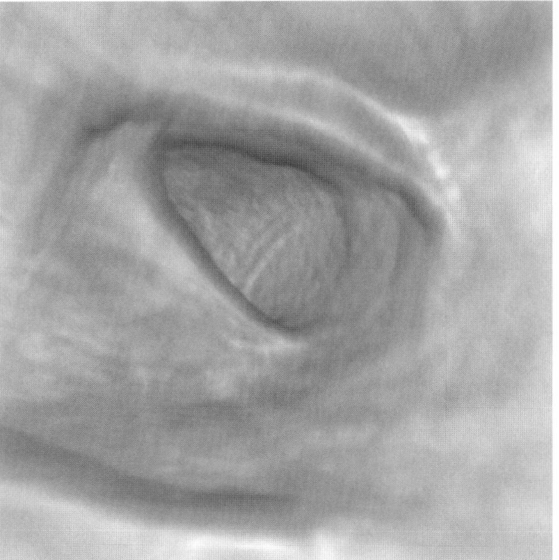

Fig. 1.16. An image of the colon with (**a**) and without (**b**) rippling artifacts

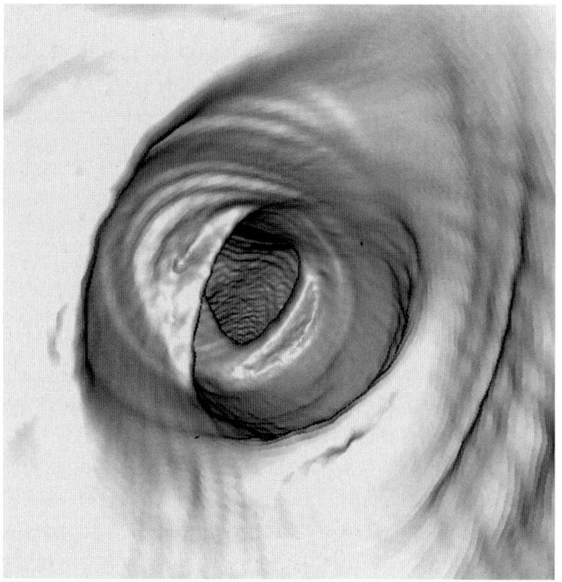

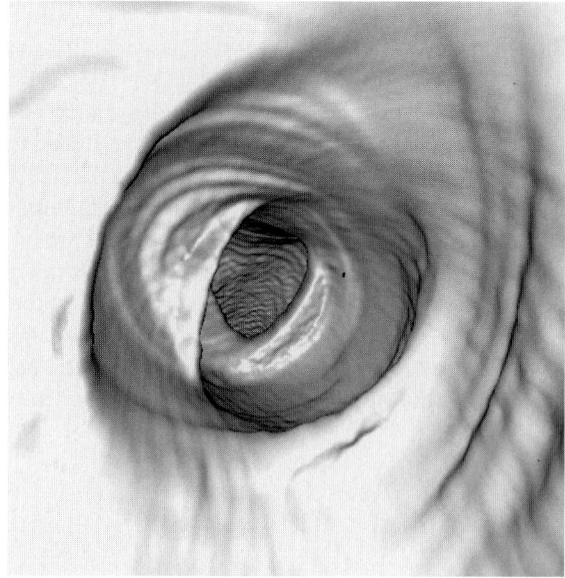

Fig. 1.17. An image of the colon with (**a**) and without (**b**) slicing artifacts

the surface wall is visualized, and it is very hard to observe depth in such images. Because branches are hardly detectable, they are easily missed. The perspective projection shows much more of the surface of tubular structures than the parallel projection. In addition the perspective distortion gives valuable depth cues.

This is illustrated in Fig. 1.18. With parallel projection, surface structures in the front block a large part of the structures behind them.

Surface shading results in images similar to true endoscopic images. This is essential for virtual endoscopy, as it shows subtle changes in surface orientation, which are not seen otherwise. The light source is normally positioned at the viewpoint, as this ensures a satisfactory illumination of all visible surfaces.

With virtual endoscopy large zoom factors are often needed. Consequently, the individual voxels become easily noticeable, especially when surface rendering is used. The reason is that only a limited amount of triangles are generated for each voxel. With the large zoom factors used, these individual (flat) triangles easily show up in images. As volume rendering generates images from the volume data itself, it allows rendering at a higher spatial resolution when zoomed-in on voxels. Therefore, volume rendered images show details not present in surface rendered images. Thus although surface rendering is capable of providing interactive frame rates, volume rendering is the preferred rendering technique for virtual endoscopy.

1.8.2 Path Planning

Navigating through the inner structures is often a problem, especially when these structures are strongly curved. With full control over a camera, it is easily moved out of this inner structure. Comparatively, a simple solution is to use a guidance path for easy

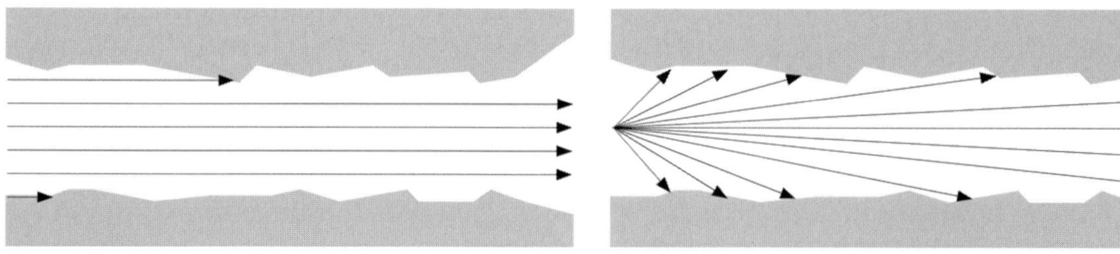

Fig. 1.18. Surface visibility for parallel and perspective projection

navigation. The path adds constraints, which are useful in guiding the viewer through the structure. An effective path needs to have certain properties:

- The path must remain inside the structure and avoid collisions with the wall.
- It should follow the centerline of the structure as closely as possible, as this provides the best visualization of the surrounding wall.
- The path should also be smooth without unnecessary kinks.

Once a path is created, navigating is simply a matter of positioning the view along the path. The viewing direction is adjusted to the local path orientation. It remains possible to look around by adjusting this viewing direction, in order to obtain a better impression of interesting features. To generate an animation, a series of images is generated along the path at small distances.

Manually specifying the path is possible by defining key points along the path. Intermediate path positions are then automatically determined by fitting a smooth curve through these manually defined points. This is a well-known technique in computer animation. But defining satisfying key points is often difficult and time consuming. Another possibility is to use a computer assisted path generation algorithm (Hong et al. 1997; Paik et al. 1998).

First, the structure of interest is segmented by applying a threshold value. A seed voxel provided by the user then selects all connected (thresholded) voxels, resulting in the structure of interest. Then the first and last point of the required path is defined by the user. These points are used to find the shortest path through the segmented structure via a distance map. This shortest path normally follows part of the surface, especially in curves. To move it towards the centerline, the outer layer of the structure is iteratively removed by an erosion step. After each iteration, the shortest path is found again using a distance map, thereby using the previous path at unconnected parts. This removal of the outer layer continues until the structure is completely removed. Finally the remaining path is smoothed to obtain a useful centralized path.

To define a view, the projection plane is positioned at a location on the path. The view direction on this position is determined by the local path orientation. The simplest view direction is along the local path direction (or tangent). But it is more natural to determine the view direction by looking towards a forward path position. An option is to locate this forward-directed position at a certain distance from the current position. Another possibility is to use the first path point that disappears behind a wall (Hong et al. 1997; Paik et al. 1998). These viewing direction possibilities are illustrated in Fig. 1.19. Looking towards the first disappearing point may result in a sudden change in viewing direction. This occurs when a partially obscured part of the path becomes totally visible. Then the disappearing point is suddenly located at another position. Thus a smoothing of the viewing direction is required to avoid sudden changes of the view orientation.

Once the viewing direction is determined, it is still possible to rotate the projection plane by changing the up direction. So the orientation of the projection plane must be carefully chosen, to avoid sudden twists when moving to another nearby path position. This requires a minimization of the relative rotation between closely positioned views. This is possible by rotating the previous projection plane towards the new view direction, followed by a translation to the new path position. A single rotation axis is sufficient, defined by the vector perpendicular to both view direction vectors. A translation of the rotated projection plane to the new path position then gives the new projection plane.

1.8.3 Conclusion

Perspective volume rendering is the preferred rendering technique for virtual endoscopy as it shows details not present in surface rendered images. A guidance path through the inner structure greatly simplifies the navigation. It provides not only an optimal position in the volume data, but also a useful viewing direction.

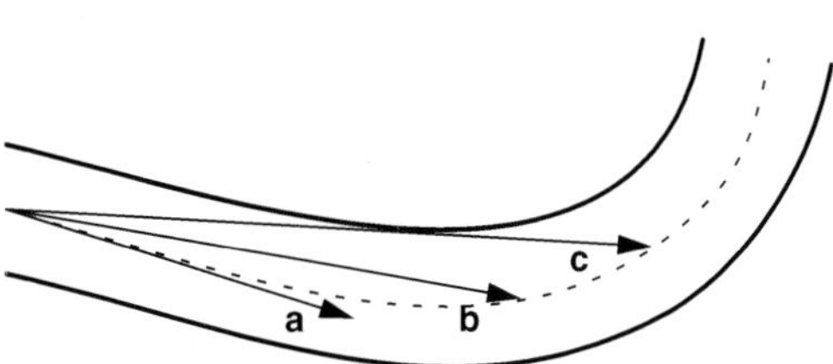

Fig. 1.19. View direction tangent to the path (**a**); towards a forward position (**b**); towards the first disappearing point (**c**)

References

Blinn JF (1977) Models of Light Reflection for Computer Synthesized Pictures. SIGGRAPH 77, pp 192–198

Bosma MK, Smit J, Lobregt S (1998) Iso-surface Volume Rendering. Proceedings of SPIE Medical Imaging '98, vol 3335:10–19

Cline HE, Lorensen WE, Ludke S, et al. (1988) Two Algorithms for the Three-dimensional Reconstruction of Tomograms. Medical Physics, 15(3), pp 320–327

Drebin RA, Carpenter L, Hanrahan P (1988) Volume Rendering. Computer Graphics, 22(4), pp 65–74

Foley JD, van Dam A, Feiner SK, et al. (1990) Computer Graphics: Principles and Practice, 2nd edn, Addison-Wesley Publishing Company, Reading

Gordon D, Reynolds RA (1985) Image Space Shading of 3-dimensional Objects. Computer Vision Graphics Image Processing 29:361–376

Herman GT, Liu HK (1979) Three-dimensional Display of Human Organs from Computed Tomograms. Computer Graphics and Image Processing, 9, pp 1–21

Herman GT, Udupa JK (1981) Display of Three Dimensional Discrete Surfaces. Proceedings of the SPIE, 283, pp 90–97

Höhne KH, Bernstein R (1986) Shading 3D Images from CT Using Grey-Level Gradients. IEEE Transactions on Medical Imaging, 5(1):45–57

Hong L, Liang Z, Viswambharan A, et al. (1997) Reconstruction and Visualization of 3D Models of Colonic Surface. IEEE Transactions on Nuclear Science, 44(3):1297–1302

Levoy M (1988) Display of Surfaces from Volume Data. IEEE Computer Graphics and Applications, 8(3):29–37

Levoy M (1990) Efficient Ray Tracing of Volume Data. ACM Transactions on Graphics, 9(3):245–261

Lorensen WE, Cline HE (1987) Marching Cubes: A High Resolution 3D Surface Construction Algorithm. Computer Graphics, 21(4):163–169

Paik DS, Beaulieu CF, Jeffrey RB, et al. (1998) Automated Flight Path Planning for Virtual Endoscopy. Med. Phys. 25(5):629–637

Parker S, Shirley P, Livnat Y, et al. (1998) Interactive Ray Tracing for Isosurface Rendering. In: (eds) IEEE Visualization '98, pp 233–238

Phong BT (1975) Illumination for Computer Generated Pictures. Communications of the ACM, 18(6):311–317

Schlick C (1994) A Fast Alternative to Phong's Specular Model. In: Heckbert P (ed) Graphics Gems IV. Academic Press, Boston, pp 385–387

Schroeder WJ, Zarge JA, Lorensen WE (1992) Decimation of Triangle Meshes. Computer Graphics 26(2):65–70

Shirley P, Tuchman A (1990) A Polygonal Approximation to Direct Scalar Volume Rendering. Computer Graphics 24(5):63–70

Terwisscha van Scheltinga JAS, Bosma MK, Smit J, et al. (1996) Image Quality Improvements in Volume Rendering. In: Höhne KH, Kikinis R (eds) Visualization in Biomedical Computing. Springer, Berlin, pp 87–92

Tuy HK, Tuy LT (1984) Direct 2-D Display of 3-D Objects. IEEE Computer Graphics and Applications, 4(10), pp 29–33

Westover L (1990) Footprint Evaluation for Volume Rendering. Computer Graphics SIGGRAPH '90, 24(4):367–376

Woo M, Neider J, Davis T (1997) OpenGL Programming Guide, 2nd edn. Addison-Wesley Developers Press, Reading

2 Virtual Endoscopy of the Nose and Paranasal Sinuses

P. ROGALLA

CONTENTS

2.1 Introduction

The origins of endoscopic paranasal sinus surgery can be traced back to HIRSCHMANN, who constructed an endoscope to inspect the nose and paranasal sinuses as early as 1903. Endoscopic paranasal sinus surgery was, however, abandoned at the beginning of the twentieth century, primarily due to severe complications (GREVERS et al. 1999; HAJEK 1904; HALLE 1906; MOSHER 1912). One of the main reasons for complications was inadequate anatomic orientation in the surgical region, which led to damage of vital structures (GUNKEL et al. 1997). The fundamental principles of functional endoscopic sinus surgery (FESS), today a technique applied worldwide, were established in the early 1970s by Professor Walter Messerklinger in Graz, Austria (MESSERKLINGER 1966), and thereafter exported from the German-speaking nations to the rest of the world by Heinz Stammberger (STAMMBERGER 1985, 1989) and David Kennedy (KENNEDY 1985; KENNEDY and KENNEDY 1985). The concept of endoscopic sinus surgery revolutionised the preceding operating standards and represented a dramatic improvement for patients in terms of diagnostic evaluation and treatment, especially because of the rapid postoperative healing after an endonasal intervention (DURSUN et al. 1998). This aspect is of utmost importance from a healthcare political point of view; in Germany, for example, approximately 40,000 patients with chronic sinusitis and 10,000 patients with acute sinusitis undergo endoscopic paranasal sinus surgery each year (FEDERAL STATISTICS OFFICE, GERMANY 1994–1996).

Until recently, inflammatory disease of the paranasal sinuses was treated surgically with radical resection, for example Caldwell-Luc radical antrostomy, intranasal ethmoidectomy or external frontoethmoidectomy. These operations have partly retained meaning today. However, amidst the general trend in medicine towards minimally invasive surgery, attempts are being made to drift away from radical, extensive procedures and rather to treat patients having benign sinus disease with more conservative structure- and mucosa-preserving microsurgery. The main advantage of minimally invasive surgery is a reduction in perioperative complications (BLOKMANIS 1994; LOBE 1991; MAY et al. 1994; SMITH and BRINDLEY 1993).

The procedure is primarily an endoscopic diagnostic strategy that assists in determining the cause of recurring and chronic sinusitis (MESSERKLINGER 1972; SENER 1994). During the endoscopic operation, the expansion pattern of the mucosal affection is followed. By normalising the secretory drainage and ventilation of the hyperplastic epithelial tissue in the maxillary, frontal and sphenoidal sinuses the operation clears the way for functional and morphological epithelial repair processes (MESSERKLINGER 1966).

The function of the paranasal sinuses still remains incompletely clarified. The first description of the maxillary sinus probably came from Leonardo da Vin-

P. ROGALLA, MD
Department of Radiology, Charité Hospital, Humboldt-Universität zu Berlin, Schumannstrasse 20/21, 10117 Berlin, Germany

ci (1452–1519) (Da Vinci 1920). From this point onwards, numerous hypotheses regarding the function of the paranasal sinuses were advanced, for example: to ease the skull, as a protective organ for the skull, as thermal isolation for the CNS, as an olfactory organ, as resonance space for the voice or for humidifying and warming the inspired air through gas exchange. Most of the hypotheses could be dismissed on the grounds of anatomical studies. It is now known that an actively controlled secretion production takes place combined with an active secretion convection in the sinuses, presumably with the goal of attaining water vapour saturation of the inspiratory air. Understanding the physiological significance of the paranasal sinuses is the key to mucosa-preserving microsurgery, in which the main goal is reestablishing conditions for physiological epithelial function.

Messerklinger built his world-renowned technique on the diagnostic information won from conventional tomography. This radiological method has been practically abandoned due to the relatively high radiation exposure and has been replaced by high-resolution computed tomography. Today, coronary CT is accepted as a standard evaluation technique (Melhem et al. 1996; Pockler et al. 1994; Zinreich 1992) and is an essential component of the diagnostic investigation of patients presenting with symptoms suggesting benign inflammatory disease of the paranasal sinuses. CT represents an ideal imaging modality for visualising the extremely thin bony leaflets of the ethmoid labyrinth. Furthermore, normal deviations (Kosling et al. 1993; Meyers and Valvassori 1998) that might potentially represent the cause of disturbed ventilation of the paranasal sinuses can be presented with adequate sensitivity. Moreover, minimal swelling of the mucosa that could be responsible for recurrent disease in the larger paranasal sinuses can be displayed. These minor mucosal changes can elude even careful endoscopy of the paranasal sinuses. This explains why the radiologist plays a key role in guiding the ENT surgeon to the correct point of interest (Mason et al. 1998).

A general consensus exists that endonasal surgery requires preoperative CT (Boguslawska-Staniaszczyk et al. 1994; Kopp et al. 1988; Mafee et al. 1993). In a diagnostic CT, all potentially dangerous locations, for example a dehiscence of the lamina papyracea, close proximity of the orbita to inflammatory foci, a septated frontal or sphenoid cavity and, most importantly, the location of the optic nerve in relation to the internal carotid artery can be determined. Systematic endoscopic evaluation of the lateral nasal boundary in combination with preoperative CT of the nose and paranasal sinuses allows for precise evaluation of the causes of a pathological condition and can help the clinician in planning adequate therapy.

2.2 Imaging Techniques

2.2.1 Computed Tomography

Preoperative CT is a standard imaging procedure (Babbel et al. 1991; Beus et al. 1995; Chakeres 1985; Chow and Mafee 1989; Som 1985). Some authors (Hosemann 1996; Suojanen and Regan 1995) favour an axial slice orientation, although the coronal imaging is generally preferred (Damilakis et al. 1998; Zinreich 1998). Axial imaging has the advantage for the patient that the supine position with an overextended neck is unnecessary. This position has proved very unpleasant, especially for elderly patients with restricted flexibility in the cervical vertebrae. Because the ENT surgeon always approaches the patient frontally, coronal reconstruction would be more helpful for anatomic correlation; however, when prepared from simple axial slices, coronal slices offer little detail resolution.

Three-dimensional reconstructions can basically be calculated from axial as well as coronal images under the condition that artefacts from metallic dental structures in the coronal slices are limited. The selection of the primary slice orientation can initially be planned according to the diagnostic question because the ability to judge anatomical details differs between the two orientations (Table 1).

Since the introduction of spiral CT in the early 1990s, the choice of a primary slice orientation has become less problematic. With spiral CT it is possible to use very thin collimation (1.0–1.5 mm thickness) in axial slice orientation, to acquire the axial slices continually with variable pitch factor, and to calculate slices from the raw data with even thinner reconstruction intervals. Through such acquisition protocols, high-quality secondary reconstructions become attainable (Suojanen and Regan 1995). Furthermore, additional reconstructions, even in other slice orientations such as the sagittal plane, may be recalculated from the same dataset. With the advent of multislice CT, allowing a primary slice thickness of 0.5 mm, coronal reconstructions can be obtained with a spatial resolution comparable with that of the originally acquired axial slices (Fig. 2.1) because the image voxels (volume elements) have an

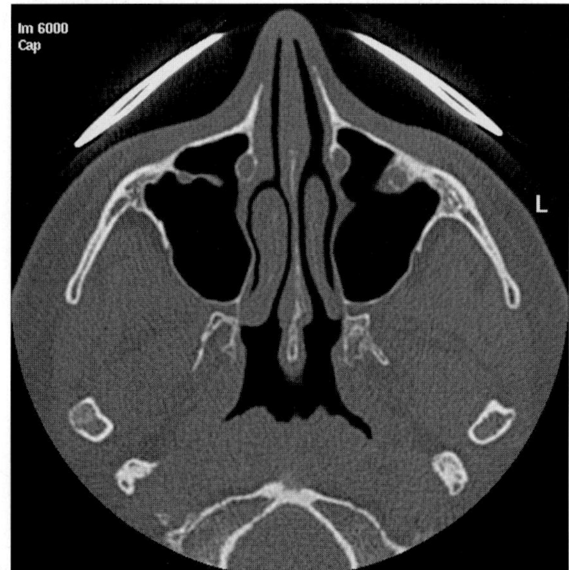

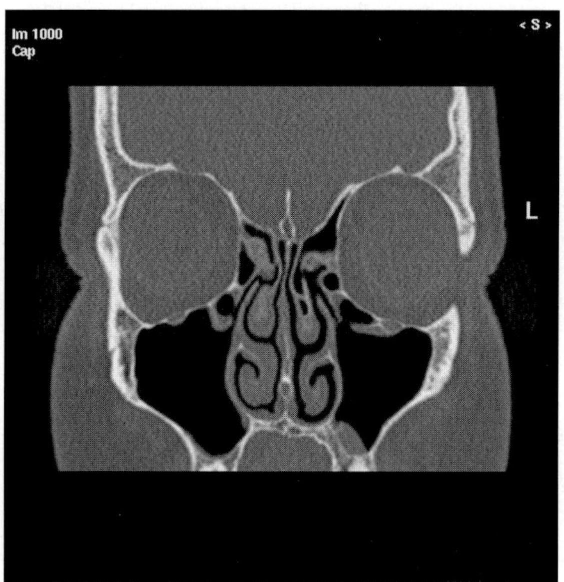

a b

Fig. 2.1. Example of **a** an axial thin-slice CT (0.5 mm slice thickness, 0.3 mm reconstruction interval) and **b** a coronal reconstruction. The spatial resolution is similar in both images because the voxels have isotropic edge lengths. Such an imaging protocol is "ideal" for three-dimensional postprocessing, because reduced resolution or poorer image quality is not expected at any viewing angle. Side finding: bilateral partially formed Haller cells (cellulae infraorbitales)

Table 2.1. Ability to assess anatomical structures on axial and coronal slices (modified from Shankar et al. 1994)

Structure	Axial	Coronal
Maxillary sinus		
Anterior wall	+	-
Posterior wall	+	-
Medial wall	+/-	+
Roof/orbital floor	-	+
Frontal sinus		
Anterior wall	+	-
Posterior wall	+	-
Floor	-	+
Sphenoid sinus		
Anterior wall	+	-
Posterior wall	+	-
Lateral wall	+	+
Septum	+	+
Floor	-	+
Ethmoid sinus		
Lateral wall	+	+
Roof	-	+
Ostiomeatal complex	-	+
Fossa pterygopalatina	+	+/-
Superior orbital fissure	-	+
Optic nerve	+	+
Cribriform plate	-	+
Turbinates	-	+

isotropic geometry. The undeniable advantage of a primary axial slice orientation is attributed additionally to the fact that metallic dental prostheses, which customarily cause beam-hardening artefacts in coronal slices, cause absolutely no disturbance in the axial image (Fig. 2.2).

An additional advantage of scanning the sinuses in an axial slice orientation is the possibility of protecting the eyes with an eye shield. The plastic shield contains the element bismuth and filters up to 40% of the radiation. Artefacts therefore arise due to beam-hardening effects; these are limited to a few millimetres beneath the shield, however, so there is no disturbing influence on the deeper-lying paranasal sinuses (Fig. 2.3).

Some examination protocols recommend intravenous administration of contrast material, preferably non-ionic agents. Basically, contrast agents can be helpful in distinguishing between active and chronic inflammatory disease states since mucosal enhancement is only visible in active inflammation (Fig. 2.4). Contrast material is also indicated by a suspected abscess and by the need to differentiate between allergic and inflammatory polyps, and can be helpful in staging tumour infiltration (Fig. 2.5). For virtual endoscopy, however, the use of contrast material is unnecessary. The natural contrast between air and soft tissue amounts to at least 700–1000 Hounsfield units, and an additional density increase of 100 HU elevates the already sufficient contrast by maximally

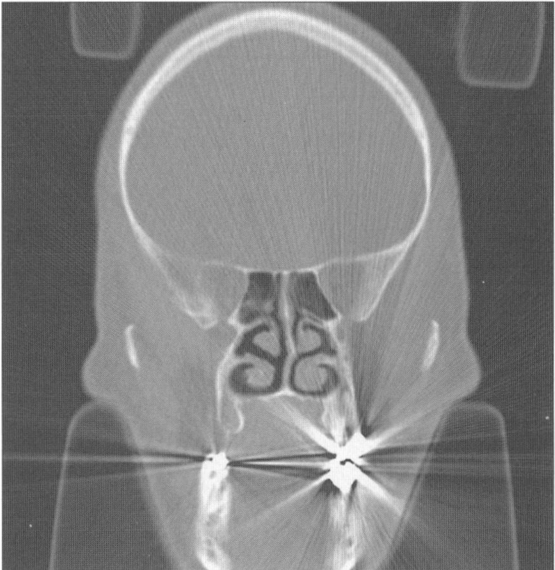

Fig. 2.2. In the coronal slice direction (patient in prone position, head dorsally reflected) dental fillings can cause strong artefacts. Therefore, a primary coronal slice orientation is not appropriate for virtual endoscopy

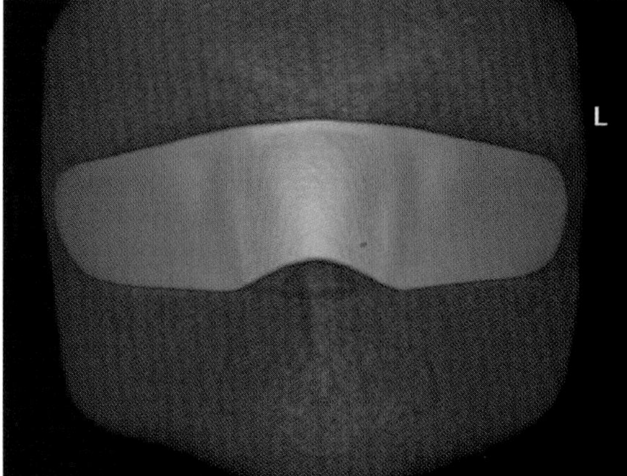

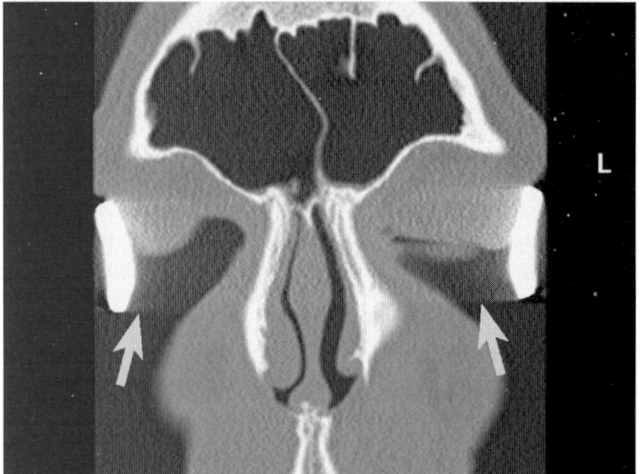

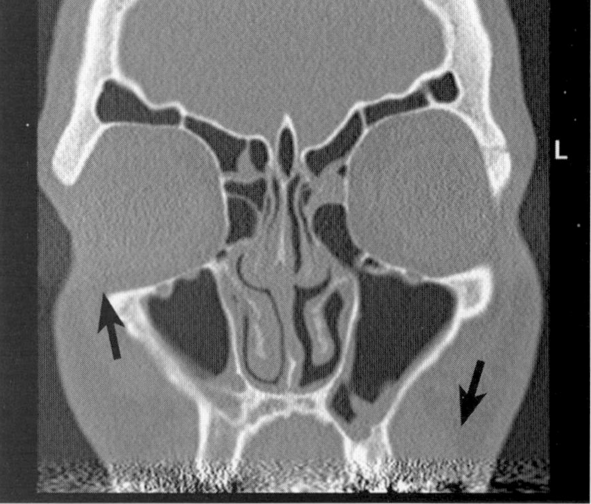

Fig. 2.3. a Three-dimensional reconstruction of a paranasal CT with a eye protector made of a rubber-bismuth mixture. **b** In the frontal slices of the coronal reconstructions the minimal hardening artefacts are depicted (*arrows*), which however do not influence the evaluation of the ventral cellulae ethmoidales. **c** The further dorsal the slice runs, the less the hardening. Only a slight band of increased noise is recognisable (*arrow*). Note additionally that the patient has many metallic fillings, which, however, produce artefacts only on the lower image border due to the primary axial slice direction (*arrow*)

10%. Virtual endoscopy is therefore not improved by administration of intravenous contrast agent.

2.2.2 Magnetic Resonance Imaging

The two most prominent advantages of MRI over CT are the absence of ionising radiation and the possibility to initially program any slice orientation, precluding the need for postprocessing. Of special significance is the issue of radiation exposure when the optical lens lies in the direct radiation field of the axial or coronal CT. The potentially resultant clouding of the lens is irreversible, and a large proportion of the patients who undergo imaging of the sinuses are very young and affected simply by a benign alteration (sinusitis). In view of these issues, radiation exposure in CT must be critically evaluated. Nevertheless, it should be mentioned that CT today, most likely carried out in low-dose technique (Gholkar et al. 1988; Rogalla et al. 1998), gives a surface dose (applicable to the lens) of approximately 3–10 mGy, while direct damage to the lens requires exposure to 1–2 Gy.

With the current MRI technique, neither cortical bone nor small metal clips or similar structures produce relevant artefacts. As standard, a routine MRI includes T1-weighted imaging in the axial orientation and T2- and proton-weighted coronal scans.

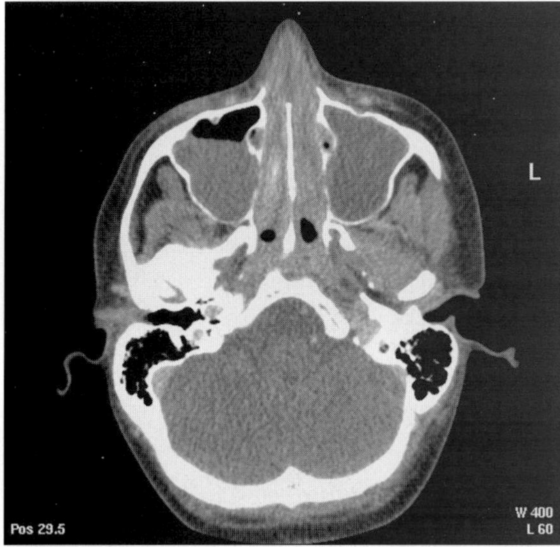

Fig. 2.4. By applying intravenous contrast agent, differentiation between inflamed mucosa (patient with acute rhinitis) and serosal secretion (maxillary sinuses) becomes very easy. For the virtual endoscopy, the administration of contrast agent is useless because the density difference between fluid and mucosa is not sufficient for a surface extraction

Sagittal slices help when evaluating the midline structures, the cribriform plate, and the sphenoid sinus and its drainage pathway. T1-weighted sequences are ideal for anatomic detail resolution and are performed in the coronal plane if this is necessary.

Since the head is a relatively motionless body part, the acquisition time of a sequence does not play such a meaningful role as it does when imaging the trunk. High-resolution sequences with 1 mm slice thickness or less (e.g. T2-weighted CISS or T1-weighted RAGE) are excellent precursors for subsequent three-dimensional postprocessing (see also Chap. 9,"Virtual Neuroscopy" and Chap. 10,"Virtual Otoscopy").

2.2.3 CT Versus MRI

Disadvantages of MRI are the well-known contraindications such as claustrophobia or the presence of pacemakers, vascular aneurysma clips or cochlear implants. CT is sensitive to even very small calcifications and subtle bony lesions. In contrast, cortical bone and calcifications cannot be detected in MRI, which means that tumours that are characterised by the pattern of calcifications, such as chondrogenic tumours and other calcifying lesions, might be misinterpreted. Both modalities, CT and MRI, currently deliver equivalently thin slices with strong contrast between the air-containing sinuses and the mucosal surface. The decision on which modality to use should be based solely upon general imaging and medical aspects (Manfre et al. 1994). The choice of modality is of secondary importance for the 3D reconstruction.

2.3 Reconstruction Techniques

Three-dimensional reconstructions of excellent quality can be calculated using thin-section MRI data or the spiral CT data mentioned in Sect. 2.2.1 due to the high spatial resolution. Under these circumstances, two basic reconstruction techniques are available: the surface rendering and the volume rendering technique. Both techniques are discussed in depth in Chap. 1 of this book; therefore, only the principal relevant aspects will be mentioned below.

2.3.1 Surface Rendering

In the surface rendering technique, a threshold value is defined. This value determines which pixels (picture elements) should be visible in the model that will be calculated, and which pixels should not appear. The choice system is binary, and intermediate definitions, such as a half-transparent pixel, are not possible. Whether a pure pixel model or a wire frame model is created from the data is a question of the software program used. Of significance is the data reduction that occurs with this technique, explaining why only limited computing power is needed and why this technique is still preferred by many today.

2.3.2 Volume Rendering

The volume rendering technique retains all pixels in the computer memory at all times. Through a classification system, the investigator attributes each voxel (volume element) to a certain characteristic, which may vary between completely transparent and completely opaque. The volume rendering technique requires notably more hardware performance; it is, however, superior to surface rendering with regard to detail resolution due to the possibility of creating stronger volume interpolations.

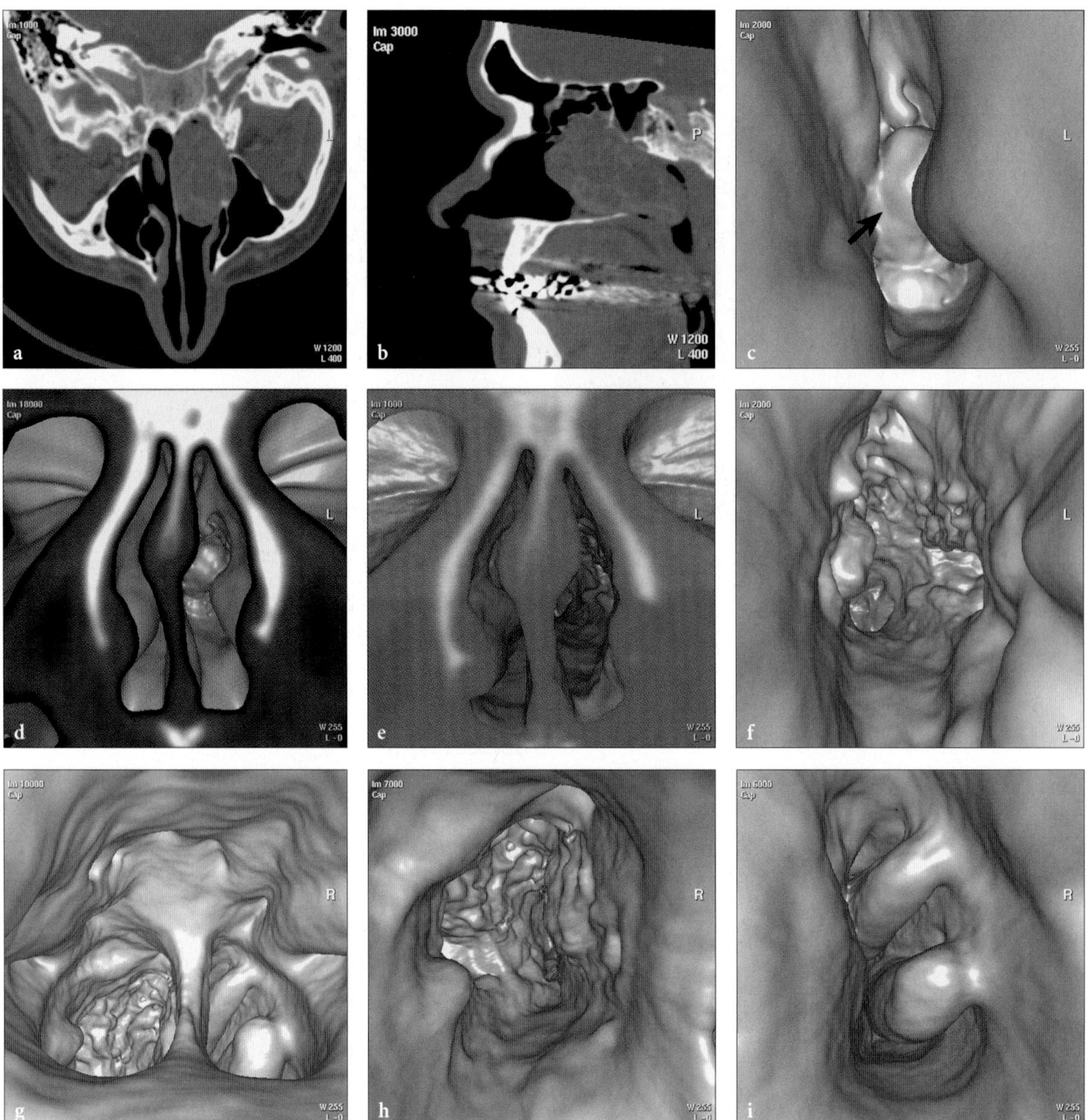

Fig. 2.5a–i. Virtual endoscopy of a young man with a histologically proven paranasal carcinoma. **a,b** Axial and sagittal views of the contrast agent enhancement in the tumour. **c,d** The tumour proliferation in the left naris has a polyp-like character *(arrow)*. **e,f** Postoperatively one can look from a left, ventral aspect far into the nasopharynx, representing the extent of the radical surgical resection. **g** The postoperative condition with a view from dorsally onto the choanae, where the large cavity on the left side is seen. **h** A focussed view left in the operated region. **i** The view to the right of the unremarkable turbinates

2.3.3 Perspective Presentations

Figure 2.6 shows a comparison between a surface rendering and a volume rendering reconstruction, based on the same dataset. Figure 2.7 represents a marked enlargement of Fig. 2.6b, which allows ample high-detail recognition despite the strong magnification. In this presentation, a perspective can then be incorporated which creates the impression that the images were obtained with a wide-angle camera. The viewing angle can be varied; however, angles larger than 120° create distortions that hinder sensible image interpretation. On the other hand, an angle that is too small limits the visual field, so that values between 80° and 120° have been chosen as most practical and as best

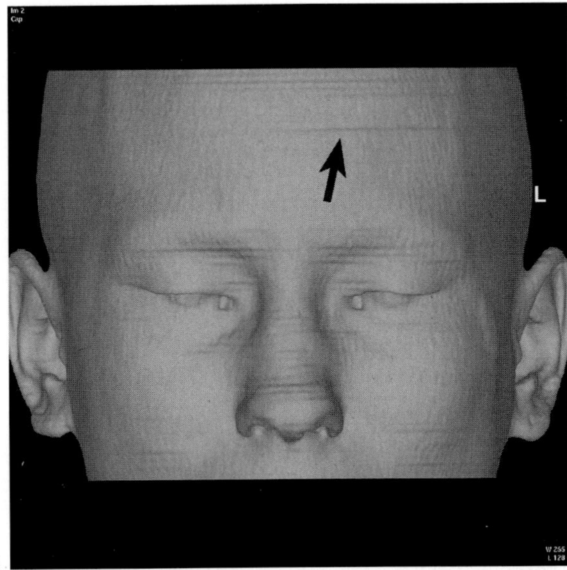

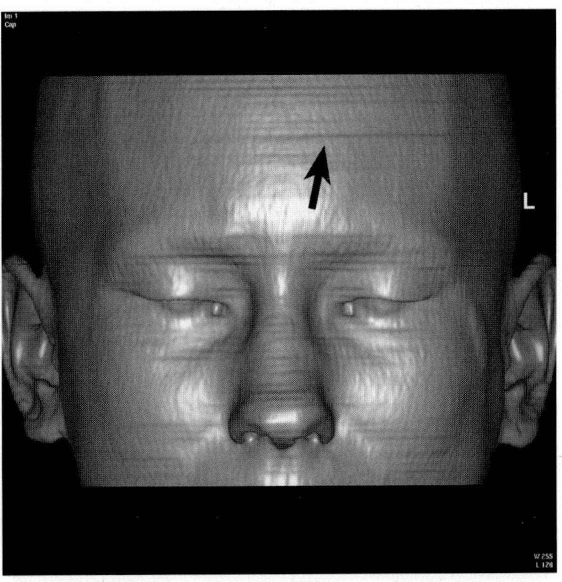

a b

Fig. 2.6a,b. Comparison of the two reconstruction techniques. **a** Surface rendering; **b** volume rendering with opaque surface classification. Both images were reconstructed from the same raw dataset of a spiral CT (scanning parameters: 1.5 mm slice thickness, 2 mm/s table feed, 1 mm reconstruction interval, 120 kV, 50 mAs, axial scanning). Note that due to the capability in volume rendering to have a smooth transition from completely opaque to completely transparent, the surface of the skin can be represented with a more natural appearance. Spiral artifacts, visible as stair stepping in the surface (*arrows*), are visible on both reconstruction techniques

supporting comparison with true endoscopic pictures. Tricks, such as calculating reflections onto the surface and attributing a colour similar to mucosa to the virtual endoscopic image can yield a shockingly "true"-appearing image.

2.3.4 Hybrid Technique

One of the obvious disadvantages of a purely endoluminal presentation is the fact that an anatomical relation to the surroundings is lacking. The hybrid technique, as described in Chap. 6, "Virtual Endoscopy of the Colon", is better suited to view anatomical relations: a cross-sectional image is viewed in which only the air-filled spaces of the paranasal sinuses contain depth information. In this case, cross-sectional information is not lost; however, black image areas are filled with three-dimensional depth information (Fig. 2.8). The advantage of this method is that the complete image information is contained in one presentation technique and that the reconstruction can be calculated without notable user interaction. Disadvantageous is only the relatively high memory requirement for the reconstructed images (approx. 2 MB/image) and if strongly enlarged, the limited resolution, even when using an image matrix of 1024×1024. Since morphological image details of 0.5 mm are not essential, this disadvantage can be clinically disregarded.

If hybrid images are laser-printed onto a film, the colour information is transformed into black and white and the resulting images might be confusing for an inexperienced viewer. Thus, for the documentation of hybrid images, colour must be recommended.

2.4 Virtual Endoscopic Examination

Since virtual endoscopic views can be calculated practically anywhere in the nose or the paranasal sinuses, an imaging algorithm producing standard views that belong to the comprehensive evaluation of the nose and neighbouring sinuses must be selected: choosing six orthogonal views in both maxillary sinuses, in the sphenoid cavity and in the nasopharynx, each having a viewing angle of 120°, has proven to be a practical approach. The result is an overlap of 30° for each viewpoint, so that pathologies cannot be overlooked due to partial representation on two neighbouring images. The frontal sinuses can be viewed similarly; however, sometimes six images

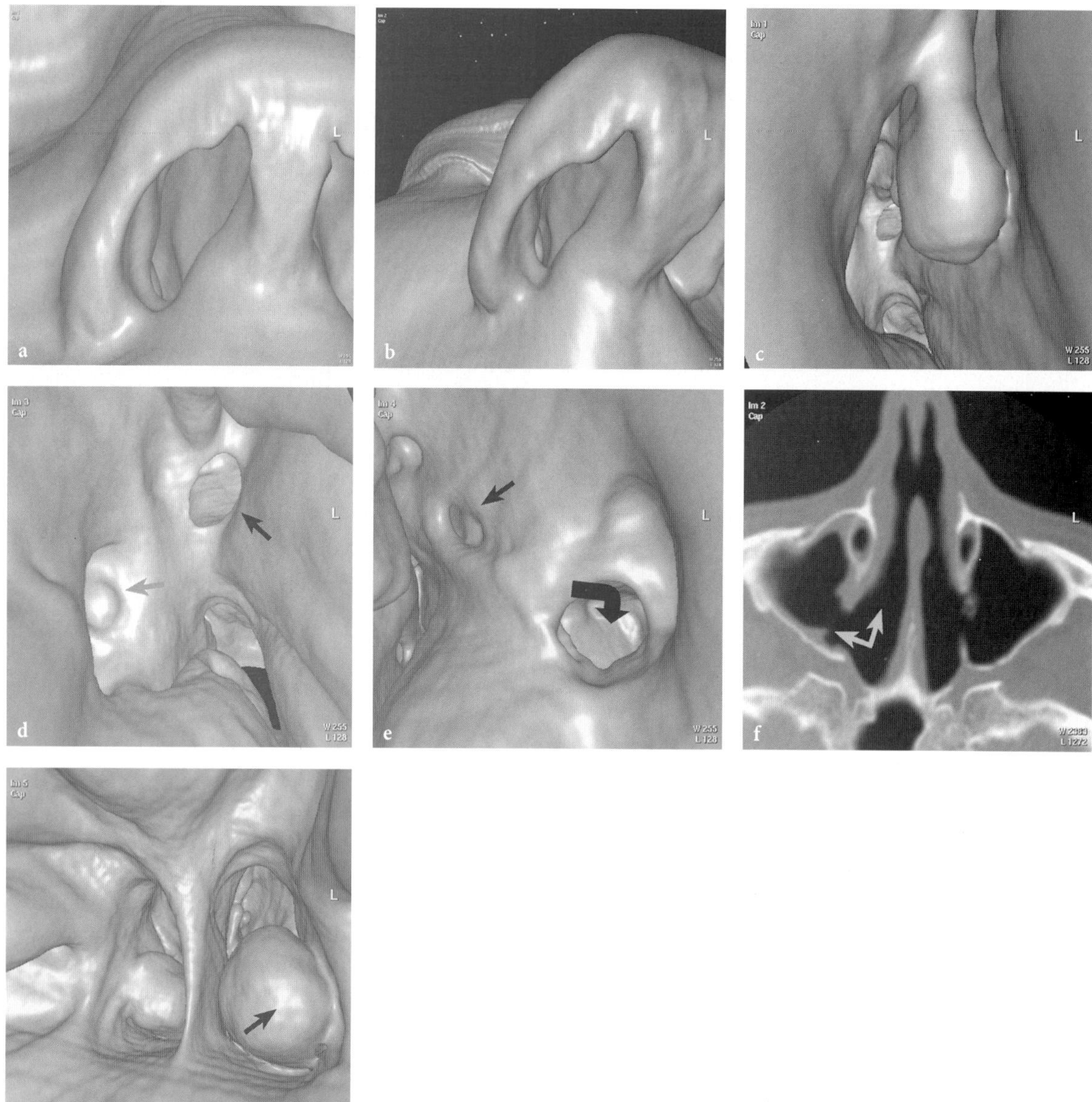

Fig. 2.7a–g. Example of a virtual endoscopy of the nose in a patient after FESS. **a** An enlargement of Fig 2.6. Note that despite the strong magnification, the volume rendering technique presents an extremely detailed information of the right nostril. **b** An image from the same viewpoint but with a 120° perspective additionally calculated. The resulting impression is similar to the view obtained with a powerful wide-angle lens. With these reconstruction parameters, the virtual endoscopic evaluation through the nose can start. **c** An image within the nose, demonstrating the inferior turbinate, which can be easily passed by the "virtual endoscope". **d** A view onto the hole (*black arrow*) that was created during the FESS to improve ventilation of the sphenoid sinus. Also the wide-open entry into the maxillary sinus is clearly seen with a remaining mucosal polyp (*grey arrow*). One of the key characteristics of virtual endoscopy is that the views can be taken in any direction. **e** A "backview" showing the natural ostium to the maxillary sinus (*straight arrow*) and the artificial ostium produced by the surgeons (*curved arrow*). **f** The corresponding axial image nicely confirms the wide-open new ostium to the sinus (the viewing direction of image **g** is indicated by the *arrows*). **g** A virtual view directed back from the nasopharynx onto the caudal ends of the inferior turbinates. These views impressively show a polyp-like swelling on the caudal end of the inferior conchae. Such a swelling of the caudal turbinate ends is the main cause for posterior rhinorrhoea

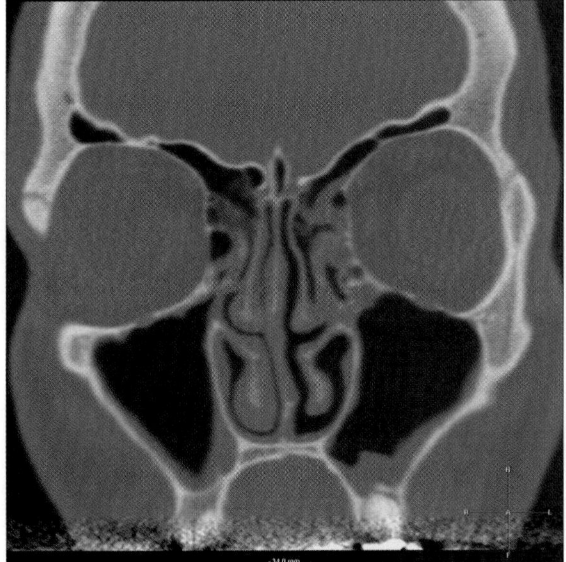

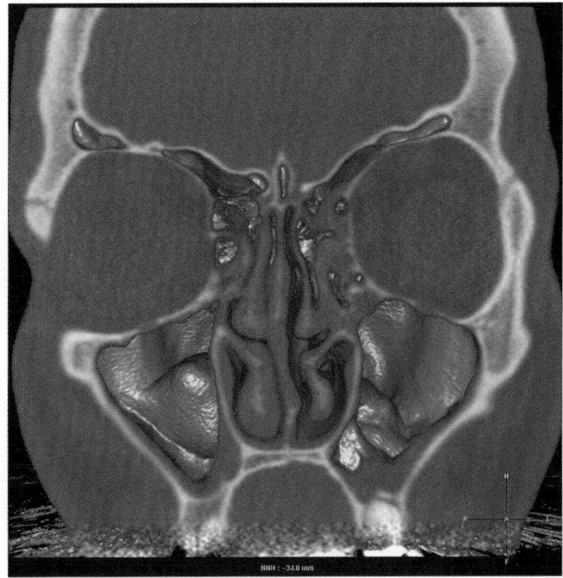

a b

Fig. 2.8a,b. Young male with recurrent sinusitis. In the hybrid technique the air-filled space that appears black in the coronal image (**a**) is "filled" with the three-dimensional information (**b**). The bilateral polypoid mucosal swelling in the maxillary sinuses are already recognisable in the hybrid image, before they are presented in the simple coronal slices

will not suffice to display all sections of the sinus due to the long anatomical structure.

In the nose, placing a path through each naris is the most favourable imaging method (Fig. 2.9). If the naris is not anatomically deviant in structure or pathologically changed, placing the path along the nasal septum between the lower and middle conchae is most promising, leading past the uncinate process and on to the ostium naturale as far as the choanae in the epipharynx. However, not infrequently the planned path is obstructed, for example by tumour masses (Fig. 2.10), swollen choanae, or simple normal variants such as septal spurs (Fig. 2.11). Due to the high variability of the main nasal cavity, the path must frequently be determined according to individual findings, so that a preliminary review of the coronary or axial slices has often already been accomplished. The need to initially view the (already diagnostic) original images prior to the reconstruction procedure represents a substantial weakness of virtual endoscopy of the paranasal sinuses.

Along the outlined path, which may also contain diverging branches, the images can be calculated by the computer. Due to the relatively short distance from the nostril to the epipharynx, 20–30 images will usually suffice to create a representative display of the naris. A reconstruction interval of the virtual images along the path of 0.5–1 mm has proven effective when the virtual images are intended to be presented as a fly-through at a later point in time. If the user is equipped with more powerful computing systems that make navigation in real-time possible, the path definition can be disregarded and direct evaluation can begin. To date, there are only few studies in which an acceptable real-time navigation has been realised, mostly for virtual endoscopy of the colon (Hoffmann et al. 1998) or of the tracheobronchial tree (Summers and Merran 1997).

2.5 Reconstruction Filter and Image Quality

Although the choice of the primary reconstruction kernel is initially only a technical parameter, it has a strong influence on the virtual endoscopy. In CT, the paranasal sinuses represent a highly contrasted area because a naturally high contrast exists between air and soft tissue. For this reason and in view of the issue of radiation protection, it is judicious to reduce the radiation dose as much as possible by choosing a lower mAs setting. The consequence is, however, that the resulting axial images show a very high noise level that renders direct evaluation of the primary slices difficult. A possible way of circumventing this

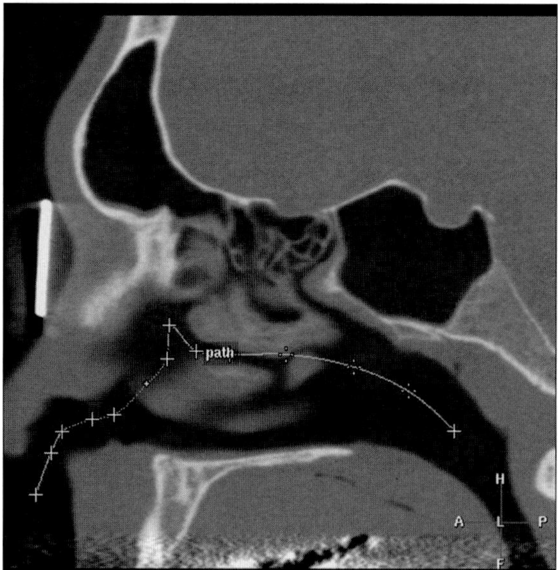

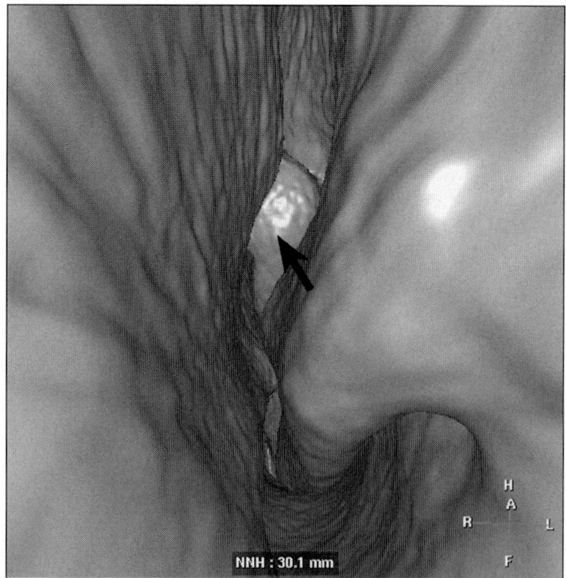

Fig. 2.9. **a** Example of a path through the left nostril. **b** Passing by the lower turbinate reaching into the nasopharynx. The *arrow* points at the middle turbinate

problem is the retrospective calculation of thicker slices, using an averaging function that is already implemented in most workstations (Fig. 2.12).

The newly calculated slabs can then be based upon any slice thickness, dependent upon how many slices were incorporated. It has already been shown that diagnostic images for evaluation of soft tissue can be created for the paranasal sinuses despite use of a low-dose technique (Diederichs et al. 1996). However, thick slabs are not suited for virtual endoscopy computation. Alternatively, in order to compensate for image noise, a soft reconstruction filter (convolution kernel) can be used, for example when imaging the abdomen. Although the resulting images are no longer acceptable for evaluation of the fine bony structure, virtual reconstructions with smooth surfaces are possible (Figs. 2.13, 2.14). An examination protocol should therefore include two primary runs: one run serving the evaluation of the osseous fine structures (bone filter with relatively high noise level), and a second run serving the virtual reconstruction. The main disadvantage is clearly the doubling of resources: twice as many slices need twice as much memory, and also the time to transfer images over the network to the workstation is doubled.

2.6 Thresholding

A further important parameter for the reconstructions, whether based on the surface or the volume rendering technique, is the choice of an appropriate threshold above which a surface should be presented as opaque. Characteristic of CT is that edges that have an abrupt density transition in reality are not presented so clear-cut, but rather with a finite gradient due to partial-pixel effects (Fig. 2.15). If the threshold defining the wall is set too high (too far towards 0 HU), air-filled lumina will appear larger than they actually are. If the threshold is set too low, the lumina appear too small and structures begin to merge (Fig. 2.16). In most cases, the calculated average between the HU-values of soft tissue and air is the optimal value to display the air-filled lumina as realistically as possible.

2.7 Clinical Evaluation

Other than the fact that virtual endoscopic images might be more attractive to the lay public and the endoscopists, evaluating the clinical value of virtual endoscopy necessitates critical evaluation of the diagnostic details that are also very important in read-

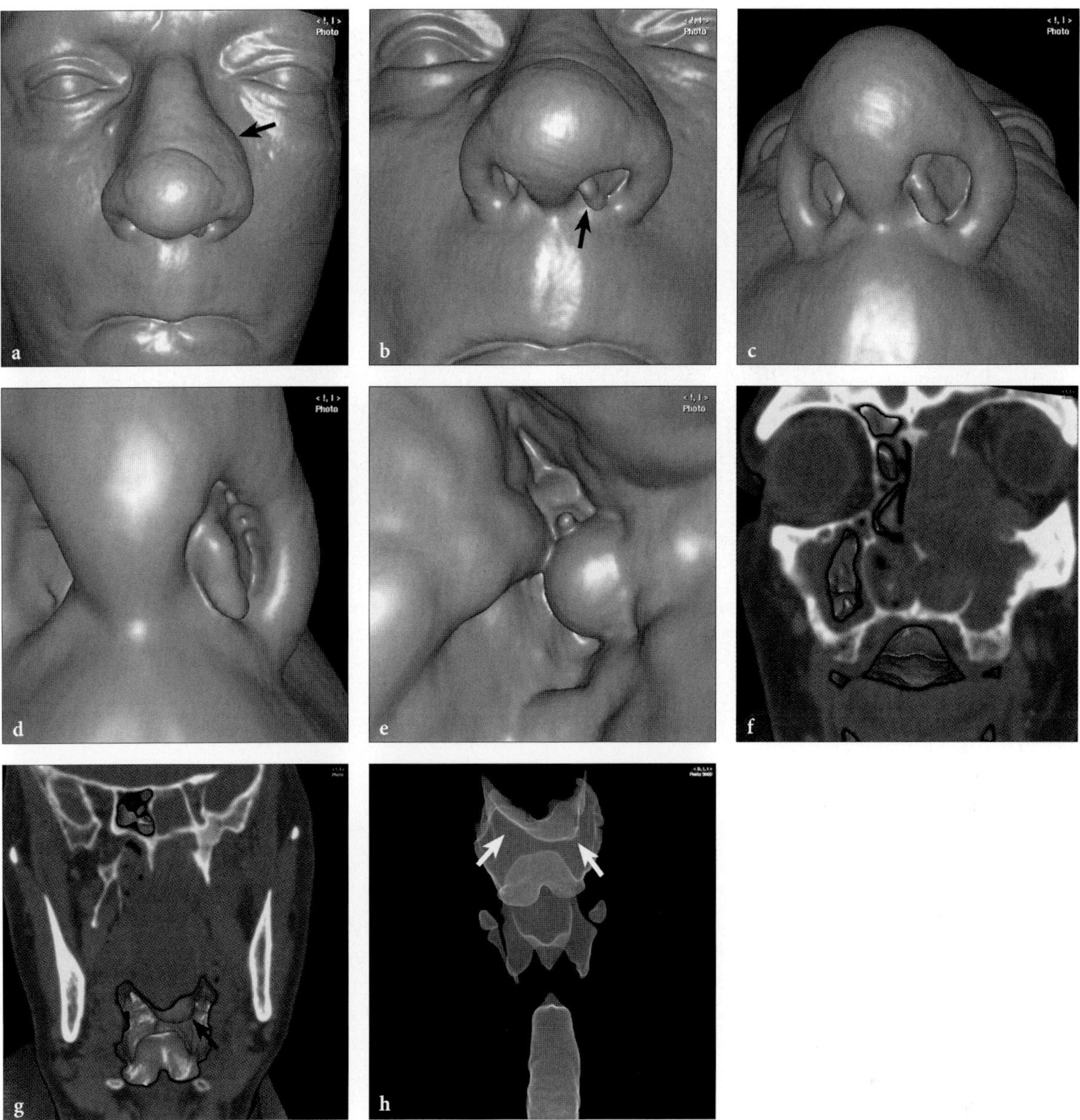

Fig. 2.10a–h. Occluding nasopharyngeal fibroma. **a–d** On the external images one can already see the tumour growing out of the nose and the bulging surface of the nasal spine (*arrow*). **e** Shortly after entering the left naris a complete occlusion of the airway is detected so that continuation of an endoscopy is impossible. **f, g** The extent of the tumour infiltration in the bones and the orbita, and the progression of the tumour tip into the oropharynx (*arrow*). **h** In the tissue transition projection (also referred to as virtual double contrast) one sees the tumour tip (*arrow*) in anatomical relation to the epiglottis

ing conventional CT or MRI examinations. In a prospective study including 45 patients suspected of having chronic or acute sinusitis, a clinical comparison of the virtual endoscopy with coronal CT slices was undertaken (Rogalla et al. 1998). The initial axially obtained CT scans (1.5 mm slice thickness, 2 mm/s table speed, 1 mm reconstruction interval, 120 kV, 50 mAs) were reconstructed coronally every 5 mm. Using a 10-point checklist (Table 2), we attempted to determine which diagnostically relevant findings could be detected with virtual endoscopy.

Especially for the evaluation of osseous deviations such as Onodi cells (Yanagisawa et al. 1998) and Haller cells (Arslan et al. 1999) as well as septal deviations, which were easily assessed on coronal scans, the virtual endoscopy allowed no diagnostic statement. The fact that only 34 of the 45 bilateral maxillary sinuses were viewable could be attributed

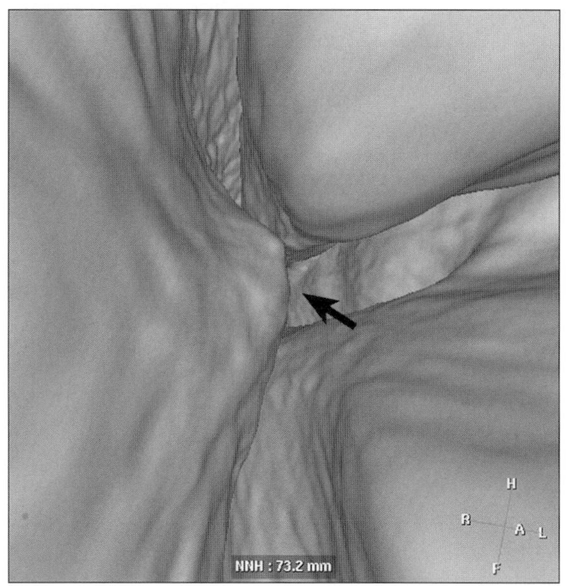

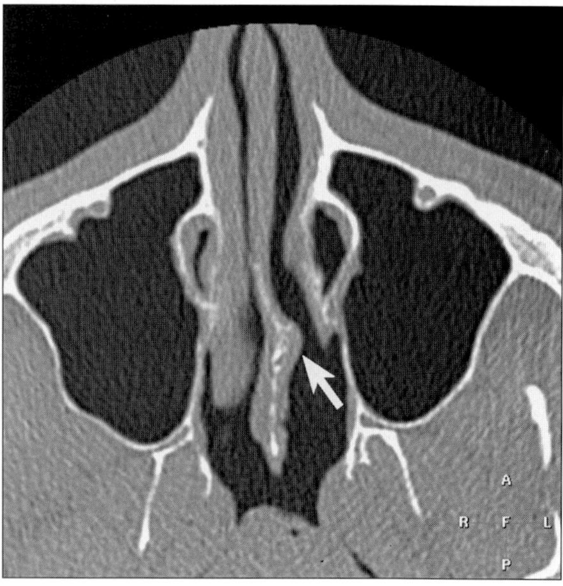

Fig. 2.11a,b. A septal spur. The findings are clearly recognisable in the virtual endoscopy (*arrow*, **a**); however, the axial slices (**b**) provide the proof. Through perspective distortion, evaluation of the extent of a spur or simply a distance measurement is not possible

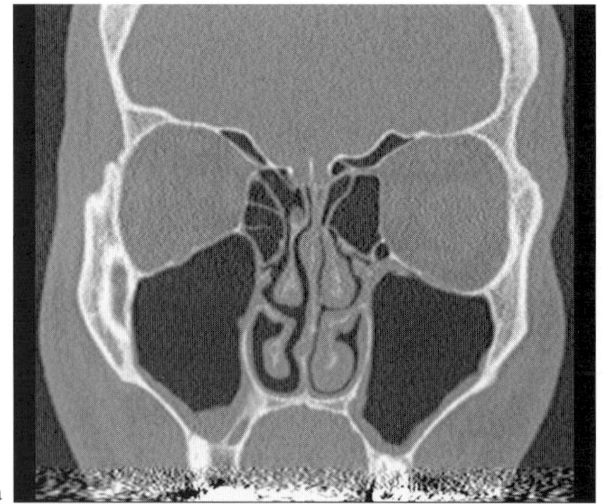

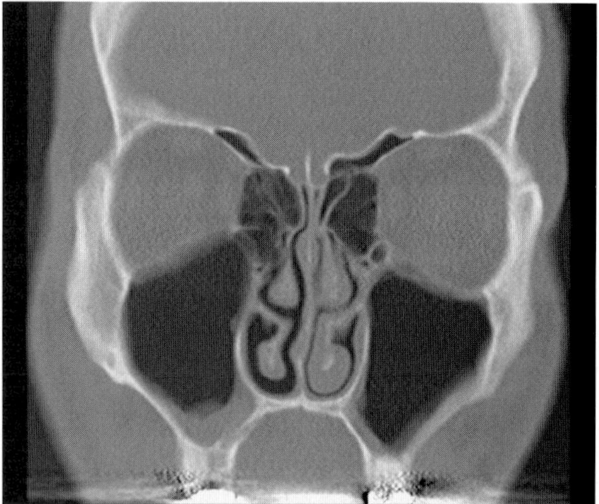

Fig. 2.12. **a** A coronal reconstruction from an isotropic dataset (0.5 mm slice thickness, 0.3 mm reconstruction interval, 25 mAs, high-frequency reconstruction kernel). Note the considerable noise, which can be reduced to a normal level by calculating a 5-mm slice thickness (**b**). However, 5-mm slice thicknesses have the trade-off of notably increased partial volume effects and are therefore not suitable for virtual endoscopy

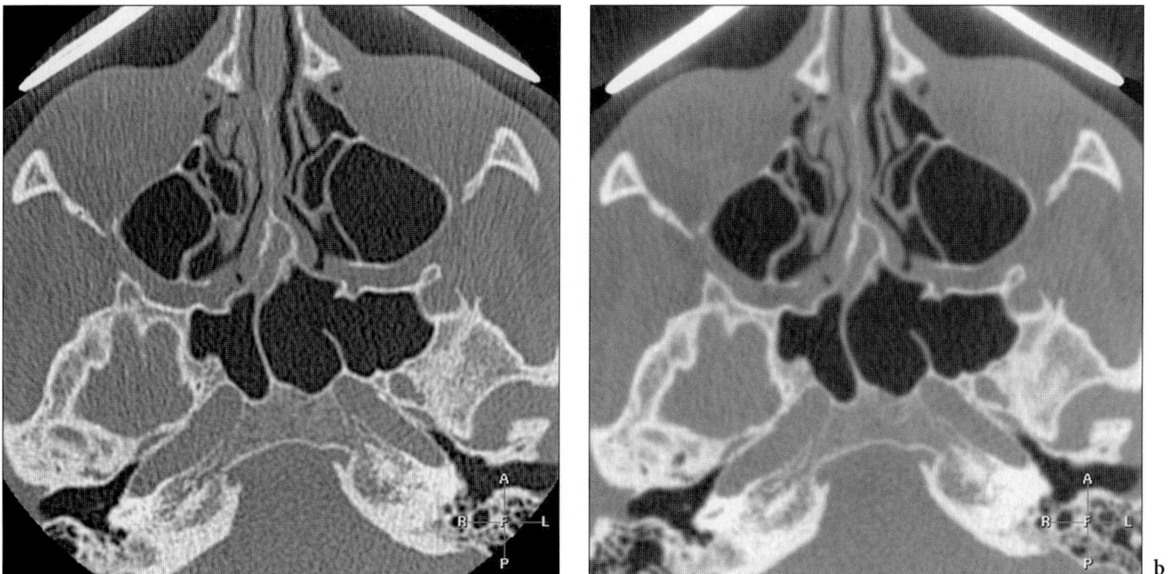

Fig. 2.13a,b. Example of two reconstruction kernels: **a** reconstructed with a bone filter (high-frequency kernel); **b** with a body filter. In this fashion it is also possible to reduce the image noise in a low-dose CT so that the virtual endoscopy shows less noise

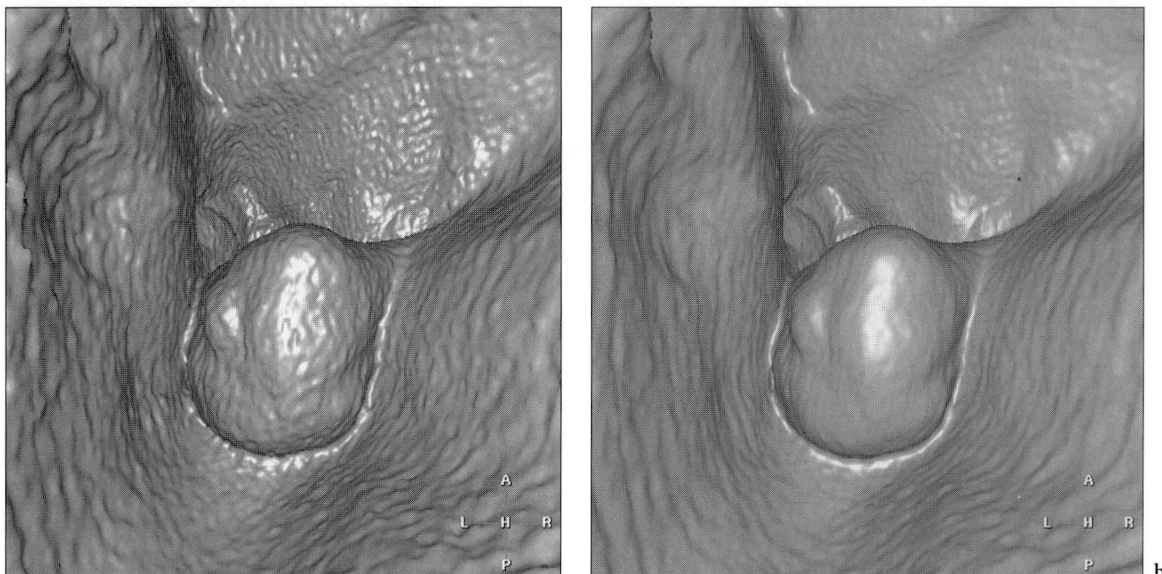

Fig. 2.14a,b. Effect of a soft reconstruction kernel on the image impression in the virtual endoscopy. The high image noise from the low-dose technique presents as an irregular surface. From a cranial viewpoint, a basal mucosal polyp is presented in the right maxillary sinus

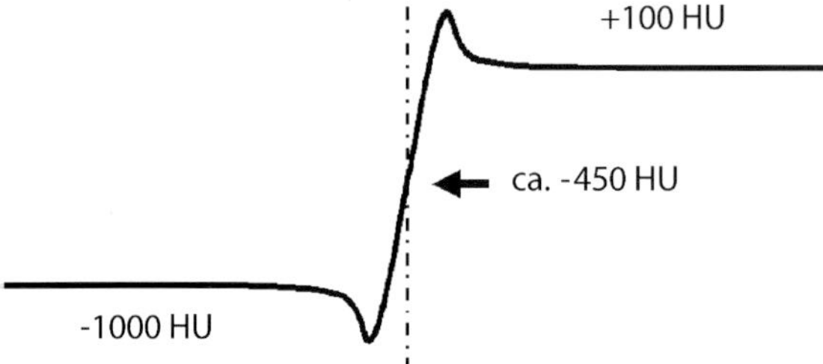

Fig. 2.15. Schematic sketch of a density profile through an ideal steep edge. Due to the reconstruction technique in CT, an abrupt density transition is presented as a density gradient. The edge exaggeration is created only by high-frequency reconstruction kernels. The ideal threshold value in the case of a density transition from air to soft tissue lies in the vicinity of –450 HU

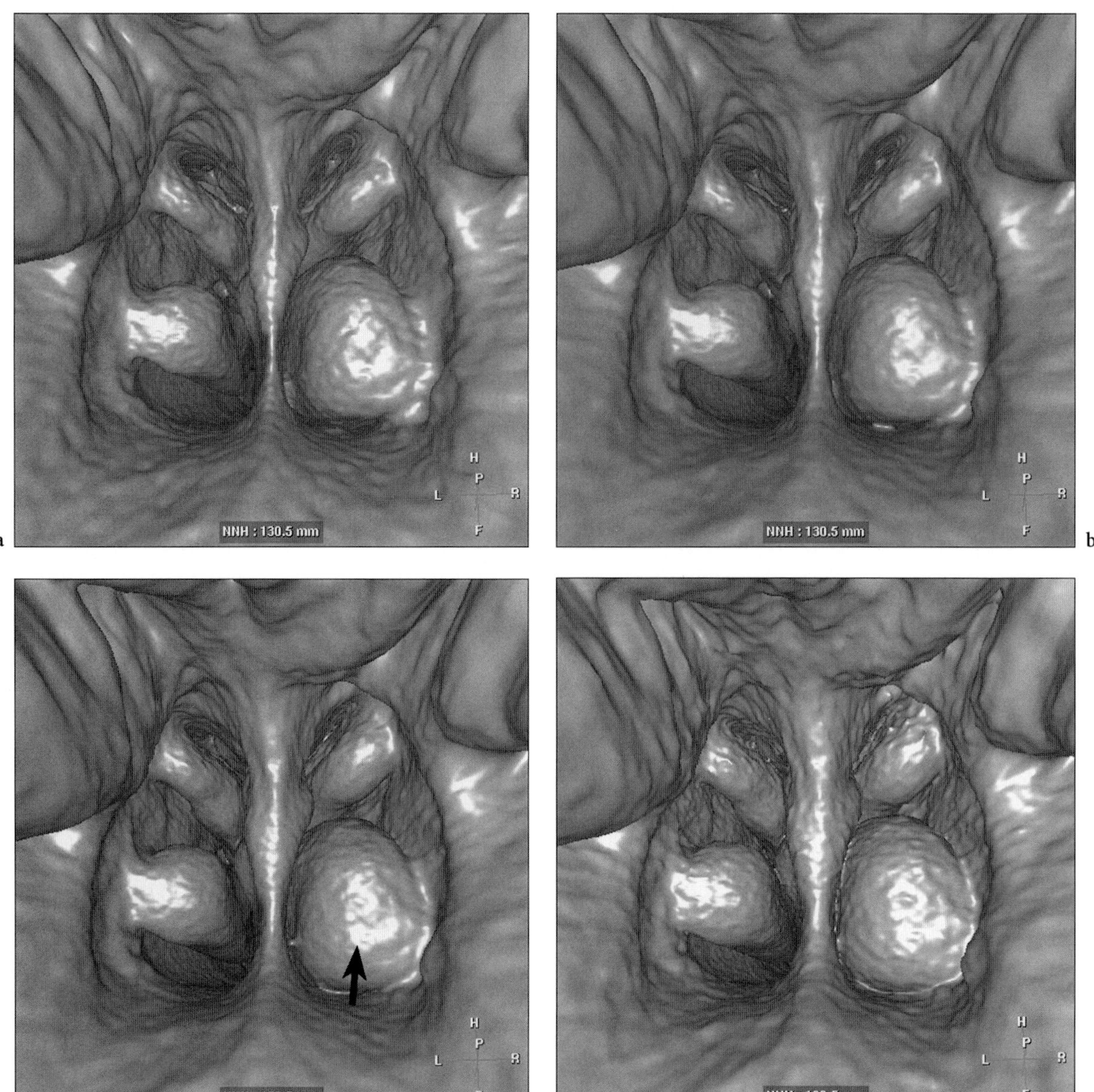

Fig. 2.16a–d. Effect of a varying threshold definition in the virtual endoscopy: At –200 HU (**a**) the lumina are displayed too wide, and at –800 HU (**d**) too narrow (**b** –400 HU; **c** –600 HU). Values around –450 to –500 HU best represent the true conditions. Findings: swelling of the caudal end of the inferior concha, right side (*arrow*), a typical finding that corresponds with the symptoms of posterior rhinorrhoea

to the fact that 11 patients had complete obstruction of the maxillary sinuses and the resulting lack of distension made virtual endoscopy impossible.

Since objective criteria for image quality in virtual endoscopy are difficult to establish, a subjective evaluation by the surgeons was used instead. For the 30 patients (67%) in this series who underwent subsequent surgery (FESS, plastic surgery of the septum etc.), the surgeons were asked to rank the degree of assistance of the virtual endoscopic images during the surgical procedure on a scale of 1 to 5, with 1 meaning very useful and 5 meaning useless. The average ranking was 1.7, and in no case did the surgeon perceive the virtual endoscopy as worthless.

The evaluation of the sphenoid cavity was not incorporated into the virtual endoscopy study since no true endoscopic images exist for comparative purposes (Fig. 2.17). However, the results of the evaluation of the other paranasal sinuses can be carried over to the sphenoid cavity. The mere ability to judge

Table 2.2. Summary of visible findings from the coronal and virtual endoscopy views

Structure	Diagnosis possible	
	Coronal views	Virtual endoscopy
Maxillary sinuses	45	34
Nasopharyngeal cavity	45	45
Conchae nasales inferiores et mediae	41	41
Conchae nasales superiores	37	25
Infundibula	43	41
Ostia naturalia	45	27
Choanae	45	45
Tubae auditivae	35	45
Septal deviation	45	22
Osseous normal variants (Onodi, Haller)[a]	45	0

With the exception of the entry to the tubae auditivae, VE provides less diagnostic information than the conventional, coronal slices.

[a]Onodi cell, cellula sphenoethmoidalis; Haller cell, cellula infraorbitalis.

the nares and sinuses as documented in the study yields no information regarding the diagnostic sensitivity or specificity of virtual endoscopy, but rather describes the initial experience in implementation. Studies documenting the diagnostic benefit and clinical correlation of virtual endoscopy alone or in comparison to conventional cross-sectional slices have not been published to date but are necessary in order to justify the technical and time investment needed for the calculation of a virtual endoscopy.

2.8 Postoperative Sinuses

A common diagnostic purpose of CT is the postoperative evaluation following FESS (Mantoni et al. 1996). Typical findings are detected on virtual endoscopy. Generally, the operation defect, that is, the surgically created access to a maxillary sinus in the level of the medial concha, is easily distinguished as long as the region of interest is not completely shadowed (Fig. 2.7). Under such conditions, the flexibility of virtual endoscopy is well demonstrated. A display in any direction is possible, including backwards-directed views through the surgical opening into the sinus cavity. A window to the sphenoid cavity can also be clearly recognised (Fig. 2.7). The accomplished window can escape detection in a pure coronal examination if it lies parallel to the sliced plane. Sometimes a single FESS procedure is insufficient to cure the chronic inflammatory mucosal swelling. In especially severe cases, a chronic infection can lead to bone affliction, and osteitis can complicate the situation (Fig. 2.18).

A history of numerous operations and re-operations leads to progressive scarring and increasingly compromises the surgeon's ability to obtain an adequate anatomic orientation. Under such circumstances, virtual endoscopy offers valuable preoperative assistance by demonstrating the anatomical situation as realistically as possible and supporting the choice of an optimal access route for a new operative intervention. Nonetheless, the coronal and sagittal slices remain imperative for the diagnostic evaluation of mucosal thickness and cannot be replaced solely by virtual endoscopy.

2.9 Posttraumatic Sinuses

The diagnostic questions following a trauma are primarily associated with detection of osseous fractures and the respective complications, for example, herniation of the inferior rectus muscle into the maxillary sinus due to fracture of the orbital floor. Fracture demonstration and tissue characterisation is a domain of cross-sectional imaging because the pathological condition can be evaluated without overlapping. Virtual endoscopy is not suited for tissue characterisation, and subtle fractures are in any case best seen on cross-sectional imaging. At most, a three-dimensional display of complex fractures of the middle face may be diagnostically relevant (Figs. 2.19, 2.20).

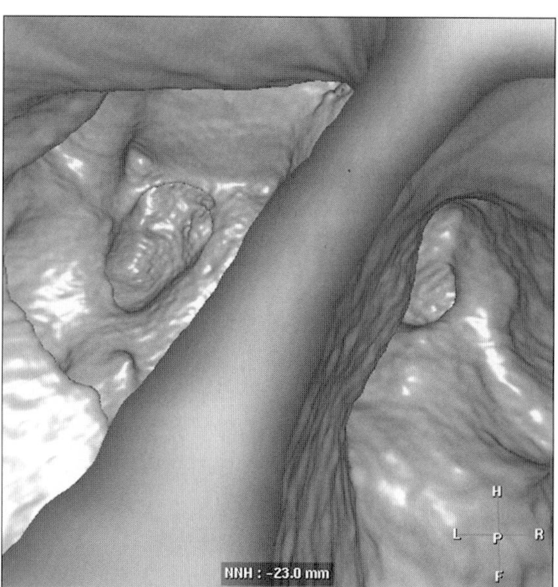

a

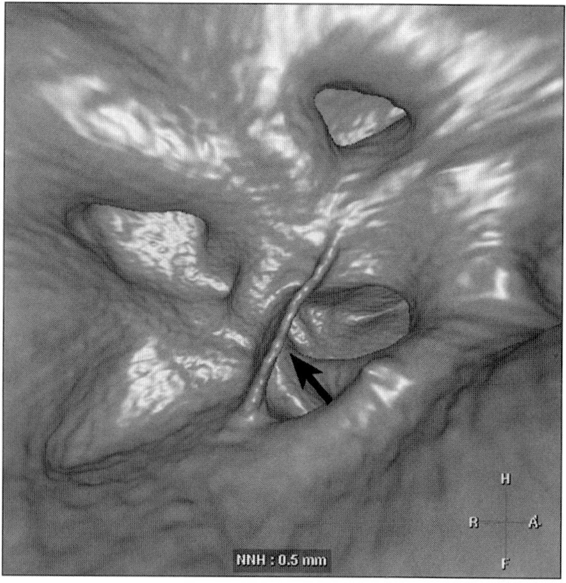

b

Fig. 2.17a,b. Unremarkable sinus sphenoidalis in a young male. **a** The septum intersphenoidale is recognisable as a middle bridge. **b** A view from the ventral to the dorsal aspect. The problem with this presentation is that no clinical correlation exists, since the sphenoid cavity is inaccessible with true endoscopy. The *arrow* points towards a partial septation that often occurs in the sphenoid cavity

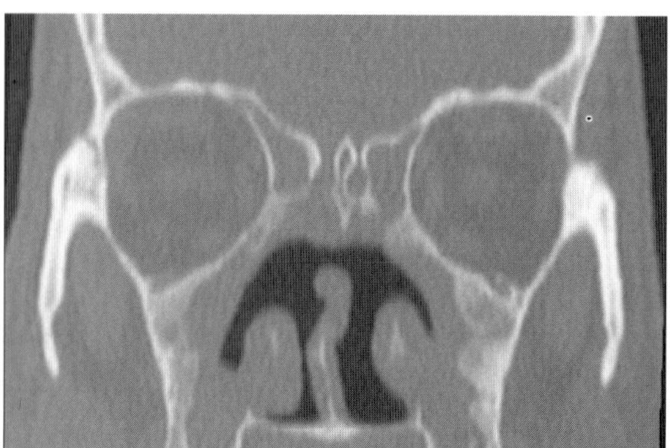

a

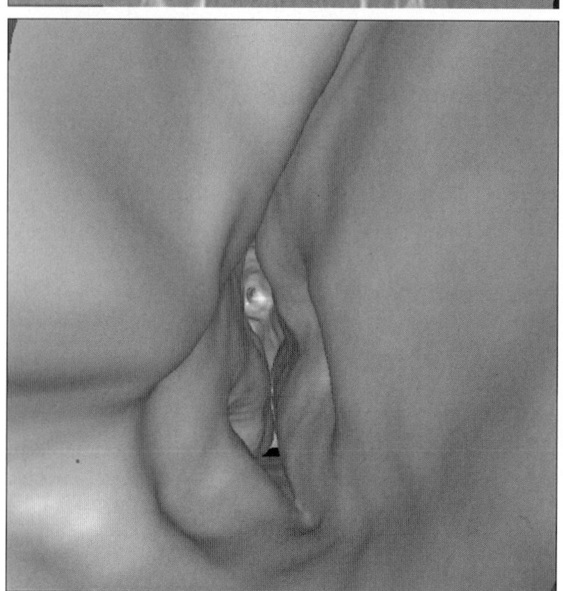

b

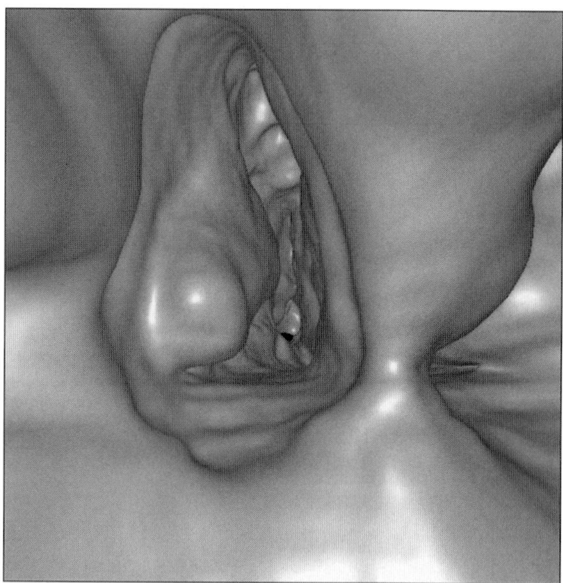

c

Fig. 2.18a–c. Example of an impressive chronic infection. The patient had already undergone multiple FESS with little success. **a** A coronal reconstruction from a spiral CT with 1.5 mm slice thickness and 1 mm reconstruction interval. Note the "chewed" appearance of the osseous boundary of the maxillary sinus and the ethmoid cells, compatible with osteitis. In the virtual endoscopy (**b** antegrade view, **c** retrograde view) the extensive mucosal changes are clearly distinguished; the osteitis, however, remains hidden behind the mucosa

2.10 Application in Paediatrics

From a clinical perspective, few indications exist for virtual endoscopy in children or newborns. The use of ionising radiation must be viewed very critically, and if CT of the paranasal sinuses is indicated (SPAETH et al. 1997), for example to evaluate a choanal atresia, than it must be carried out in low-dose technique. Due to the small paediatric occipital volume, even with a minimal electrical current of 10–25 mAs no notable noise occurs in the images compared to adult examinations; hence the virtual reconstructions are of good quality (Fig. 2.21). A prerequisite is, however, that small children remain motionless during the imaging time in the spiral or multislice CT. Additional difficulty is encountered when trying to explain to young children that they should not swallow during the examination because swallowing artefacts make the impression of a membrane in the virtual endoscopy. In most cases, scanning through the axial slices permits differentiation between true anatomical structures and motion artefacts.

2.11 Value of Virtual Endoscopy for the Sinuses

Virtual endoscopy of the nose and paranasal sinuses represents one of many applications of this new technique (GILANI et al. 1997; MORRA et al. 1998). The paranasal sinuses are well suited for virtual endoscopy because they contain air as a natural contrast material and thus represent a high-contrast object

a
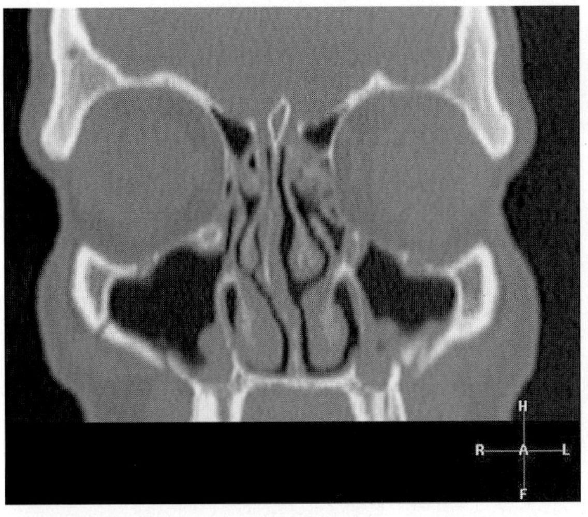

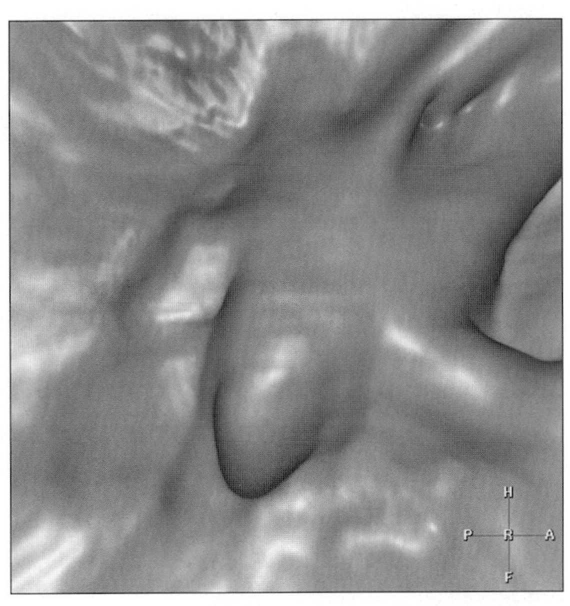

b

Fig. 2.19a,b. Young patient with a LeFort fracture. Since the mucosa remained intact despite the multiple fractures (**a**), the fracture cleft is not displayed in the virtual endoscopy (**b**)

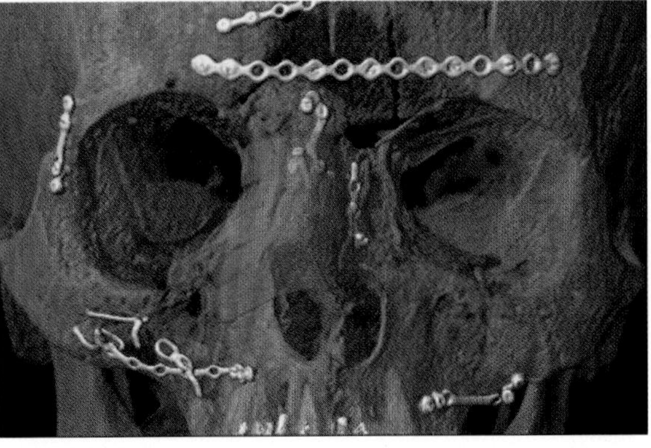

Fig. 2.20. An alternative to the virtual presentation in complex osseous questions is surface reconstruction with different colours for different tissue types. This young patient had a motorcycle accident with extreme facial injuries. Using three-dimensional reconstruction, the ENT and plastic surgeons could repair the osseous defect with a segment of the iliac bone. Note the enormous detail resolution; even the indentations in the screw heads are clearly seen. Multislice CT, 0.5 mm slice thickness, 0.3 mm reconstruction interval, 50 mAs, 120 kV. Three thresholds for tissue characterisation: bone, metal, and titanium (nose reconstruction). Bones and titanium are presented as slightly transparent

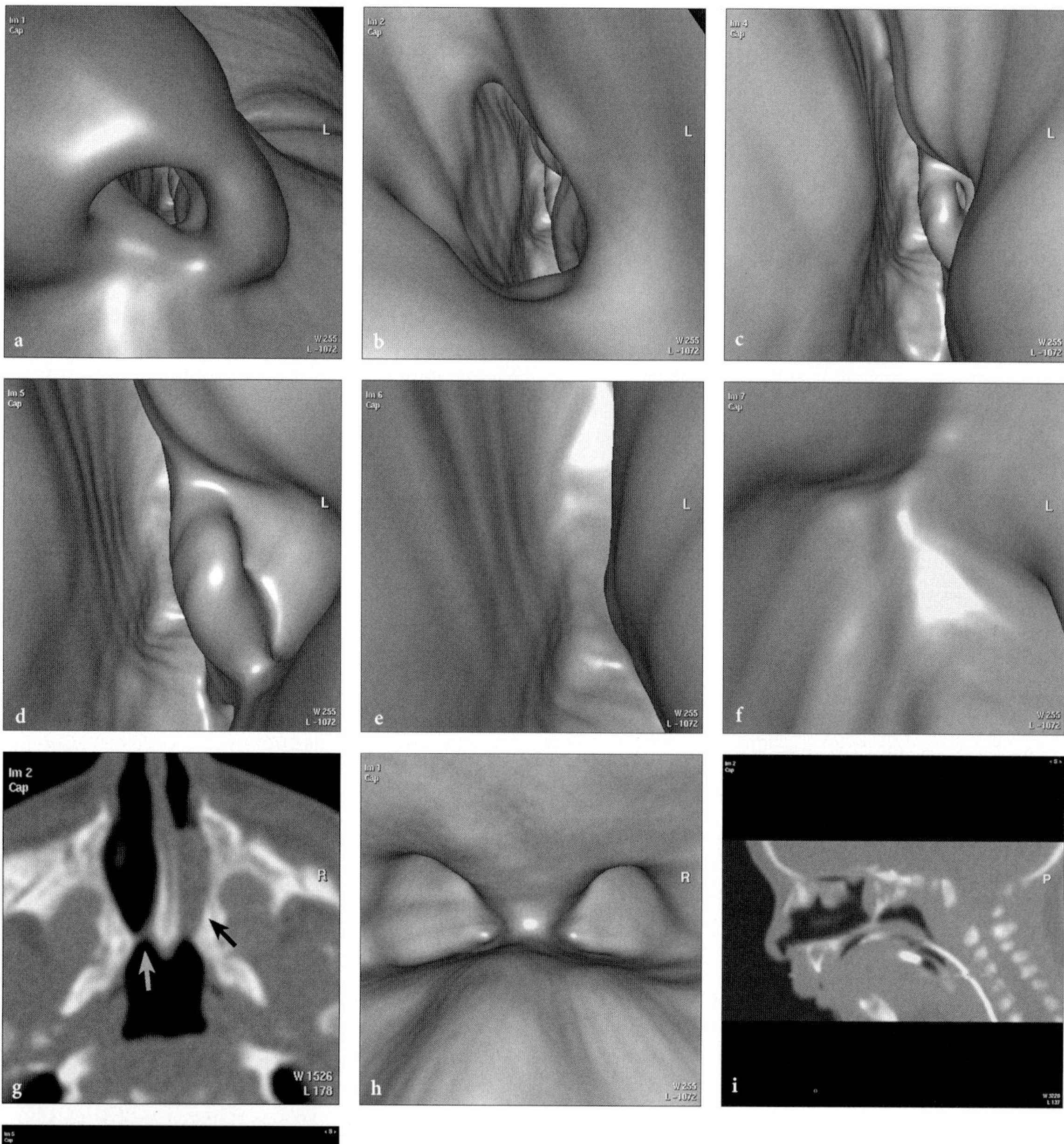

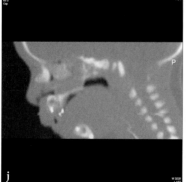

Fig. 2.21a–j. Virtual endoscopy in a 5-day-old infant. Clinically, choanal atresia was suspected. Important is whether only a thin membrane or an osseous occlusion exists. **a–f** Fly-through in the left naris, passing the early inferior choanal structure and reaching an occluding membrane. There is no connection to the nasopharynx. A similar impression exists on the right side. **g** An axial slice from above, in which a thin membrane on the left and a thick occlusion on the right can be seen (*arrows*). **h** The virtual view from the nasopharynx impressively shows the bilateral occlusion. **i,j** In the sagittal reconstruction, it can be additionally demonstrated that although the left side has a thin membrane, it contains an osseous component. On the right side, a voluminous mucosal plug lies in front of the osseous membrane

for CT. Most sections of the nose and paranasal sinuses are also accessible with the true endoscope, and FESS is an operation technique that has received enormously increased recognition in recent years. The question that remains is: What role can and will virtual endoscopy play?

Diagnostic Value. For simple diagnostic questions, the clinical value of virtual endoscopy must be viewed critically, not only because the procedure is time-consuming and thus indirectly very costly, but also because the expected diagnostic gain in comparison to axial or coronal cross-sectional images is not very conspicuous. Virtual endoscopy with an intensive reconstruction technique is better suited for answering questions regarding osseous normal deviations. If mucosal inflammation is so extreme that the necessary air is no longer present in the nose or sinuses as contrast, then virtual endoscopy is no longer feasible. Nonetheless, once the virtual endoscopy is calculated practically automatically, with limited guiding steps by a technologist or a radiologist, meaning the procedure can be carried out routinely, its clinical value will increase. With few views, a good anatomical presentation is possible, which is otherwise difficult to perceive from the axial or coronal slices without a trained eye. A very promising presentation form is the hybrid technique since the calculation of images can proceed in near-automated fashion.

Teaching Device. A second potential function of virtual endoscopy is as a teaching device, both for the radiologist and for the ENT surgeon (Plinkert and Lowenheim 1997; Yanagisawa and Christmas 1999). It is not yet possible to interactively manipulate images on commonly marketed workstations, for example, to remove polyps from the virtual endoscopic image. However, an interactive function that could certainly facilitate learning of endoscopic operation techniques (Edmond et al. 1997; Rudman et al. 1998) will be widely available in the near future and will attain clinical significance. Initial experiments on preoperative site-tagging based on virtual reality have already been conducted and have achieved promising results (Hopper et al. 1999).

Image-Guided Surgery. Intraoperative guidance will become practical only when high-performance computers that enable an instantaneous reconstruction of virtual or 3D images are accessible (Gunkel et al. 1997). Under such circumstances, the existing position of the surgical instruments (scalpel, drainage tubes, etc.) must be transferred to the computer in three-dimensional coordinates. The first experiments were carried out in 1996 and then tested in routine practice (Kruckels et al. 1996).

Image accuracy of 1–2 mm is technically possible to date (Freysinger et al. 1997; Hopper et al. 1999; Metson et al. 1999). However, considerable intraoperative image discrepancies may appear in comparison to the preoperative CT because anti-inflammatory agents for the intranasal mucosa must be given intraoperatively, and also for an FESS, to facilitate surgical access; a procedure that, in most cases, is not essential for CT. Nonetheless, for the calculation of a virtual endoscopy in CT, the preliminary administration of anti-inflammatory medication in the nose is sensible because the navigational area is enlarged and the virtual endoscopy can be calculated with fewer manual interventions. The extent to which general administration of anti-inflammatory agents is justified will not be discussed here. Initial results from a study with real-time intraoperative navigation have already been presented (Yamashita et al. 1999), and this is undoubtedly the future direction of computer-assisted surgery (CAS).

Information Compression, Clinical Communication. The fourth function lies in the main feature of virtual endoscopy itself: with a single view it is possible to demonstrate an anatomical relation or pathology to clinicians, which is otherwise laborious when using axial and coronal images. In this respect, virtual endoscopy represents a data- or, more correctly, an information-compression tool which facilitates the communication between radiologists and ENT specialists, hence indirectly improving medical care.

References

Federal Statistics Office, Germany (Statistisches Bundesamt) (1994–1996)

Arslan H, Aydinlioglu A, Bozkurt M, Egeli E (1999) Anatomic variations of the paranasal sinuses: CT examination for endoscopic sinus surgery. Auris Nasus Larynx 26:39–48.

Babbel R, Harnsberger HR, Nelson B, Sonkens J, Hunt S (1991) Optimization of techniques in screening CT of the sinuses. AJNR Am J Neuroradiol 12:849–854.

Beus J, Kauczor HU, Schwikkert HC, Mohr W, Mildenberger P (1995) [Coronal paranasal sinus CT: using the spiral technique]. Aktuelle Radiol 5:189–191.

Blokmanis A (1994) Endoscopic diagnosis, treatment, and follow-up of tumours of the nose and sinuses. J Otolaryngol 23:366–369.

Boguslawska-Staniaszczyk R, Krzeski A, Samolinski B (1994) [The usefulness of CT studies for the needs of endoscopic surgery of the nose and paranasal sinuses]. Otolaryngol Pol 48 Suppl 17:63–75.

Chakeres DW (1985) Computed tomography of the ethmoid sinuses. Otolaryngol Clin North Am 18:29–42.

Chow JM, Mafee MF (1989) Radiologic assessment preoperative to endoscopic sinus surgery. Otolaryngol Clin North Am 22:691–701.

Da Vinci L (1920): In Skillern RH (ed), Accessory sinuses of the nose, 2nd edn. Philadelphia: Lippincott.

Damilakis J, Prassopoulos P, Mazonakis M, Bizakis J, Papadaki E, Gourtsoyiannis N (1998) Tailored low dose three-dimensional CT of paranasal sinuses. Clin Imaging 22:235–239.

Diederichs CG, Bruhn H, Funke M, Grabbe E (1996) [Spiral CT with reduced radiation dose]. Rofo Fortschr Geb Rontgenstr Neuen Bildgeb Verfahr 164:183–188.

Dursun E, Bayiz U, Korkmaz H, Akmansu H, Uygur K (1998) Follow-up results of 415 patients after endoscopic sinus surgery. Eur Arch Otorhinolaryngol 255:504–510.

Edmond CV, Jr., Heskamp D, Sluis D, et al. (1997) ENT endoscopic surgical training simulator. Stud Health Technol Inform 39:518–528.

Freysinger W, Gunkel AR, Thumfart WF (1997) Image-guided endoscopic ENT surgery. Eur Arch Otorhinolaryngol 254:343–346.

Gholkar A, Gillespie JE, Hart CW, Mott D, Isherwood I (1988) Dynamic low-dose three-dimensional computed tomography: a preliminary study. Br J Radiol 61:1095–1099.

Gilani S, Norbash AM, Ringl H, Rubin GD, Napel S, Terris DJ (1997) Virtual endoscopy of the paranasal sinuses using perspective volume rendered helical sinus computed tomography. Laryngoscope 107:25–29.

Grevers G, Menauer F, Leunig A, Caversaccio M, Kastenbauer E (1999) [Navigation surgery in diseases of the paranasal sinuses]. Laryngorhinootologie 78:41–46.

Gunkel AR, Freysinger W, Thumfart WF (1997) 3D anatomoradiological basis of endoscopic surgery of the paranasal sinuses. Surg Radiol Anat 19:7–10.

Hajek M (1904) Zur Diagnose und intranasalen chirurgischen Behandlung der Eiterungen der Keilbeinhöhle. Arch Laryngol Rhinol 16:105–108.

Halle W (1906) Externe oder interne Operation der Nasennebenhöhleneiterungen. Berl Klin Wochenschr 43:1369–1372, 1404–1407.

Hirschmann A (1903) Über Endoskopie der Nase und der Nasennebenhöhlen. Eine neue Untersuchungsmethode. Arch Laryngol Rhinol 14:195–202.

Hoffmann KR, Samara Y, Fiebich M, Lan L, Doi K, Dachmann A (1998) Workstation for rapid interpretation of CT colon studies. Proceedings of the first international symposium on virtual colonoscopy, Boston, Oct. 1998 :97.

Hopper KD, Iyriboz AT, Wise SW, Fornadley JA (1999) The feasibility of surgical site tagging with CT virtual reality of the paranasal sinuses. J Comput Assist Tomogr 23:529–533.

Hosemann W (1996) [Endonasal surgery of the paranasal sinuses–concepts, techniques, results, complications and revision interventions]. Eur Arch Otorhinolaryngol Suppl 1:155–269.

Kennedy DW (1985) Functional endoscopic sinus surgery. Technique. Arch Otolaryngol 111:643–649.

Kennedy DW, Kennedy EM (1985) Endoscopic sinus surgery. Aorn J 42:932, 934, 936.

Kopp W, Stammberger H, Fotter R (1988) Special radiologic imaging of paranasal sinuses. A prerequisite for functional endoscopic sinus surgery. Eur J Radiol 8:153–156.

Kosling S, Wagner F, Schulz HG, Heywang-Kobrunner S (1993) [Osseous variations in the coronary CT of the paranasal sinuses]. Rofo Fortschr Geb Rontgenstr Neuen Bildgeb Verfahr 159:506–510.

Kruckels G, Korves B, Klimek L, Mosges R (1996) Endoscopic surgery of the rhinobasis with a computer-assisted localizer. Surg Endosc 10:453–456.

Lobe LP (1991) [Indications for transnasal endoscopic and microscopic and external paranasal sinus operations. A critical intermediate report]. HNO 39:233–235.

Mafee MF, Chow JM, Meyers R (1993) Functional endoscopic sinus surgery: anatomy, CT screening, indications, and complications. AJR Am J Roentgenol 160:735–744.

Manfre L, Ferlito S, Conticello S, Pero G, Cardinale AE (1994) [A comparative study of the pterygopalatine fossa by computed tomography and magnetic resonance]. Radiol Med (Torino) 88:183–189.

Mantoni M, Larsen P, Hansen H, Tos M, Berner B, Orntoft S (1996) Coronal CT of the paranasal sinuses before and after functional endoscopic sinus surgery. Eur Radiol 6:920–924.

Mason JD, Jones NS, Hughes RJ, Holland IM (1998) A systematic approach to the interpretation of computed tomography scans prior to endoscopic sinus surgery. J Laryngol Otol 112:986–990.

May M, Levine HL, Mester SJ, Schaitkin B (1994) Complications of endoscopic sinus surgery: analysis of 2108 patients–incidence and prevention. Laryngoscope 104:1080–1083.

Melhem ER, Oliverio PJ, Benson ML, Leopold DA, Zinreich SJ (1996) Optimal CT evaluation for functional endoscopic sinus surgery. AJNR Am J Neuroradiol 17:181–188.

Messerklinger W (1966) [On the drainage of the human paranasal sinuses under normal and pathological conditions. 1]. Monatsschr Ohrenheilkd Laryngorhinol 100:56–68.

Messerklinger W (1972) [Technics and possibilities of nasal endoscopy]. HNO 20:133–135.

Metson R, Cosenza M, Gliklich RE, Montgomery WW (1999) The role of image-guidance systems for head and neck surgery. Arch Otolaryngol Head Neck Surg 125:1100–1104.

Meyers RM, Valvassori G (1998) Interpretation of anatomic variations of computed tomography scans of the sinuses: a surgeon's perspective. Laryngoscope 108:422–425.

Morra A, Calgaro A, Cioffi V, Pravato M, Cova M, Pozzi Mucelli R (1998) [Virtual endoscopy of the nasal cavity and the paranasal sinuses with computerized tomography. Anatomical study]. Radiol Med (Torino) 96:29–34.

Mosher P (1912) The applied anatomy and the intranasal surgery of the ethmoid labyrinth. Trans Am Laryngeal Assoc 34.

Plinkert P, Lowenheim H (1997) Trends and perspectives in minimally invasive surgery in otorhinolaryngology-head and neck surgery. Laryngoscope 107:1483–1489.

Pockler C, Brambs HJ, Plinkert P (1994) [Computed tomography of the paranasal sinus prior to endonasal surgery]. Radiologe 34:79–83.

Rogalla P, Nischwitz A, Gottschalk S, Huitema A, Kaschke O, Hamm B (1998) Virtual endoscopy of the nose and paranasal sinuses. Eur Radiol 8:946–950.

Rudman DT, Stredney D, Sessanna D, et al. (1998) Functional endoscopic sinus surgery training simulator. Laryngoscope 108:1643–1647.

Sener Y (1994) [Paranasal sinus endoscopy]. Soins Chir 164:7–8.

Shankar L, Evans K, Hawke M, Stammberger H (1994): An atlas of imaging of the paranasal sinuses. London: Martin Dunitz Ltd, The Livery House, 7–9 Pratt Street, London NW1 OAE.

Smith LF, Brindley PC (1993) Indications, evaluation, complications, and results of functional endoscopic sinus surgery in 200 patients. Otolaryngol Head Neck Surg 108:688–696.

Som PM (1985) CT of the paranasal sinuses. Neuroradiology 27:189–201.

Spaeth J, Krugelstein U, Schlondorff G (1997) The paranasal sinuses in CT-imaging: development from birth to age 25. Int J Pediatr Otorhinolaryngol 39:25–40.

Stammberger H (1985) [Personal endoscopic operative technic for the lateral nasal wall–an endoscopic surgery concept in the treatment of inflammatory diseases of the paranasal sinuses]. Laryngol Rhinol Otol (Stuttg) 64:559–566.

Stammberger H (1989) History of rhinology: anatomy of the paranasal sinuses. Rhinology 27:197–210.

Summers RM, Merran S (1997) Navigational aids for real-time virtual bronchoscopy [Virtual imaging: applications to virtual endoscopy]. AJR Am J Roentgenol 168:1165–1170.

Suojanen JN, Regan F (1995) Spiral CT scanning of the paranasal sinuses. AJNR Am J Neuroradiol 16:787–789.

Yamashita J, Yamauchi Y, Mochimaru M, Fukui Y, Yokoyama K (1999) Real-time 3-D model-based navigation system for endoscopic paranasal sinus surgery. IEEE Trans Biomed Eng 46:107–116.

Yanagisawa E, Christmas DA (1999) The value of computer-aided (image-guided) systems for endoscopic sinus surgery. Ear Nose Throat J 78:822–824, 826.

Yanagisawa E, Weaver EM, Ashikawa R (1998) The Onodi (sphenoethmoid) Cell. Ear Nose Throat J 77:578–580.

Zinreich SJ (1992) Imaging of the nasal cavity and paranasal sinuses. Curr Opin Radiol 4:112–116.

Zinreich SJ (1998) Functional anatomy and computed tomography imaging of the paranasal sinuses. Am J Med Sci 316:2–12.

3 Virtual Laryngoscopy

A.J. Aschoff and E.M. Merkle

CONTENTS

3.1 Introduction

Laryngoscopy is one of the clinically performed endoscopic evaluations that has not drawn much attention in terms of virtual imaging so far. This is rather surprising as virtual laryngoscopy (VL) is in many ways similar to bronchoscopy. It deals with an air-containing hollow organ that essentially forms the upper airways. Virtual bronchoscopy, on the other hand, has already been thoroughly explored by a number of researchers (Buthiau et al. 1996; Ferretti et al. 1996; Fleiter et al. 1997; Rodenwaldt et al. 1997; Silverman et al. 1995; Summers et al. 1996; Vining et al. 1996). They usually attempted to cover the entire tracheobronchial tree in one examination and optimized their imaging parameters for this purpose.

Requirements for virtual laryngoscopy differ from those used for bronchoscopy. The larynx itself is smaller; accordingly the pathology tends to be smaller as well. This explains why higher spatial resolution is required.

The larynx is divided into three anatomical regions. The supraglottic larynx includes the epiglottis, false vocal cords, ventricles, aryepiglottic folds, and arytenoids. The glottis includes the true vocal cords and the anterior and posterior commissures. The subglottic region begins approximately 1 cm below the true vocal cords and extends to the lower border of the cricoid cartilage or the first tracheal ring. Virtual laryngoscopy is applicable for examining all three anatomical regions.

A.J. Aschoff, MD; E.M. Merkle MD
Department of Radiology, University Hospital of Ulm, Germany

3.2 Pathology

There are numerous pathologic entities suitable for virtual laryngoscopy, including laryngeal tumors and subglottic stenoses. The detection and staging of laryngeal cancer using virtual laryngoscopy might come to be of clinical benefit. The estimated number of new cases of laryngeal cancer in the United States in 1999 is 8600 for men and 2000 for women (Landis et al. 1999). The estimated number of laryngeal cancer deaths during the same time period is 3300 for men and 900 for women. Similarly, the estimated number of new cases of pharyngeal cancer in the United States in 1999 is 6100 for men and 2200 for women, while the estimated number of pharyngeal cancer deaths in 1999 is 1500 for men and 600 for women. Thus, laryngeal and pharyngeal cancer together account for approximately 1.5% of all estimated new cancer cases.

Histologically, the vast majority of laryngeal cancers are of the squamous cell type. Squamous cell subtypes include keratinizing and nonkeratinizing as well as well differentiated to poorly differentiated grades. There are also a variety of nonsquamous cell laryngeal cancers (Sessions et al. 1997). The staging system is clinical and is based on the best possible estimate of the extent of disease before treatment. Assessment of the primary tumor is based on inspection and palpation when possible, and by both indirect mirror examination and direct endoscopy when necessary. The tumor must be confirmed histologically, and any other pathological data obtained on biopsy may be included. Head and neck magnetic resonance imaging (MRI) or computed tomography (CT) should also be performed prior to therapy in order to supplement inspection and palpation (THABET et al. 1996).

Small, superficial cancers without laryngeal fixation or lymph node involvement are usually treated successfully by radiation therapy or surgery alone, including laser excision surgery. Radiation therapy may be selected to preserve the voice mechanism, reserving surgery for salvaging failures. The location and size of the primary tumor determine the radiation field and dose. A variety of curative surgical procedures, some of which preserve vocal function, are also recommended for laryngeal cancers. The most appropriate surgical procedure must be considered for each patient, given the individual's anatomical circumstances and performance status, and the clinical expertise of the treatment team. Advanced laryngeal cancers are often most successfully treated by combining radiation and surgery (SILVER 1981; WANG 1990; THAWLEY et al. 1986; SESSIONS et al. 1997).

The most important adverse prognostic factors for laryngeal cancers include increasing T-stage and/or N-stage (YILMAZ et al. 1998). Patients treated for laryngeal cancers have the highest risk of recurrence during the first 2–3 years. Recurrences after 5 years are rare and usually represent new primary malignancies. Close, regular follow-up is crucial in order to maximize the chance for salvage. Careful clinical examination and repetition of any abnormal staging study should be included in the follow-up. However, because of clinical problems related to smoking and alcohol use in this patient population, many patients succumb to intercurrent illness rather than to the primary cancer.

To our knowledge, all published work on virtual laryngoscopy to date focuses on helical CT and not on MRI for data acquisition (ASCHOFF et al. 1998; FRIED et al. 1999; RODENWALDT et al. 1996). This may be due to the fact that CT is routinely used in the diagnostic work-up of laryngeal tumors (WILLIAMS 1997; ZBAREN et al. 1996) and stenosis (HERMANS et al. 1995), while the combination of (conventional) laryngoscopy and CT is known to yield significantly improved staging accuracy (ZBAREN et al. 1997).

3.3 Data Acquisition

Our own experience is based on a protocol using 1 mm collimation to provide the necessary high spatial resolution required for virtual laryngoscopy (ASCHOFF et al. 1998). Using a double helix CT scanner (Elscint Twin Flash, Haifa, Israel), scan time can be kept down to under 30 s, during which the whole larynx and proximal trachea is examined. We used a table speed of 3 mm/s and an increment of 0.5 mm (120 kV, 133 mAs, no contrast medium). After the first scan, a second scan was performed using a standard larynx protocol (5 mm collimation, pitch 1.5:1, 5 mm reconstruction increment, 120 kV, 199 mAs, scan start 95 s after injecting 100 ml of an iodine-containing contrast agent with a flow rate of 1.5 ml/s). The images from this second scan were used for the clinical work-up. The images (up to 300) from the first scan were then transferred via a network to a workstation (Indigo 2 Maximum Impact, Silicon Graphics, Mountain View, USA). Both the surface detection and the real-time rendering were performed using commercially available software (Explorer, Silicon Graphics). We applied the "marching cubes" algorithm for surface detection (LORENSEN and CLINE 1987; CLINE et al. 1988).

The time required for transferring the images, selecting a proper threshold, and creating the initial 3D data set was approximately 1 h. Once the data preparation has been completed, virtual laryngoscopy can be performed at any time without further delay in real time.

A crucial step in the data preparation is the selection of an appropriate threshold for the surface detection. This is especially true when quantitative assessment of the grade of a stenosis is desirable. This quantification is very difficult because selecting a threshold that is too low will cause underestimation of a stenosis, while a threshold that is too high will lead to overestimation.

3.4 Clinical Application

Acquiring images during breath-hold usually leads to closed vocal cords, which prevents the classic fly-through. Therefore, it is usually preferable to acquire images during slow breath expiration.

Swallowing leads to major movements in the laryngeal area, which may prohibit successful image reconstruction for virtual laryngoscopy purposes. Although patients are asked in advance not to swallow, involuntary swallowing can make successful image reconstruction impossible in up to 35% of examinations.

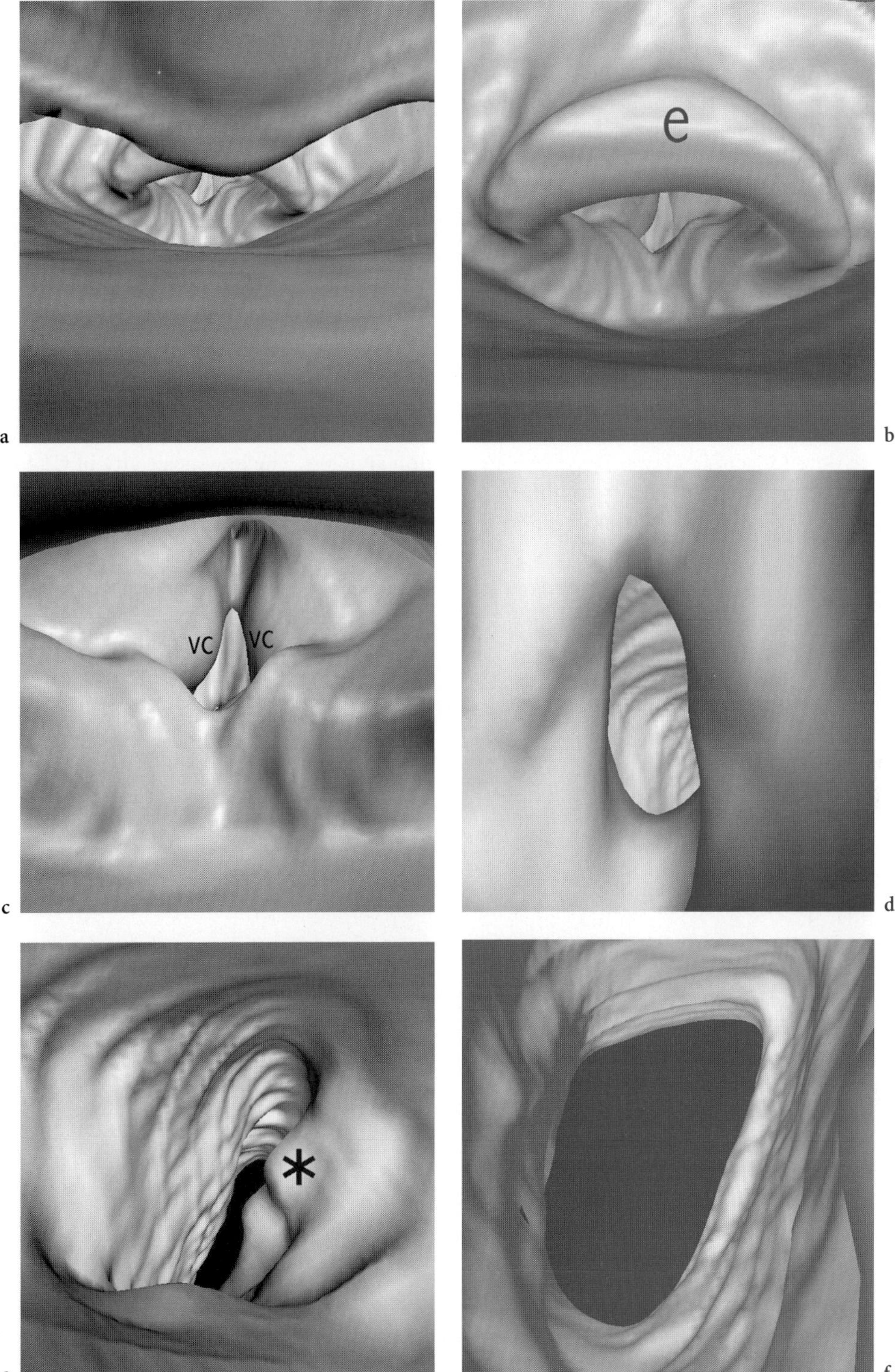

Fig. 3.1a–f. Patient with 3-month history of coughing. Virtual fly-through offers views on different pharyngeal/tracheal levels with excellent spatial resolution. The epiglottis (*e*) is best seen on **b**; **c** shows the vocal cords (*VC*), which are just about to be passed in **d**. A small submucosal tumor can be made out in image **e** (*asterisk*). Of note is the reconstruction artifact in the tracheal wall of image **f** caused by the specific threshold selection used (*small black triangle, lower left*)

Patients examined in our study using virtual laryngoscopy were suffering from laryngeal tumors and subglottic stenoses. In these cases, as well as in other studies, the endoscopic impressions and results achieved using CT-based virtual laryngoscopy were comparable to those obtained using fiberoptic endoscopy (Aschoff et al. 1998; Fried et al. 1999; Rodenwaldt et al. 1996). As with most virtual endoscopies, the main advantages over fiberoptic endoscopy cited include its noninvasive character, repeatability, and the possibility of passing even high-grade stenoses. The cross-sectional images used to calculate the endoscopic views might also provide additional information regarding the extent of an infiltration that is not visible on endoscopic views. Disadvantages of this technique include its inability to obtain biopsy specimens or to detect slight changes in the color of the laryngeal surface that might indicate underlying pathology.

We could not find any significant information using virtual laryngoscopy that could not be detected in cross-sectional images, although the reconstructed views using the workstation made it easier to estimate the grade of a stenosis, especially for physicians not experienced in the use of CT (Figs. 3.1, 3.2).

Virtual laryngoscopy does not seem to be suitable for detecting small tumors of the vocal cords. The main reason is its poor sensitivity, which is due to the fact that the vocal cords lie anatomically at a tangent to the z-axis of the patient, and to the additional risk that the vocal cords continue to vibrate beyond the voluntary control of the patient, leading to motion artifacts. The low sensitivity of CT for the diagnosis of small vocal cord tumors has already been documented (Kazkayasi et al. 1995).

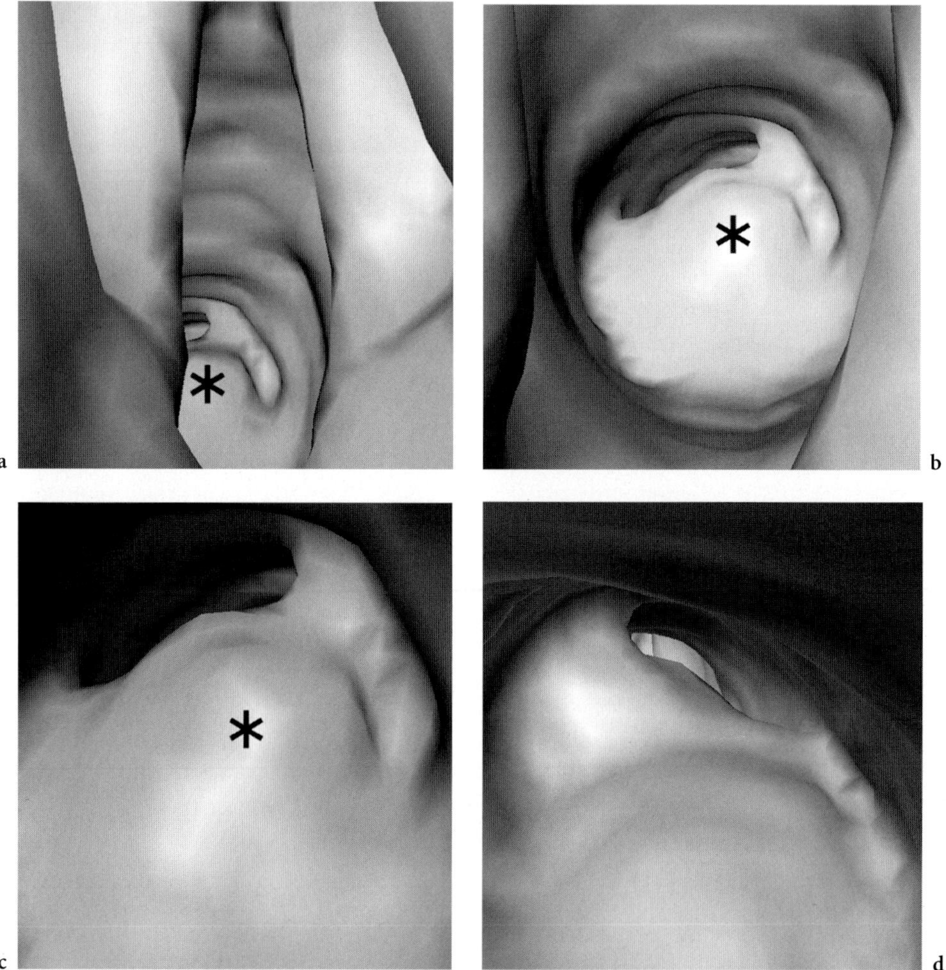

Fig. 3.2a–d. Patient with stridor. Virtual laryngoscopy reveals a subtotal stenosis caused by a dorsally located endotracheal tumor (*asterisk*) that could not be passed in fiberoptic endoscopy. **a** Just above the vocal cords. **b, c** Close-up of the tumor. **d** Retrograde view of the tumor, having passed the stenosis with the virtual endoscope

3.5 Summary

In conclusion, high-resolution virtual laryngoscopy is feasible using helical CT. It is capable of visualizing laryngeal tumors and stenoses. Excellent visualization of anatomic details is provided, including the epiglottis, false vocal cords, ventricles, aryepiglottic folds, arytenoids, and the anterior and posterior commissures, as well as the subglottic region. As mentioned above, the major problem affecting the quality of virtual laryngoscopy and its results are motion artifacts resulting from involuntary swallowing.

Although virtual laryngoscopy does not seem able to provide additional diagnostic information, as discussed previously, it may be useful in demonstrating the pathology to clinicians untrained in reading cross-sectional images as well as for educational purposes.

References

Aschoff AJ, Seifarth H, Fleiter T, Sokiranski R, Görich J, Merkle EM, Wunderlich AP, Brambs HJ, Zenkel ME (1998) [High-resolution virtual laryngoscopy based on helical CT data sets] Radiologe 38:810–815

Buthiau D, Antoine E, Piette JC, Nizri D, Baldeyrou P, Khayat D (1996) Virtual tracheo-bronchial endoscopy: educational and diagnostic value. Surg.Radiol.Anat. 18:125–131

Cline HE, Lorensen WE, Ludtke S, Crawford CR, Teeter BC (1988) Two algorithms for the threedimensional reconstruction of tomograms. Med.Phys. 15:320–327

Ferretti GR, Vining DJ, Knoplioch J, Coulomb M (1996) Tracheobronchial tree: three-dimensional spiral CT with bronchoscopic perspective. J.Comput.Assist.Tomogr. 20:777–781

Fleiter T, Merkle EM, Aschoff AJ, Lang G, Stein M, Gorich J, Liewald F, Rilinger N, Sokiranski R (1997) Comparison of real-time virtual and fiberoptic bronchoscopy in patients with bronchial carcinoma: opportunities and limitations. AJR.Am.J Roentgenol. 169:1591–1595

Fried MP, Moharir VM, Shinmoto H, Alyassin AM, Lorensen WE, Hsu L, Kikinis R (1999) Virtual laryngoscopy. Ann.Otol.Rhinol.Laryngol. 108:221–226

Hermans R, Verschakelen JA, Baert AL (1995) Imaging of laryngeal and tracheal stenosis. Acta Otorhinolaryngol. Belg. 49:323–329

Kazkayasi M, Onder T, Ozkaptan Y, Can C, Pabuscu Y (1995) Comparison of preoperative computed tomographic findings with postoperative histopathological findings in laryngeal cancers. Eur.Arch.Otorhinolaryngol. 252:325–331

Landis SH, Murray T, Bolden S, Wingo PA (1999) Cancer statistics, 1999. Cancer J Clin 49:8–31

Lorensen WE, Cline HE (1987) Marching Cubes: A High Resolution 3D Surface Construction Algorithm. Computer Graphics, 21(4):163–169

Rodenwaldt J, Kopka L, Roedel R, Grabbe E (1996) [Three-dimensional surface imaging of the larynx and trachea by spiral CT: virtual endoscopy]. Fortschr. Röntgenstr. 165:80–83

Rodenwaldt J, Kopka L, Roedel R, Margas A, Grabbe E (1997) 3D virtual endoscopy of the upper airway: optimization of the scan parameters in a cadaver phantom and clinical assessment. J.Comput.Assist.Tomogr. 21:405–411

Sessions RB, Harrison LB, Forastiere AA (1997) Tumors of the larynx and hypopharynx. In: DeVita VT Jr, Hellman S, Rosenberg SA, eds.: Cancer: Principles and Practice of Oncology. Philadelphia, Pa: Lippincott-Raven Publishers, 5th ed., 802–829

Silver CE (1981) Surgery for Cancer of the Larynx and Related Structures. New York: Churchill Livingstone

Silverman PM, Zeiberg AS, Sessions RB, Troost TR, Davros WJ, Zeman RK (1995) Helical CT of the upper airway: normal and abnormal findings on three-dimensional reconstructed images. Am.J.Roentgenol. 165:541–546

Summers RM, Feng DH, Holland SM, Sneller MC, Shelhamer JH (1996) Virtual bronchoscopy: segmentation method for real-time display. Radiology 200:857–862

Thabet HM, Sessions DG, Gado MH, et al. (1996) Comparison of clinical evaluation and computed tomographic diagnostic accuracy for tumors of the larynx and hypopharynx. Laryngoscope 106:589–594

Thawley SE, Panje WR, Batsakis JG, et al. (1986) Comprehensive Management of Head and Neck Tumors. New York: W.B. Saunders Company.

Vining DJ, Liu K, Choplin RH, Haponik EF (1996) Virtual bronchoscopy. Relationships of virtual reality endobronchial simulations to actual bronchoscopic findings. Chest 109:549–553

Wang CC, Ed. (1990) Radiation Therapy for Head and Neck Neoplasms: Indications, Techniques and Results. Littleton, MA: John Wright-PSG, Inc., 2nd ed.

Williams DW (1997) Imaging of laryngeal cancer. Otolaryngol.Clin.North Am. 30:35–58

Yilmaz T, Hosal S, Gedikoglu G, Turan E, Ayas K (1998) Prognostic significance of depth of invasion in cancer of the larynx. Laryngoscope 108:764–768

Zbaren P, Becker M, Lang H (1996) Pretherapeutic staging of laryngeal carcinoma. Clinical findings, computed tomography, and magnetic resonance imaging compared with histopathology. Cancer 77:1263–1273

Zbaren P, Becker M, Lang H (1997) Staging of laryngeal cancer: endoscopy, computed tomography and magnetic resonance versus histopathology. Eur. Arch. Otorhinolaryngol. Suppl. 1:S117–S122

4 Virtual Endoscopy of the Trachea and Bronchi

P. Rogalla and N. Meiri

CONTENTS

P. Rogalla, MD
Department of Radiology, Charité Hospital, Humboldt-Universität zu Berlin, Schumannstrasse 20/21, 10117 Berlin, Germany
N. Meiri, RD
Department of Radiology, Charité Hospital, Humboldt-Universität zu Berlin, Schumannstrasse 20/21, 10117 Berlin, Germany

4.1 Introduction

Studying the internal organs of a living body has fascinated physicians around the world throughout history and has always been of elementary significance for the physiologists and clinicians who explore the healthy and ill human being. The bronchoscopy technique has existed since 1897, when Gustav Killian pioneered examination of the lower trachea and bronchi by means of a laryngoscope. Today, bronchoscopy represents probably one of the most frequently used invasive procedures (Sackner 1975). According to a survey conducted by the American College of Chest Physicians, 53,639 bronchoscopies were carried out in the USA in 1989. This number demonstrates the clinical importance attained by bronchoscopic examination. In light of the technical advances of the past decade, the clinical value of bronchoscopy has further increased (Jover et al. 1978; Liebler and Markin 2000; Mitchell et al. 1980). Even in the hands of the clinically experienced pulmonologists, the potential risks for the patient created by the high invasiveness of the procedure must still be considered. Not only should those who operate this instrument be well versed in its use; equally important is that the indication is carefully considered, ascertaining that this useful technique is neither overused nor inappropriately used (Guidelines for competency and training in fiberoptic bronchoscopy 1982; Standards for training in endoscopy 1976).

The goal of developing virtual bronchoscopy is by no means to replace true bronchoscopy, which has distinct advantages arising from direct inspection of the mucosa (Burke et al. 2000). On the other hand, chest imaging is a domain practically reserved for CT, and this is unlikely to change substantially in the near future. Thus, the risks of CT, including radiation exposure and, if necessary, intravenous administration of contrast agent, must be weighed against the risk of an invasive bronchoscopy.

A CT examination also requires a clinical indication, and the indication is dependent upon the expected outcome. The calculation of virtual images from a clinically indicated CT considerably increases the diagnostic value, provided that the CT is carried out with an examination protocol that permits the calculation of high-quality virtual endoscopies.

4.2
Why CT?

Computed tomography, as already mentioned, currently represents the standard examination technique of the thorax when a diagnosis cannot be reached with conventional radiography. In CT, a natural contrast exists between air and soft tissue, explaining why the trachea and the tracheobronchial tree are perfectly suited for the generation of a virtual endoscopy. A further advantageous property of the strong intrathoracic contrast is that correspondingly less radiation is needed for a clear anatomical depiction.

Lower tube energy in CT correlates linearly with lower radiation exposure. In addition, the thorax, with its relatively large proportion of air, for example in comparison to the abdomen, contains less absorbing soft tissue, which also beneficially influences the chosen dose. After considering all the differences between the various CT machines, the radiation quality, the geometry, etc., an energy-time product of 10–75 mAs can be realistically clinically achieved.

CT is robust, widely available, intermediately priced and relatively simple to use. The CT characteristics of soft tissue and contrast media are well established and artefacts can be clearly distinguished. The prevailing three CT procedures are incremental CT, spiral CT and multislice CT. The next section discusses the technical aspects of the examination protocols.

4.2.1
Incremental CT

In incremental CT, a slice is imaged in the axial or paraxial orientation, after which the table shifts to the next position in order to image the next slice. CT devices using the incremental technique, although still in use, are no longer being manufactured. Three-dimensional (3D) reconstructions can be calculated from incremental data only when the subject lies so still that no motion occurs during the whole examination. These conditions are met, for example, when examining the sphenoid bone, if the patient is well stabilised on the examination table. For the calculation of a virtual bronchoscopy, incremental data are of little use.

4.2.2
Spiral CT

Spiral CT was discovered in the late 1980s (Mori 1986), and quickly proved superior to incremental CT. The continuous table advancement during the gantry rotation (tube-detector system) has made examinations of large anatomical regions during one breathhold possible. Only with the advent of the spiral CT has it become possible to continually examine the thorax without anatomical misregistration – an indispensable prerequisite for 3D reconstructions.

Until the next milestone in the development of CT, the multislice CT, 0.75 to 1 revolution per second was standard in single-detector spiral CT. This translates into a primary slice thickness of 5–7 mm, generally also in combination with a higher table advancement (pitch factor greater than 1:1), for example 10 mm/s, in order to complete the examination of the thorax in a reasonable time.

Modern CT units commonly have an image matrix of 512×512 picture elements (pixels). With an average field of view of 30–40 cm, a 0.6- to 0.8-mm-long edge of the pixels in the *x*/*y*-axis results. In the *z*-axis, the longitudinal axis of the patient, one pixel has an edge corresponding to the slice thickness of 5–7 mm, or at least 5–10 times that of the *x*/*y*-axis. The *z*-axis resolution in spiral CT is considerably worse than the in-plane resolution. However, as every reconstruction of the trachea requires a frontal view, the poorer image resolution in the *z*-axis determined by the restricted spatial resolution becomes the limiting factor, especially for the presentation of smaller details such as the 3rd- and 4th-order branches of the bronchial tree.

For the above-mentioned reasons, one can reduce the slice thickness in spiral CT to 1 or 1.5 mm. With a breathhold of 30 s and a pitch factor of 2:1 (with 1 mm slice thickness, the table advances at 2 mm/s with a gantry revolution time of 1 s), a total of 6 cm of the thorax may be examined. This exemplifies why only specific regions of the thorax can be examined with high-resolution techniques; should greater coverage be desired, a larger primary slice thickness must be chosen, compromising the *z*-axis resolution.

4.2.3 Multislice CT

The introduction of multislice CT (Klingenbeck-Regn et al. 1999) has largely solved the "coverage problem" of spiral CT. The multislice CTs that are currently available are 8 times faster than a 1-s scanner: four simultaneous slices are imaged in 0.5 s rotation time. For imaging of the chest and trachea the increased time effectiveness can be taken advantage of in two basic manners. The primary slice thickness can remain identical to that used in spiral CT, which means the chest examination will be completed in one eighth of the time, or 4 s. Otherwise, the examination time can be kept constant at 30 s, allowing a reduction in slice thickness to 1 mm. A combination of both possibilities can be chosen. One-millimetre slices can also be calculated with an overlapping slice reconstruction, for example every 0.5 mm, an option known from spiral CT. The result is an image consisting of isotropic volume elements (voxels) with edges of 0.8 mm in all three directions (see also Sect. 4.3.1). Thinner slices contain notably more image noise than thick slices if the radiation dose is not simultaneously increased. When judging mediastinal structures the noise can be problematic; possible solutions are discussed in Sect. 4.4.4.

Multislice CT is an ideal imaging modality because it offers the prospect of calculating a virtual bronchoscopy from a routine CT "free of charge", that is, without additional radiation exposure. The many benefits of multislice CT will support its establishment as a standard examination procedure in the near future.

4.2.4 Electron-Beam CT

Originally developed for cardiac imaging, electron-beam CT (EBT) can also be implemented for general diagnosis of the thoracic and abdominal cavities. By completely eliminating any mechanically rotating elements, an exposure time of 50 ms for one slice is made possible. This singular technical possibility has essentially made EBT the gold standard for cardiac imaging in CT. With its short exposure time, EBT can also be used for pulmonary diagnosis (Rogalla et al. 1998; Schoepf et al. 1998). Imaging the chest with acceptable image quality requires exposure times of 100–200 ms. In other words, with a primary slice thickness of 1.5 mm, the thorax can be examined in 17 s. However, when using such a protocol, overlapping reconstructions are not possible with EBT so that the resultant image points have 3 times poorer resolution in the z-axis than in the axial plane (x/y-axis).

In comparison to spiral CT, very few EBTs have been installed worldwide; in Germany, for example, only five units were in use at the time of writing. Thus, the technical details are not further elaborated in this book.

4.3 Examination Protocols

Achieving high-quality 3D reconstructions requires the thinnest possible slices with comprehensive volume coverage. Spiral CT and especially multislice CT deliver the necessary data during one breathhold. The natural contrast between air and soft tissue is already present in the native CT examination, so that additional administration of i.v. contrast material for the virtual bronchoscopy would be superfluous. If a complete thorax examination is simultaneously requested in spiral CT, a dedicated thin-slice spiral acquisition that covers the region to be virtually examined is additionally required, since adequate detail resolution is not present in the commonly used 5- to 7-mm slices. A selected examination protocol for spiral CT is shown in Table 4.1.

Table 4.1. Examination protocol for spiral CT

First examination (entire chest):	
Slice thickness	5–7 mm
Pitch factor	1:1 to 1.5:1
Scanning direction	Bottom to top
Non-ionic contrast material (if indicated)	ca. 80 ml
Reconstruction kernel	Sharp
Tube load (according to indication)	50–200 mAs
Breathhold	Inspiration
Field-of-view	Full
Select area of interest	
Second examination (dedicated for virtual bronchoscopy):	
Slice thickness	1–2 mm
Pitch factor	1:1 to 2:1
Scanning direction	Bottom to top
Non-ionic contrast material	–
Reconstruction kernel	Medium
Tube load	25–50 mAs
Breathhold	Inspiration
Field-of-view	(Enlargement)

If the radiation dose is minimised by selecting a low mA for the second, dedicated spiral acquisition, the image noise will be very high because the slice is also very thin, which means few photons reach the detector. Although, as already mentioned, little radiation is necessary for the presentation of a highly contrasted object, the image noise can become so extreme that the surface of a virtual reconstruction appears ruffled. Therefore, the choice of an edge-emphasising reconstruction filter should be avoided and a somewhat softer filter, although not too soft (e.g. body filter), should be used (see also the explanation in Sect. 2.5). The scanning direction is not of primary significance for the dedicated spiral acquisition; however, the general rule applies that if the patient cannot hold her or his breath for the entire examination, the respiratory movements are less disturbing in cranial slices than in slices located further caudally. A slight enlargement of the structures of interest or the choice of a smaller field of view over the trachea and the central bronchi can raise the spatial resolution in the axial plane (*x*/*y* axis); since the *z*-axis resolution represents the limiting factor, however, significant improvements cannot be expected. Rather, one runs the risk that the most interesting regions of the bronchi will be cut out and thus will no longer appear in the virtual bronchoscopy.

For the multislice CT, a slightly altered protocol is recommended. Due to the ability to prospectively plan very thin slices and still cover the entire thorax in one breathhold, a second examination dedicated to the virtual depiction is no longer necessary. An examination protocol for the chest using multislice technology is shown in Table 4.2.

Table 4.2. Examination protocol for multislice CT

Slice thickness	1–2 mm
Image thickness	5–7 mm
Pitch factor	4:4 to 6:4
Scanning direction	Bottom to top
Non-ionic contrast material (if indicated)	ca. 60 ml
Reconstruction kernel	Sharp
Tube load (according to indication)	50–200 mAs
Breathhold	Inspiration
Field-of-view	Full
Instead of a second spiral acquisition, use raw data for a second reconstruction:	
Image thickness	1–2 mm
Reconstruction index	0.5–1 mm
Reconstruction kernel	Medium
Field-of-view	(Enlargement)

Using the suggested protocol, the first reconstruction series will produce images that closely resemble the images of a spiral CT; the descriptions of findings are as usual. Also, the number of images is no greater than in spiral CT. A second, dedicated acquisition may be dispensed with; instead, the raw data should be reconstructed to slices with 1 or 2 mm thickness every 0.5–1 mm representing a 50% overlap. These reconstructions, which also can be slightly enlarged, easily result in 700–1000 images per patient – a new burden for the networks, workstations and digital archives.

As for spiral CT, the reconstruction filter must be chosen so that noise does not dominate the image (see also Fig. 5.5), but should not be so soft that spatial resolution is lost. Since the *z*-axis is no longer inferior in multislice CT, the choice of an improper filter leads to deterioration of image quality.

4.3.1 Isotropic Voxel Geometry

One of the unique features of multislice CT is that during one breathhold, an entire anatomical region can be contained in the volume data whose volumetric image points (voxels) display edges of practically identical length in all three spatial directions. In an isotropic dataset, secondary reformations have the same spatial resolution as the original axial slice images. An examination of the thorax with a 1-mm slice thickness and a slice reconstruction every 0.5 mm (overlapping reconstruction) results in a voxel measuring circa 0.8×0.8×0.8 mm by a given image matrix of 512×512 and a FOV of 30–40 cm. According to the Nyquist theorem, structures with a diameter of 2 mm or more should become clearly visible with this voxel size.

Problems in isotropic imaging occur primarily due to the extensive image noise, which, at its peak, can extend beyond the magnitude of the density difference to be displayed (see Fig. 5.5). For highly contrasted objects such as the trachea, this point is reached much later, so that the examination is also possible with low radiation exposure and thin slices; however, image noise represents an important problem in low-contrast areas and can make application of an isotropic data acquisition unfeasible.

For virtual endoscopy, an isotropic data set is the ideal prerequisite because the spatial resolution is identical in all planes of the 3D reconstruction. However, the large number of images can create a problem, as they often overload the inadequate storage capacity of currently available workstations. The calculation and processing time also becomes so long that clinical application may not be realistic.

4.3.2 Artefacts

One problem has not been solved even with multislice technology and isotropic data acquisition: cardiac motion cannot be suppressed despite an acquisition time of 0.5 s per slice. Only a prospective or retrospective trigger, as employed for cardiac imaging, could provide assistance. Currently, substantial problems, which cannot be further elaborated here, impede routine application of cardiac gating for the chest.

Cardiac motion extends predominantly to the directly neighbouring pulmonary parenchyma, especially the lingula. As a result, cogwheel-like artefacts can be expected in the coronal slices, which then appear as irregularities in the respective bronchial wall. Much more striking is the portrayal of the aortic pulsations transmitted to the trachea and the main bronchi: they are displayed as ring-like structures in the 3D virtual endoscopy. These artefacts initially appear very similar to cartilage rings (Fig. 4.1); however, they can be distinguished from tracheal cartilage relatively easily since they always appear horizontal in the slice direction and are clearly discernible on both main bronchi. Nonetheless, knowledge of these artefacts is necessary in order to avoid misinterpretations.

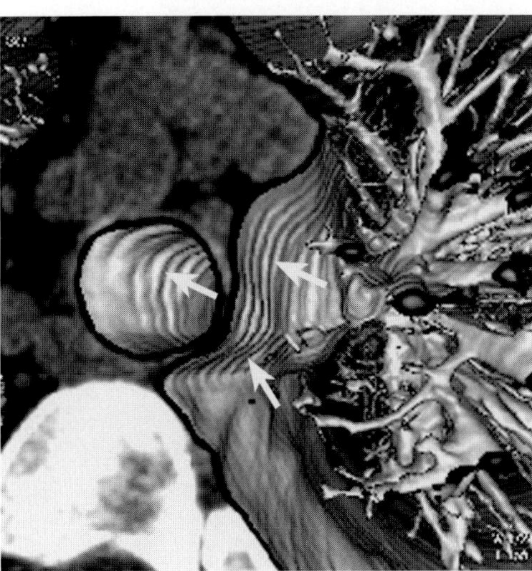

Fig. 4.1. Display of pulsation artefacts (*arrows*), carried over from the left ventricle and from the arteries (mostly the aorta) onto the mediastinum and thus the trachea. These pseudo-ring formations should not be confused with the natural tracheal ring cartilage

Furthermore, if the patient is unable to maintain a breathhold for the length of the examination, artefacts can result from breathing motions. This problem occurs especially during virtual bronchoscopy in children. Sudden, abrupt movements nearly create the impression of a complete dislocation of the trachea. Thorough evaluation of both the axial as well as the coronal slices prevents such misinterpretations. Additional artefacts common to CT caused by metallic implants do not differ from the well-known effects of beam hardening in the chest cavity. Even the shoulder girdle can lead to hardening artefacts that create the impression of an irregular wall in the virtual endoscopy.

4.4 Visualisation Techniques

The trachea can be presented in many fashions. Practically all of the postprocessing techniques available can be used for the tracheobronchial tree and each has its own advantages. In the following section, the principles behind each technique and the most relevant imaging characteristics will be explained. Furthermore, the processing time and thus the time required for reconstructions are discussed, factors that play a significant role in deciding whether the application can be defended from a clinical and economical standpoint.

4.4.1 Original Scans

The "mother" of all imaging techniques in CT is the observation of axially reconstructed original slices. Currently, the only possible calculation from the raw data is into axial images (a direct reconstruction of coronal images from the raw data is not yet realisable, but can be expected in the near future with the multislice technology) and thus, the complete diagnostic information is contained in the axial slices. In other words, there is no substitute for evaluation of the original slices. A review of the literature concerning 3D reconstruction and virtual endoscopy reinforces the importance and necessity of viewing the original slices (Remy et al. 1998; Rodenwaldt et al. 1997)

Especially, although not initially, since the introduction of the multislice technology, it has become necessary to view hundreds of axial images, for example, up to 700–1000 images for a chest CT with isotropic voxel geometry. Viewing every single image is not even sensible because the minimal distance advanced limits the eye's ability to perceive any changes from one image to the next. One solution is the often-cited observation in the movie mode, where the viewer can interactively flip or page through the images with a mouse or a dial.

So why make a 3D reconstruction? The following example should emphasise the advantages. Figure 4.2a shows an axial slice through an object. With this single slice, the object cannot be apprehended. By observing many slices, also in the movie mode on the monitor (the data set is comprised of 900 axial slices), it is surely possible to identify it as a flower. But who would have enough certainty to name the type? In contrast, a single 3D reconstructed image says everything needed and the flower can be named without doubt. Detailed questions such as how and where the flower buds are positioned require laborious evaluation of the axial slices but can also be answered with a single presentation as a computed volume projection. In this image, the detailed questions that remained open after viewing the 3D reconstruction can easily be answered. This example should make it clear that every imaging possibility has advantages, and deciding upon a visualisation technique requires consideration of the question to be answered.

4.4.2 Multiplanar Reformations

The best-known postprocessing technique is the calculation of simple secondary reformations (LACROSSE et al. 1995). This technique requires compar-

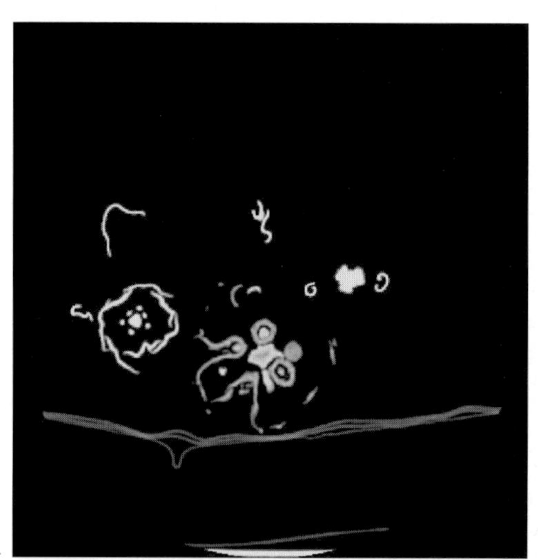

a

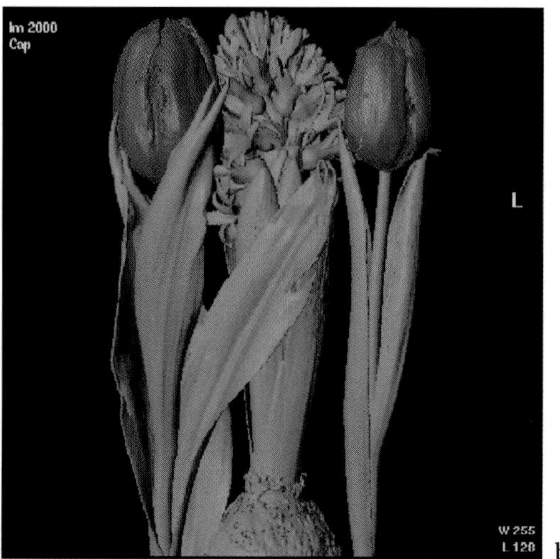

b

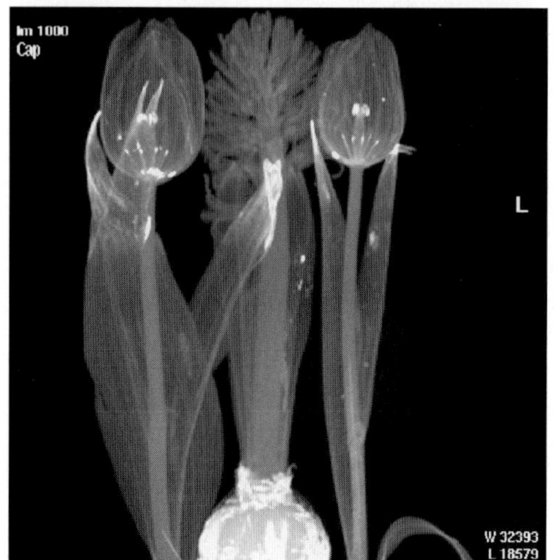

c

Fig. 4.2. **a** Axial slice, **b** 3D surface reconstruction and **c** computed volumetric projection (CVP) of three flowers (multislice CT, 0.5 mm slice thickness). Judging the shape of the object solely based upon the axial scans presupposes excellent imaginative talent and the time to view 900 images. In contrast, a single 3D image can show the object in its entirety. However, in the surface representation the information within the tulip is lost; in this case, CVP displays the structures within the flower through transparent petals

atively little computing power and can be interactively used on most workstations. Ordinarily, workstations use reformatted slice thickness of one image point, which does not represent a problem in spiral CT with relatively little image noise due to the comparatively thick slices. In multislice CT, secondary reformations (MPRs) have the same noise level in isotropic voxel geometry as the unprocessed original slices. As long as images are only viewed in the pulmonary window (e.g. window/level: 1300/–500), the image noise plays no relevant role. Particularly in a soft tissue window (window/level: 400/50), the noise can be recognised to the full extent.

In coronally positioned MPRs, both the cardiac and the aortic pulsations are especially well depicted. The disadvantage of simple MPRs can be seen in the trachea because the branches seldom remain at one level, and the same image problem results as seen in axial slices, namely structures wandering out of the imaging plane.

4.4.3 Curved MPR

Somewhat more intensive preparation is required for calculation of secondary planes along a predefined path. The path can be curved in all directions and dimensions and is repressed in a given plane when chosen as a viewing plane. Thus, true 3D proportions are maintained in the viewing plane. This technique is especially suited for displaying vasculature (see Chap. 8) and is also suited for the trachea: if a specific bronchus is the target of investigation, a path can be placed from the trachea through the main bronchus into the targeted bronchus. The bronchus then appears in the reconstruction in its full length, measurements can be directly determined and evaluation of the entire bronchus is possible (Fig. 4.3). An enormous disadvantage is, however, that the path is only applicable for the single, chosen bronchus. For every other proportional presentation of another bronchus, a new path must first be placed. If, however, a tumour has already been identified, with the assistance of a curved path the affected bronchus can be depicted with a high degree of accuracy.

4.4.4 Slab MPR, Averages, Computed Volume Projection

Image noise occurring in MPRs has been mentioned on numerous occasions. For the secondary reformation, a relatively simple possibility is to use a full block instead of only a single row of pixels (Fig. 4.4). Choosing the thickness of the reconstructed slice is then unrestricted. This technique reduces the image noise reciprocally (slice thickness doubled = square root of noise), but increases partial volume effects. The term "slab MPR" or "averages" has been established to describe a slice thickness of up to about 10 mm.

But what argument exists against broadening the slice thickness to 20 mm, or even 100 mm? The ensuing images slowly begin to resemble a conventional X-ray image. Similarity to the previously used conventional tomography is also undeniable. Clinical partners who have experience with conventional tomography will value these presentations. Although significant partial volume effects result with such thick reconstructions, it is possible to display the trachea together with the main bronchi and further branches in one image. Since the image preparation is completed on a workstation, the reconstructed object can be freely rotated and tilted in every direction. When using the entire volumetric data set for reconstructions (full slab), the computed images resemble chest X-rays. However, since the image is cal-

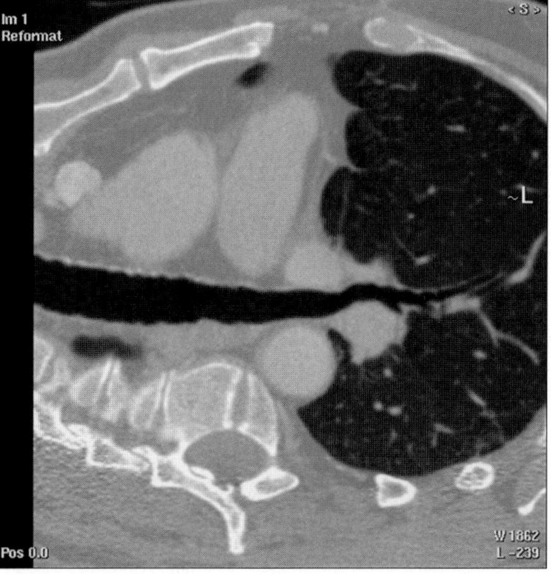

Fig. 4.3. Multiplanar reformation through an upper lobe bronchus. Aside from the fact that such a presentation strongly distorts the anatomy and requires adjusting time, a further disadvantage is that many paths must be laid for comprehensive evaluation of the tracheobronchial tree. Only with automatic path finding can the use of a curved MPR be considered efficient

a

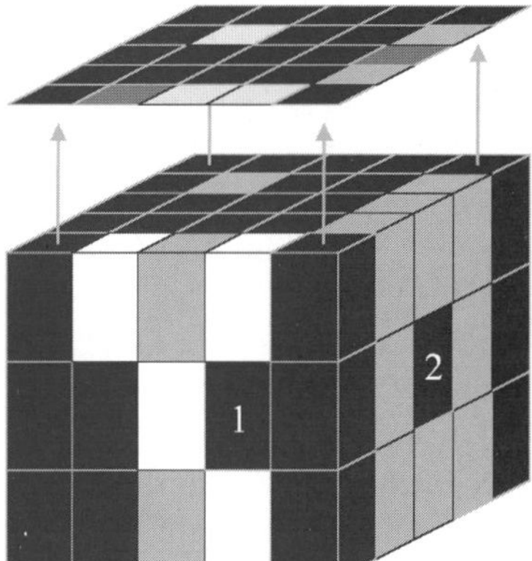

b

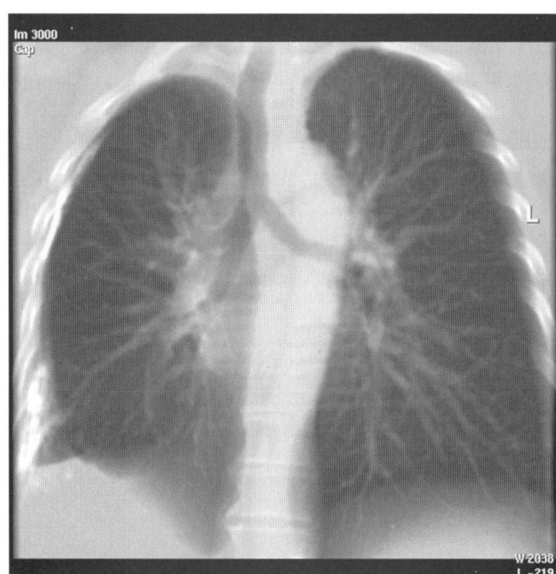

Fig. 4.4. a Model illustration of an "average projection". In general, the density of all voxels in a projection plane are averaged. In this projection technique the classic partial volume effects appear proportional to the thickness of the lumen that should be projected. If the volume is set at a thickness of 2–5 cm, the images take on the character of a conventional tomogram (**b**; multislice CT, 1 mm primary slice thickness, 0.5 mm reconstruction interval). Average-projection images are distortion-free, as in MIP (Fig. 4.5) and mIP (Fig. 4.6), and allow adequate presentation of the trachea by skilful selection of the target volume. The advantage of this technique is that by doubling the thickness of the target volume the image noise is also reduced by the square root of 2. The disadvantage is that with increasing thickness of the volume, the contrast decreases and thus small density differences might be disguised. Note the voxels *1* and *2*. Voxel *2* is in portrayed with a greater density in the projection, but can still be disassociated from the surroundings; voxel *1*, on the other hand, can no longer be identified in the projection because as a result of the averaging with denser voxels, the density value became greater than a neighbouring voxel

culated with the computer, the reconstructions are termed computed volume projections (CVP).

4.4.5 Maximum Intensity Projections

The maximum intensity projection (MIP) diagram (Fig. 4.5) is a symbolic representation of the principles behind an MIP. In the direction of the projection, only the brightest image points are used to calculate the resulting image. An important characteristic of this technique is the contrast amplification (without notable noise reduction), especially appropriate for vessels with little contrast. For the trachea, there is hardly a worthwhile application because the trachea always contrasts negatively with the surrounding structures.

4.4.6 Minimum Intensity Projections

More sensible is the presentation of a minimum intensity projection (mIP). Instead of using the brightest points in a volume set, only the darkest points are used to calculate an image in the direction of projection. The mIP also creates a contrast amplification that clearly depicts the trachea (Fig. 4.6). The danger behind an MIP or mIP is that with the loss of depth information, stenoses in the mIP and protrusions (e.g. diverticula) in the MIP can be overlooked, the extent depending naturally upon the chosen slice thickness of the projection. Nonetheless, mIPs are well suited for obtaining a general overview of a large part of the tracheobronchial tree with relatively limited computation effort.

a

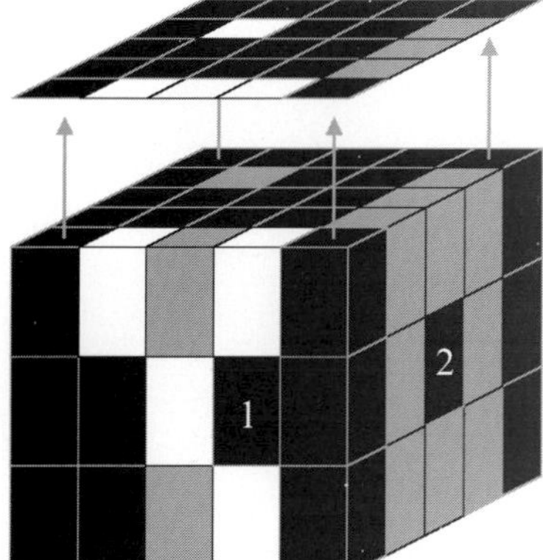

b

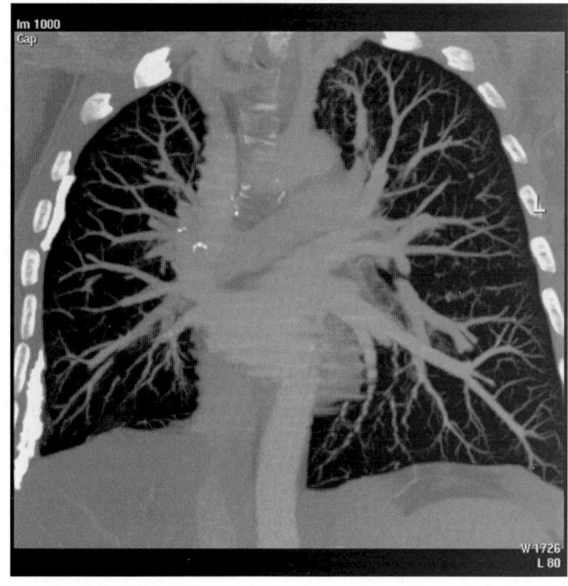

Fig. 4.5. a Model illustration of a maximum intensity projection (MIP). Only the brightest points (points with the greatest intensity) are used for image computation. The MIP is a projection technique. The thickness of the volume projected in one plane can vary. Two characteristics can be shown on the simplified illustration: both voxels *1* and *2* are no longer visible in the projection because brighter voxels lie in front of them. A dark trachea is thus not depicted (**b**)

4.4.7
Surface Rendering

The surface reconstruction of the trachea requires an initial definition of a threshold value. In general, the grey scale for all image points is reduced to a binary system: after the transformation according to a threshold value, only opaque and transparent voxels are viewed. A precise explanation of this technique is contained in Chap. 1, Technical Background.

Figure 4.7 shows a 3D surface reconstruction of a trachea. The impression that one is looking into the trachea is achieved through strong enlargement and a cranial viewpoint. It quickly becomes obvious, however, that the spatial resolution, the illumination effects, and the absence of perspective distortions prevent useful interpretation of the image. By calculating a wire-frame model (Fig. 4.8), presentations with significantly improved surface texture are created. However, the principal disadvantage of the method remains unchanged. The spatial resolution is defined by the calculation of the polygons by which the model is constructed and the quality is highly dependent upon the initially chosen threshold value; corrections at a later time require a completely new calculation of the model. The process of defining the threshold to produce a binary volumetric data set is called *segmentation*. Segmentation generates a significant reduction in the data volume, explaining why the surface rendering method, although it requires notably more hardware capacity than a simple MPR or MIP, can still be considered to have moderate hardware requirements, so that images can be effortlessly attained with most workstations. Predominantly this factor has made surface rendering the most widely used 3D presentation type.

a

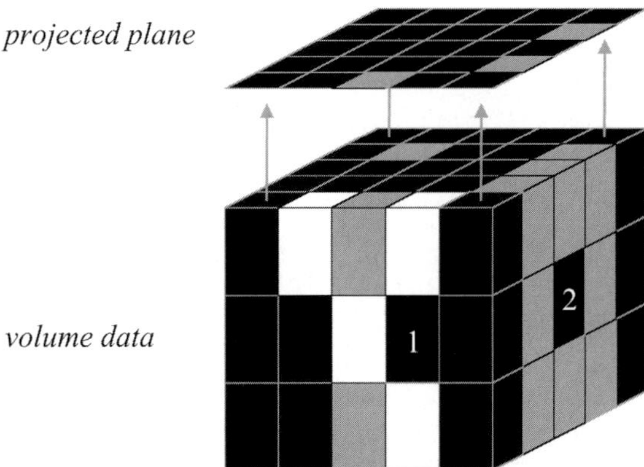

b

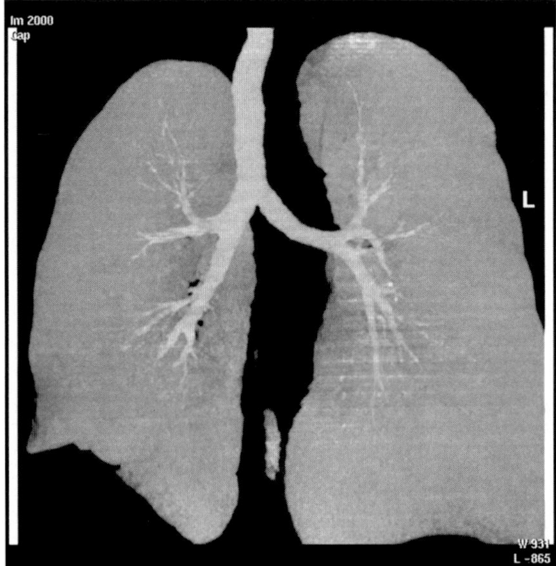

Fig. 4.6. a Model illustration of a minimum intensity projection (mIP). This technique is based upon the same principles as MIP, with the exception that the darkest points, rather than the brightest points, are presented in the projection plane without distortion. Once again, note voxels *1* and *2*: both become visible in the projection because the brighter voxels in front of them are not used to create the image. This example clarifies why, for example, the sternum must not be manually separated although located in front of the trachea in the projection direction (**b**, image inverted). The brighter points of the bones are not depicted in the mIP. Problems are more likely to be caused by both lung lobes, which, with a narrow mediastinum, are very close to one another and ventral to the trachea, and as a result of their inflated nature obstruct the view of the trachea

4.4.8 Volume Rendering

The principles behind the volume rendering technique have also been explained in detail in Chap. 1. Unlike the surface rendering technique, segmentation is not necessary; rather, the density values of all image points in a volume are stored at all times. The viewer designates density values to image attributes ranging from completely transparent to completely opaque. Every transition and every repetition of the attributes are possible. This process is called *classification.* It is already obvious that a classification does not correspond with a reduction in data; rather, a classification is a guideline indicating how the entire volume should appear in the image. Thus, the volume rendering technique presupposes a considerable increase in computing power and entered the pool of medical imaging techniques relatively late. Even today, volume rendering is not implemented on all workstations. The issue of increased capacity becomes especially problematic in combination with the multislice CT: 700–1000 images alone require 350–500 MB RAM; only a limited number of workstations can meet these demands.

Volume rendering entails complete freedom when assuming a view-adapted interpolation in order to improve the spatial resolution (super-resolution), and when implementing mirror effects and shading. All virtual endoscopies in this chapter are, if not explicitly stated otherwise, created with the volume rendering technique.

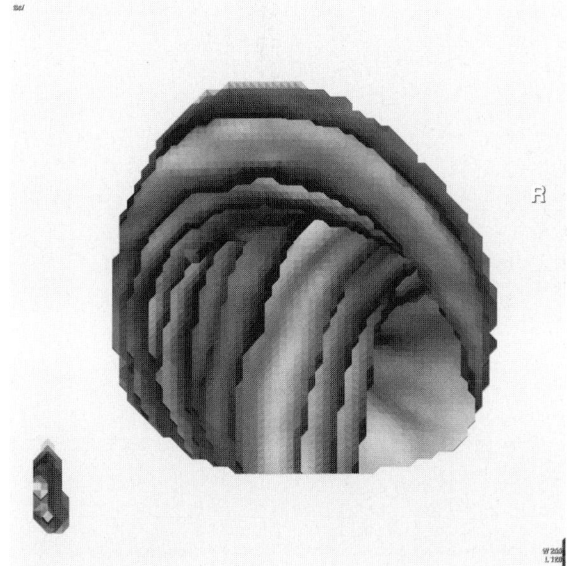

a

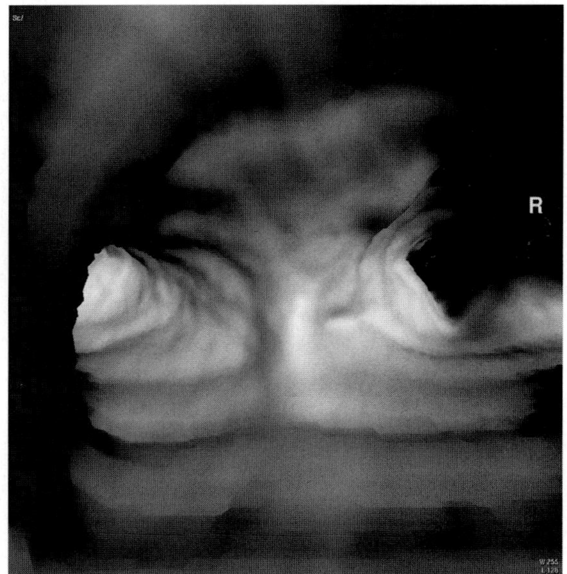

b

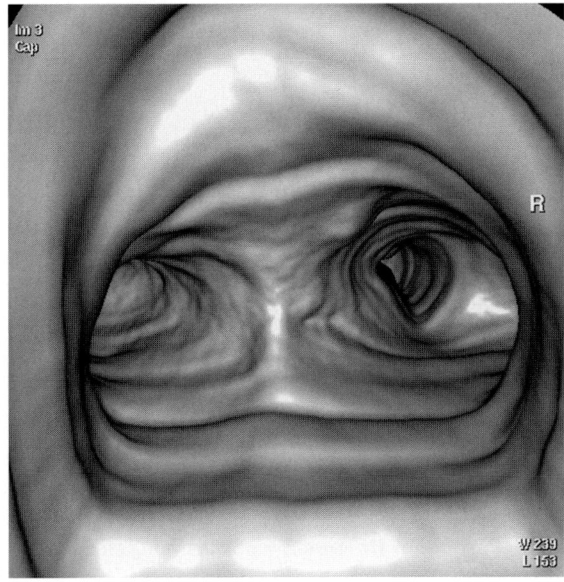

c

Fig. 4.7. An example of the difference between a pixel-based, non-interpolated surface reconstruction (**a,b**) and a volume rendering-based reconstruction (**c**). **a** A surface reconstruction of the trachea without perspective distortion and without pixel interpolation. The separate steps in the reconstruction are clearly viewed. Even with perspective distortion (**b**), although the carina can be recognised, the fact that the single pixels can be seen due to step artefacts is disturbing. The pixel model is calculated according to a segmentation process so that further interpolation is not possible. Programming a stronger enlargement would only intensify the pixel presentation. **c** A volume rendering-based image from the same perspective. The original dataset from the CT (1.5 mm slice thickness, 3 mm table feed, 1 mm reconstruction interval) is identical. Note the enormous quality difference between the presentations, especially the absence of separate pixel steps and thus a more natural surface presentation. Findings: Infiltrating mass below the carina with tracheal wall infiltration

4.4.9 Tissue Transition Projection

Tissue transition projection (TTP) is a projection technique that generates a transparent demonstration of the imaged area. A prerequisite for this presentation type is variation in density levels of the tissues to be displayed. On tissue interfaces, these density differences must lead to clear transitions in the density, which have been termed density gradients. The TTP technique only demonstrates the density transitions, that is, the tissue gradients, explaining why the technique may also be termed gradient imaging. The ensuing images closely resemble a conventional bronchography, in which also only a thin and thus transparent layer exists around the trachea and the bronchi, which then can be displayed in the fluoroscopy.

The TTP display, like all other 3D techniques, is created by computer calculations, which means objects can be equally viewed from all sides. Adding a function for depth encoding that darkens objects farther away from the viewer enhances the 3D effect. The additional calculation of a viewing perspective between 15° and 30°, a viewing angle common to conventional bronchography, can make the images

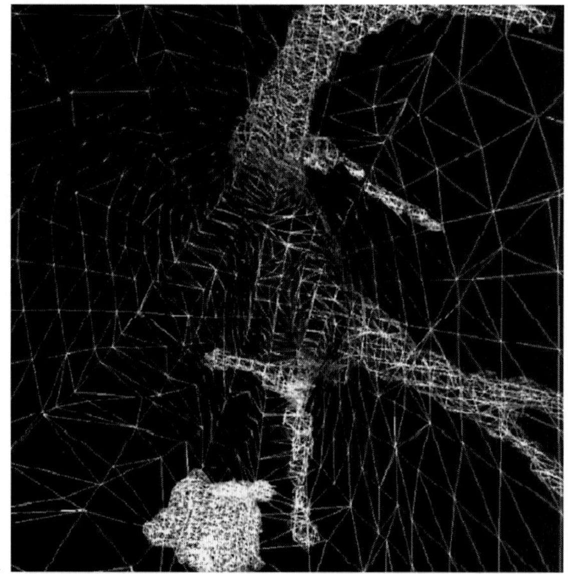

a

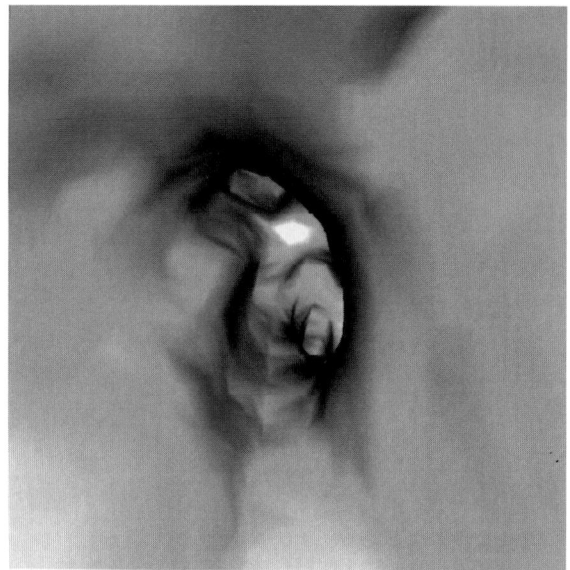

b

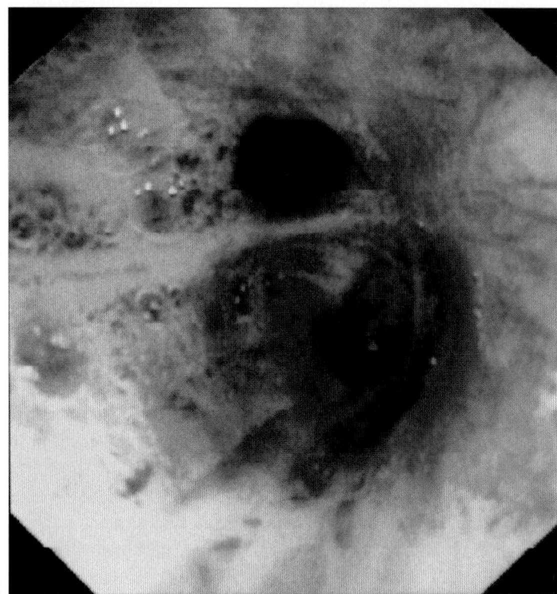

c

Fig. 4.8a–c. Presentation of a bifurcation of the right upper lobe with ostia to segments 2 and 3. **a** The calculation of a wire frame, composed of many small triangles. The volumetric information is lost by the segmentation process. However, one can see through the wire frame and identify the intrapulmonary tumour beneath, which becomes impossible when the surface is textured with a mucosa-like appearance (**b**). Scanning was performed with 2 mm slice thickness. **c** The true-endoscopic correlation, in which the intrapulmonary round lesion was, expectedly, also not conspicuous. (Images kindly provided by Dr. H. Moriya of Fukushima Medical College, Japan)

even more alike. However, the perspective calculation requires additional computing power, and since the calculation of a gradient presentation is already computationally very expensive, the additional perspective function is generally omitted.

Given the need for interpolation to the second degree, the spatial resolution is considerably worse than in the original axial slices. Nonetheless, TTP represents an interesting projection technique because the transparency still permits recognition of the anatomical form but the deeper-lying structures are not completely hidden.

4.4.10 Virtual Endoscopy

Virtual endoscopy represents one of the most recent developments in 3D visualisation techniques (Summers 1997). The novel technique combines established principles (surface or volume rendering methods) and interpolation techniques with a very strong enlargement function and – the critical difference – a perspective distortion (Fig. 4.9). The fundamental technical and acquisition characteristics are described here in detail.

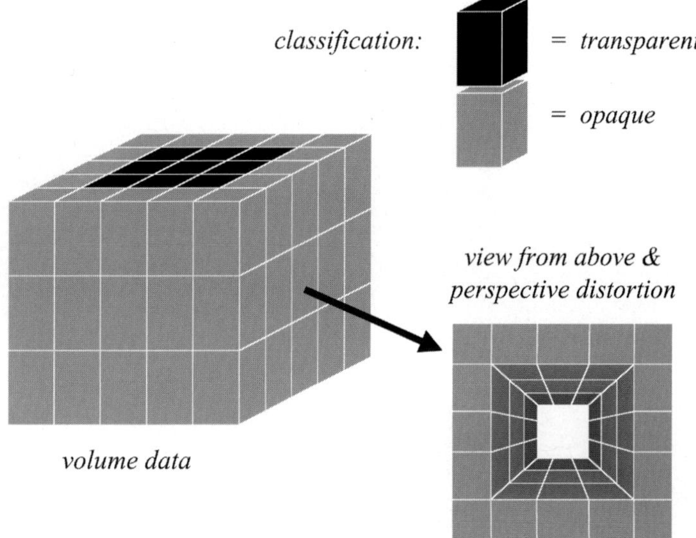

Fig. 4.9. Principle of the virtual presentation simplified in a few voxels. In a user-defined classification, the black image voxels that represent the air in the trachea are classified as transparent and the tracheal wall as opaque. In the virtual reconstruction, the once black voxels are no longer apparent and the view into a hollow room is created. By calculating perspective distortion and decreasing brightness intensity with increasing distance from the viewer, the virtual view into a tube results

4.4.10.1 Magnification, Slice Thickness and Spatial Resolution

A "normal" 3D reconstruction from computed tomographic image data uses an image matrix consisting of 512×512 points; an optical increase in resolution can be attained only by interpolation. If the 3D image is strongly enlarged, the calculated image points also become larger and eventually the isolated points will be visible. In order to maintain a surface whose appearance is as smooth and as natural as possible, also in structures that are composed of relatively few pixels, the interpolation degree of the virtual endoscopy must be significantly higher than with a non-enlarged 3D reconstruction. The smaller the already imaged pixels are, the less necessary it is to interpolate and the more natural the anatomical appearance. Since the image matrices in the CT scanning level are created, almost without exception, in a 512×512 pixel format (the previously used matrix of 320×320 pixels is no longer of practical value), the chief resolution problem lies in the z-axis, the longitudinal axis of the patient. The resolution in the longitudinal direction can be improved solely by choosing thinner slices (see Sect. 4.3.1). The effect of increased slice interpolation with thicker slices on the authenticity of the depiction of smaller objects in virtual endoscopy is illustrated in Fig. 4.10, which shows a series of 3D reconstructions of a small figure with differing slice thicknesses. Although all 3D reconstructions have the same pixel resolution (in this case 512×512 pixels), the detail resolution becomes worse with increasing slice thickness, because less sampling data is available for the reconstruction. An overlapping slice reconstruction partly improves the 3D reconstructions by increasing the amount of sampling data. The principal parameter influencing the quality of the reconstruction remains, however, the primary slice thickness (Rodenwaldt et al. 1997), not only since using thin slices increases the sampling rate but also because the physical partial volume effects are minimised (Fig. 4.11).

4.4.10.2 Pitch Factor

The dimensionless pitch factor is determined with the following equation:

$$\frac{\text{table feed (mm/s)}}{\text{slice thickness (mm)} \times \text{revolutions per second}} : \text{no. of detector rows}$$

The standard written format, which also takes the number of detector rows in multislice CT into consideration, is for example 6:4 when four slices are obtained simultaneously. This factor would be equivalent to a pitch factor of 1.5 in conventional spiral CT. The pitch factor directly influences the slice sensitivity profile in spiral CT, which becomes wider with an increasing pitch factor. The slices become "smeared". For the virtual reconstructions, the pitch factor in spiral CT is less influential than the primary slice thickness (Neumann et al. 2000), which is why a thin slice collimation with

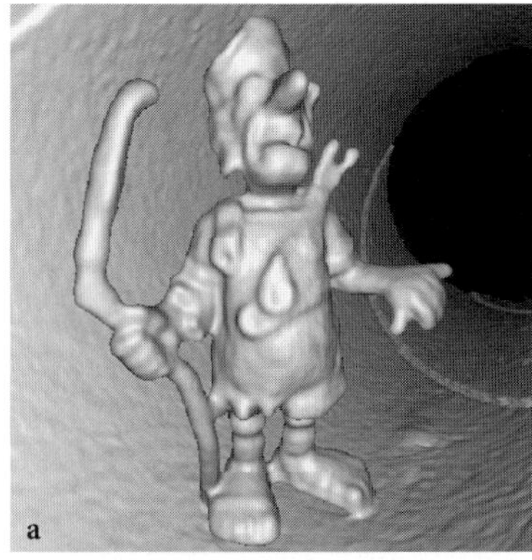

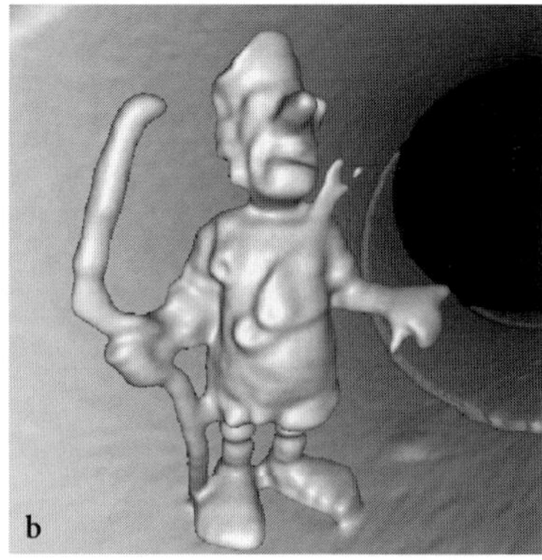

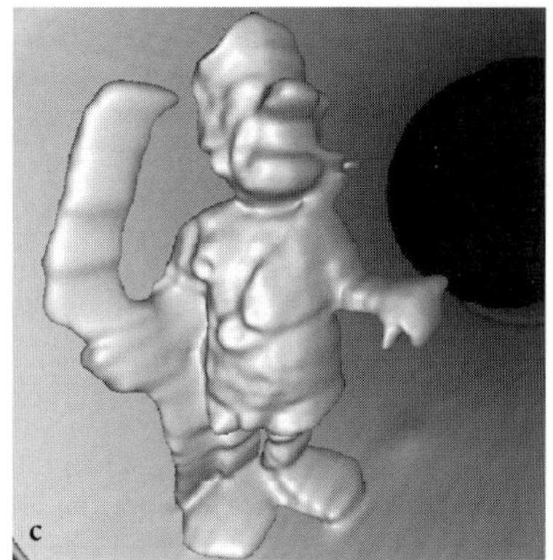

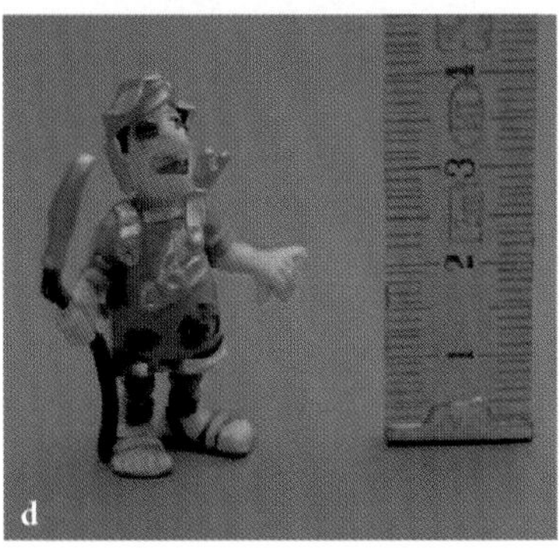

Fig. 4.10a–d. Dependence of the detail presentation on the primary slice thickness: **a** 0.5 mm; **b** 1.5 mm; **c** 4.5 mm. In all cases, the reconstruction interval was 40% of the primary slice thickness, i.e. 0.2, 0.6 and 1.8 mm, respectively. As expected, the reconstruction using 0.5 mm slice thickness gives the highest detail resolution, e.g. the demonstration of the individual fingers. Examination with tripled slice thickness (1.5 mm) also produces an acceptable reconstruction with sufficient detail resolution in the millimetre range. A further tripling (to 4.5 mm) reduces the *z*-axis resolution strongly, so that partial volume effects may cause associated objects to appear disconnected. A slice thickness of 4–5 mm does not suffice for the computation of a virtual bronchoscopy. **d** Photograph of the imaged figurine

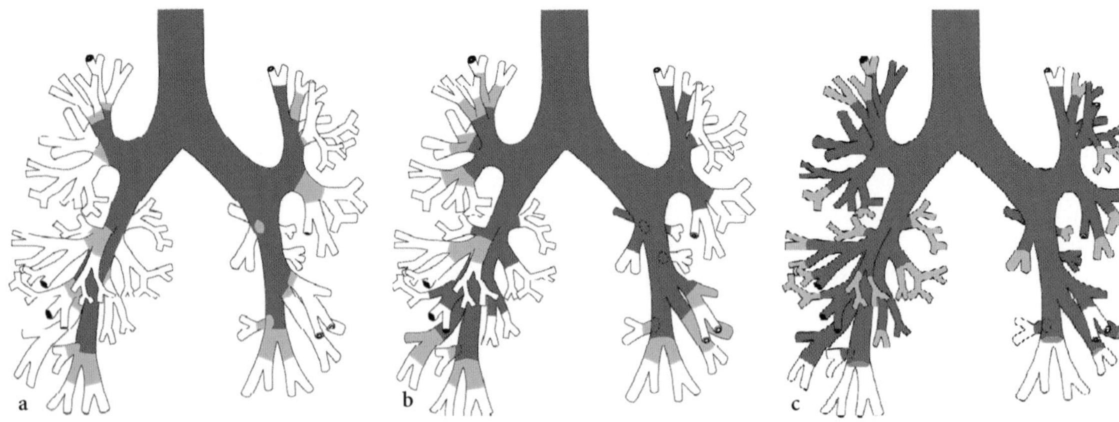

Fig. 4.11a–c. Model illustration of the tracheobronchial tree showing the regions visualised with various virtual techniques: **a** 5 mm slice thickness, surface rendering technique; **b** 5 mm slice thickness, volume rendering technique; **c** 2 mm slice thickness, surface rendering technique. *Red* means that the bronchi are always visible, while the *yellow* bronchi are only partly visible. It can be readily appreciated that more details will be depicted with the volume rendering technique than with the surface rendering technique. Furthermore, the choice of the primary slice thickness implicitly influences the visibility of the bronchi – in image **c** subsegmental bronchi are ascertainable (Images provided by Dr. H. Moriya of Fukushima Medical College, Japan)

higher pitch factors is generally preferred over a thicker slice collimation with a lower pitch factor. An acceptable compromise can be reached at a pitch factor of 1.5–1.7 (Rodenwaldt et al. 1997). In spiral CT, the pitch factor has no influence on image noise.

The situation is somewhat different with multislice technology (Wang and Vannier 1999): due to the reconstruction algorithm, higher pitch factors barely influence the slice sensitivity profile, but influence image noise almost proportionally. This holds true if the pitch factor ranges between 1:1 and 2:1. With higher pitch factors, anatomical distortions come increasingly into play and can, as in spiral CT, diminish image quality. However, a linear correlation between the pitch factor and the reduction of radiation exposure exists both in spiral and in multislice CT.

4.4.10.3 Perspective Distortion

Virtual bronchoscopic images are created when a 3D reconstruction is strongly enlarged followed by a perspective computation. A perspective distortion is necessary in order to choose a projection plane, representing the frontal opening of the lens in the true bronchoscopy, that is small enough to fit into the bronchus and still allow a wide overview. The effect of a perspective simulates a wide-angle objective in photography. The computation of perspective distortion results in a more natural appearance of the objects, but has a considerable disadvantage for imaging in general. From a modality like CT that is prized for its absence of distortions and its realistic dimensions, images are generated in which structures can no longer be measured due to lacking depth information (Fig. 4.12). The diameter cannot be defined in the virtual, perspective-distorted endoscopy. This situation is somewhat absurd in light of the efforts in bronchoscopy to tackle exactly this weakness by implementing laser-measurement techniques (Dorffel et al. 1999).

The absence of exact depth information helps explain, for example, the difficulty encountered in making a statement from a virtual endoscopy pertaining to the form of a tubular structure that had been endoscopically examined. Figure 4.13 shows a virtual view into a tube that looks like a funnel due to the perspective distortion. For comparative purposes, a virtual view into a funnel with the same opening point is also shown. The single imaging difference is that for the shot through the tube a stronger perspective distortion was included than for the funnel. Disregarding the type and extent of artefacts and light reflections, it is impossible for the viewer, when solely making use of the virtual endoscopic images, to differentiate between the funnel and the tube.

4.4.10.4 Thresholding

An important parameter for the reconstructions based on surface or volume rendering technique is

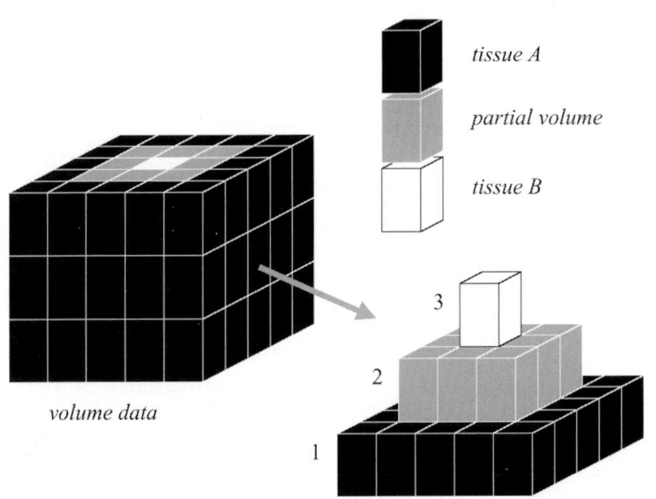

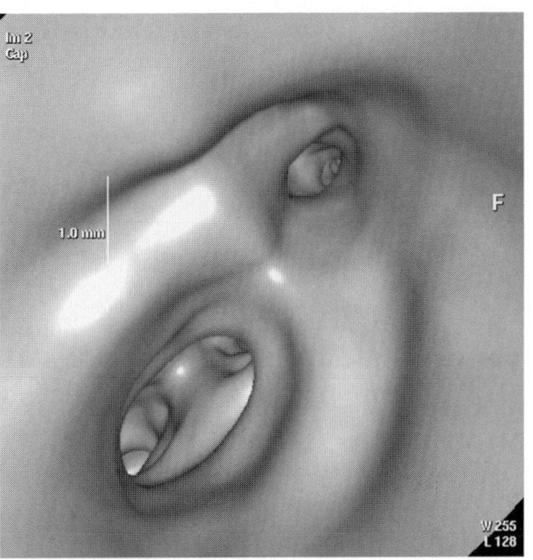

Fig. 4.12a,b. The choice of a threshold both for surface rendering and for volume rendering can substantially influence the size presentation of a 3D reconstruction. **a** An example to demonstrate this relationship. A simplified, bright linear structure surrounded by darker tissue is presented. Through partial volume effects in the axial plane, a sharp boundary between the two distinct tissues is not depicted, but rather transition voxels with intermediate density exist. If the threshold for the 3D extraction of the white structure is set too low, surrounding tissue is also included in the 3D representation (*1*). A threshold that lies between the two values (surrounding tissue and targeted tissue) leads to a relatively large depiction of the 3D image (*2*). If the threshold is set too high, the result is a reconstruction of only the core of the targeted structure. The diameter in the 3D presentation has shrunk even further (*3*). This example should explicitly demonstrate that 3D presentations that are dependent upon a threshold value that is freely defined at any point during processing are not suited for making measurements. **b** A virtual endoscopy of bronchi. The inserted ruler may appear anywhere. Due to the absence of depth information, the calculated distance is of no value

the selection of an appropriate threshold, above which a surface should be presented as opaque representing the mucosa (Fig. 4.12). In a comparative study, it was shown that for the surface rendering technique, the threshold should be placed in the density region of the soft tissue in order to create an optimal virtual image of the mucosa. For the volume rendering technique the authors obtained the best results when the threshold for classification was halfway between the density values (HU) of air and soft tissue (Hopper et al. 2000). For further information on this subject, see Chap. 2.

4.5 Pathology – What Can Be Seen?

Despite the availability of virtual bronchoscopy in recent years, usage has been focused only on those cases where from the clinical indication the ability to address the diagnostic question seemed feasible. As explained in Sect. 4.3, in spiral CT a second scan must be dedicated to a qualitatively assessable virtual bronchoscopy – and this additional radiation exposure must be clinically justifiable. Since the introduction of multislice CT, the situation has changed because from essentially one routine CT examination, the virtual bronchoscopy can be calculated. Thus, a new spurt in postprocessing of the tracheobronchial tree can be anticipated.

4.5.1 The Normal Tracheobronchial Tree

Figure 4.14 shows the most important standard views that should be calculated by a virtual bronchoscopy. Similar standard settings are not only intended to help the radiologist get acquainted with the bronchoscopy, but also, importantly, to facilitate communication with clinicians and, if pathology is present, it assists in drawing a sketch of the detected changes and preparing a demonstration for one's clinical partners. Each of the image sequences in Fig. 4.14 shows a correlation between the true, fibreoptic bronchoscopy and the virtual bronchoscopy. The respective position of the endoscope is indicated with an arrow in the sketch.

Table 4.3 gives a simplified overview of the standard nomenclature of the tracheobronchial tree.

Table 4.3. Standard bronchial nomenclature

Right lung
Upper lobe
Segment 1 (apical)
Segment 2 (posterior)
Segment 3 (anterior)
Middle lobe
Segment 4 (lateral)
Segment 5 (medial)
Lower lobe
Segment 6 (superior/anterior[a])
Segment 7 (medial basal)
Segment 8 (anterior basal)
Segment 9 (lateral basal)
Segment 10 (posterior basal)
Left lung
Upper lobe
Segment 1+2 (apicoposterior)
Segment 3 (anterior)
Lingula
Segment 4 (superior)
Segment 5 (inferior)
Lower lobe
Segment 6 (superior/anterior[a])
Segment 8 (anterior basal)
Segment 9 (lateral basal)
Segment 10 (posterior basal)

[a]Some differences exist between the European and the North American nomenclature: in the USA "superior" is preferred in order to avoid confusion with the anterior upper lobe bronchus.

4.5.2 Benign Tumours

Granuloma, resulting from sarcoidosis in one third of cases, is the most common pulmonary lesion, followed by entities such as tuberculosis, histoplasmosis and coccidioidomycosis. True benign tumours in the lung are less common than malignant neoplasms. The most frequent such tumour is hamartoma (originating from lung tissue), the third most common lung lesion overall (6%). Hamartoma is followed, in descending order, by lipoma (fat tissue, most commonly in the form of pleural lesions), fibroma (fibrous tissue), leiomyoma (muscle tissue), schwannoma, neurofibroma, paraganglioma (all neural tissue), intrapulmonary lymph node (lymph tissue), amyloid, splenosis, endometrioma and extramedullary sites of haematopoiesis (deposits). One of the rare amyloid tumours is shown in Fig. 4.15. It can generally be said that all pulmonary or mediastinal lesions can be seen on virtual endoscopy only when a morphological alteration of the tracheal or bronchial wall has taken place. For the most part, virtual and

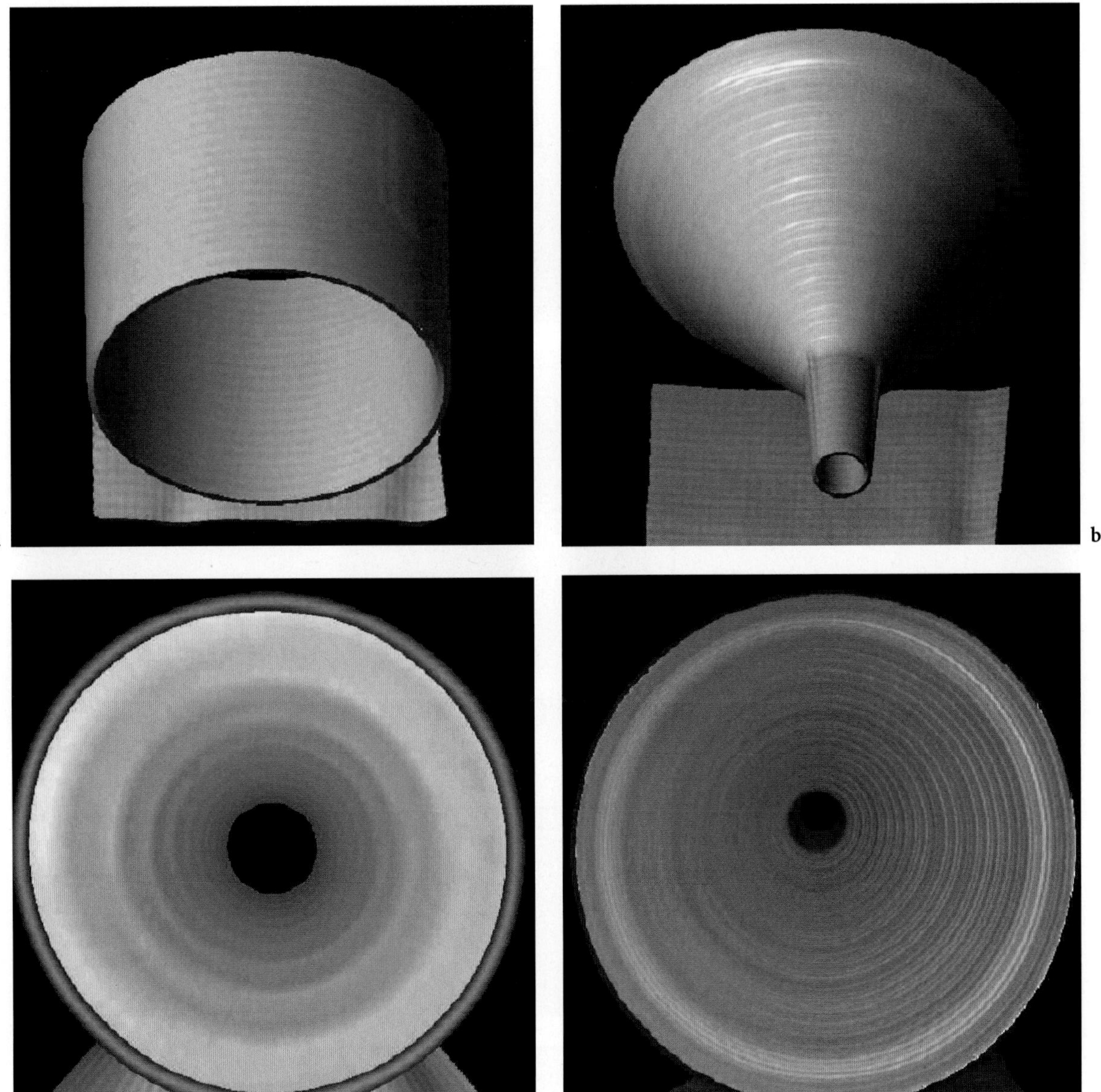

Fig. 4.13a–d. Representation of a significant problem in virtual endoscopy: because of the calculated perspective distortion it is hardly possible to recognise luminal changes along the viewing direction. **a** The 3D presentation of a plastic tube; **b** that of a funnel. **c** The consequent virtual endoscopy of the tube with a perspective distortion of 90°; **d** the view into the funnel with a 30° viewing angle. Note that without information of the 3D surface reconstruction it would be impossible to describe the shape of the phantom solely based on the virtual views. Some minor stair-stepping artefacts in **d** may indicate that the spiral acquisition was obtained over a diagonal surface, but such symmetrical shapes would not occur in human organ examinations. Virtual endoscopy presents a problem when judging luminal changes in the trachea

true bronchoscopy do not differ in this respect. However, one exception exists: virtual endoscopy lacks natural pigmentation, which can clearly indicate pathology on true endoscopy.

Furthermore, the inability to perform biopsies gives virtual endoscopy the role of a detection and much less a characterisation technique. The tissue type can naturally be characterised in the cross-sectional diagnostics much earlier, and even this is difficult or impossible in many cases. Consequently, virtual bronchoscopy should not be expected to contribute substantially to characterisation of tumours. The example in Fig. 4.15 shows that the calcified nature of the mediastinal lesion is only clearly

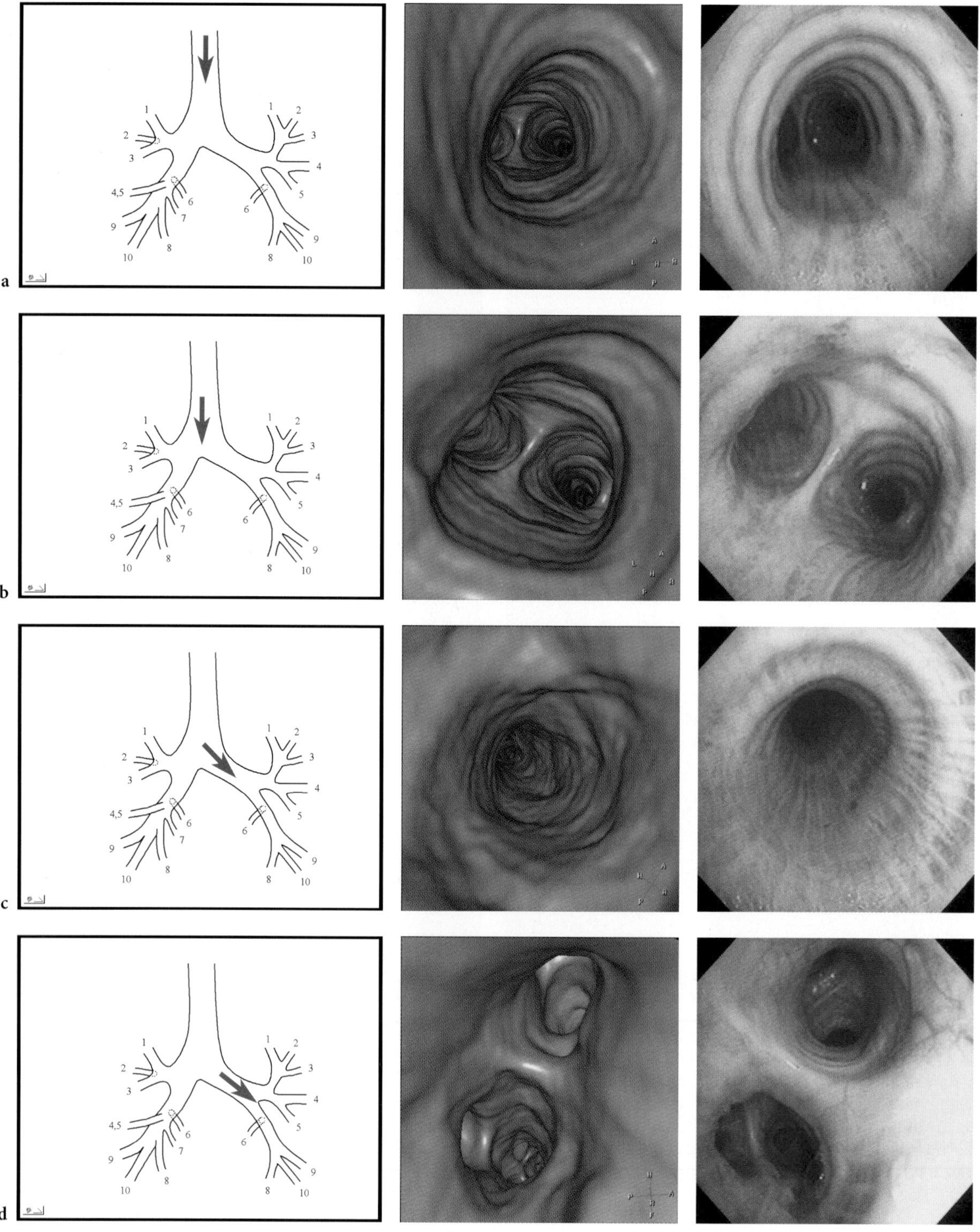
a
b
c
d

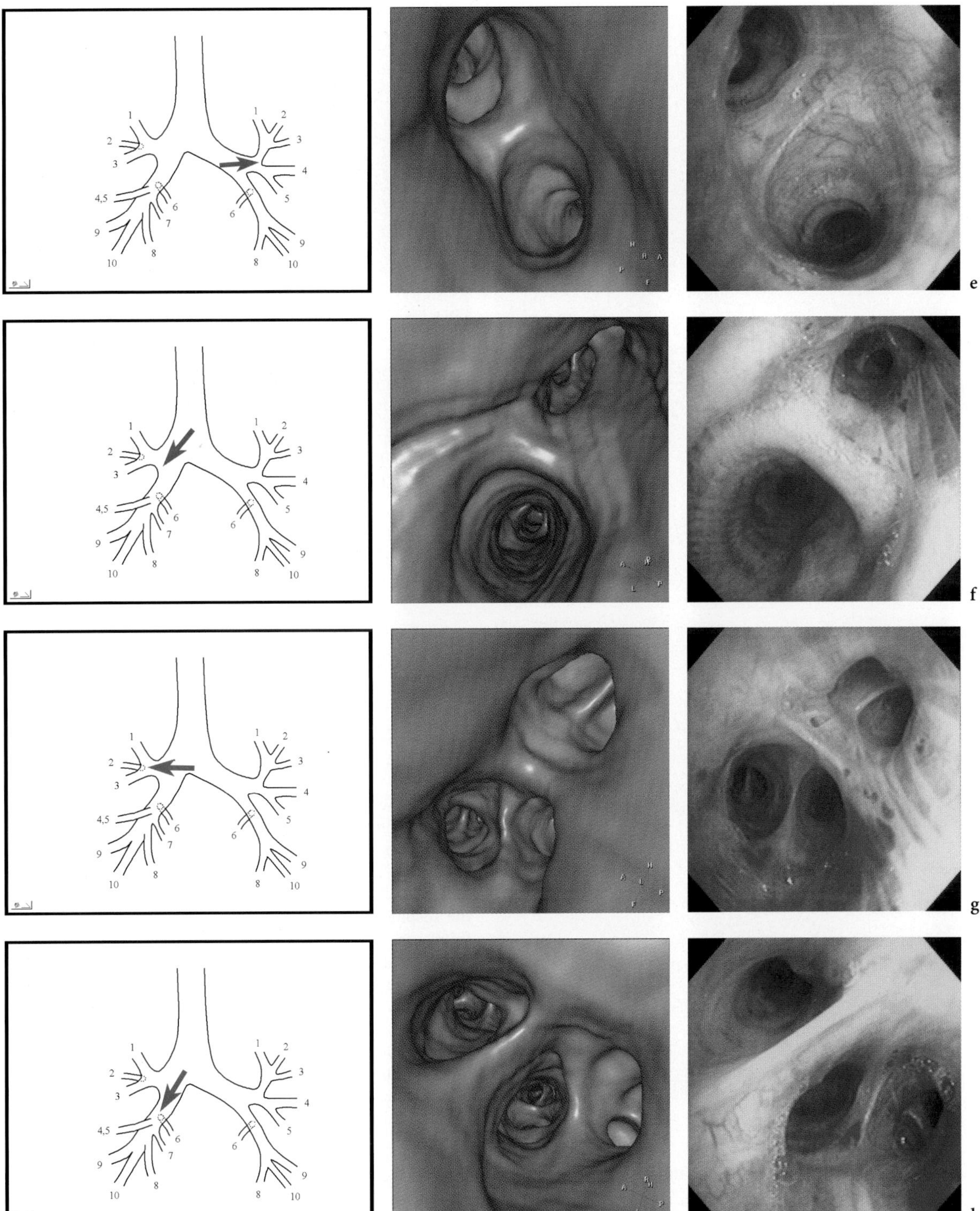

Fig. 4.14a–h. Standard views of a normal finding in the virtual and true bronchoscopy. By assuming the following basic settings, the transmission of findings to clinicians, and possibly correlation of findings, is made easier since the pulmonologist also uses the same settings. A 57-year-old patient with pleuritis calcarea. **a** View into trachea onto carina; **b** general view of carina; **c** main left bronchus; **d** left main carina with view into lower lobe bronchus (segments 6–10); **e** left upper lobe bronchus (segments 1–3 and 4, 5); **f** right upper lobe carina with view into bronchus intermedius; **g** z; **f** right upper lobe bronchus (segments 1–3); **h** right lower lobe carina with view into middle and lower lobe. Summarised, other than a vulnerable mucosa in the distal main carina and a mild reddening of the mucosa, no pathological findings were identified. The subsequent bronchoalveolar lavage was also unremarkable. There was no suspicion of a neoplasm. (True bronchoscopic images provided by Bernd Schmidt, MD, Dept. of Pulmonology, Charité Hospital, Berlin)

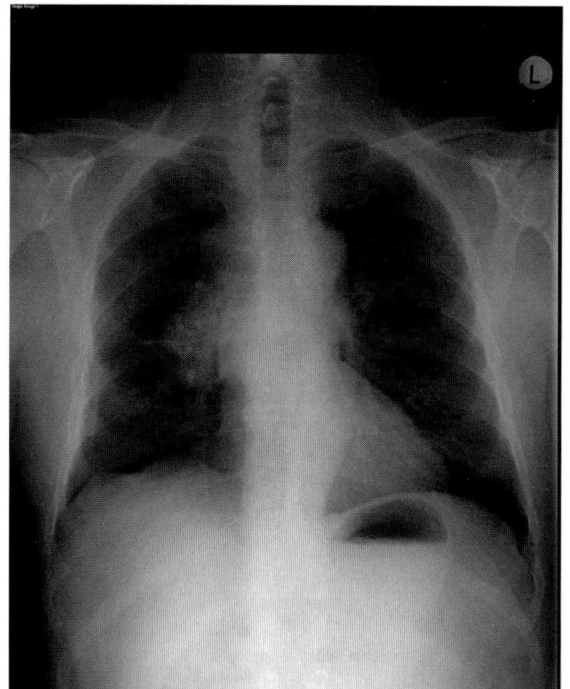

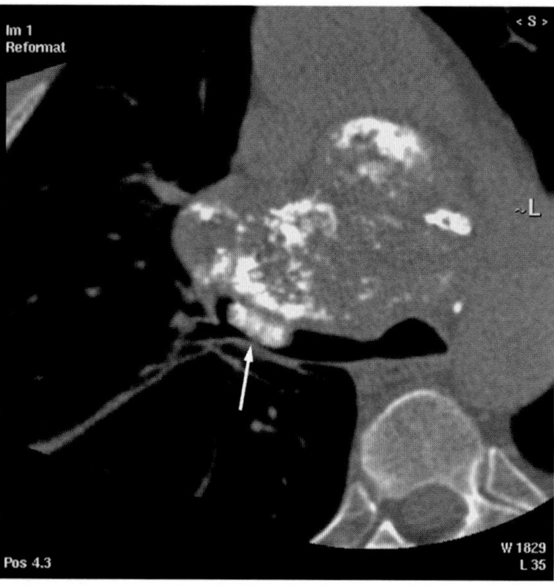

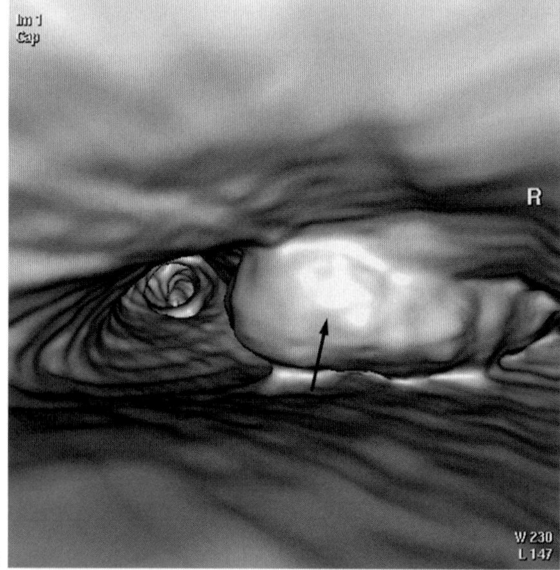

Fig. 4.15a–c. Primary mediastinal amyloid tumour with extended infiltration into the right main and upper lobe bronchus. **a** On the conventional chest X-ray, a calcifying mass projecting on to the mediastinum was detectable; together with the clinical symptoms (slight dyspnoea), this aroused the suspicion of a bronchial carcinoma. **b** CT (1.5 mm slice thickness, 3 mm/s table feed, 1 mm reconstruction interval, dedicated spiral scan) shows the extensively infiltrating tumour with extension into the right bronchus. The virtual bronchoscopy clearly shows the intraluminal tumour fragment that, most importantly, has obstructed the upper lobe ostium. The attempt to surgically remove the tumour had to be abandoned because, despite its benign nature, it could not be detached from the vessels intraoperatively

recognised in the cross-sectional modality. Figure 4.16 is a virtual endoscopy of a patient who underwent bronchoscopy to clarify reported breathing difficulties. From the start, virtual endoscopy showed a protrusion into the larynx as the cause, initially creating the suspicion of a malignant lesion. However, axial CT showed that a small, dislocated bony structure led to the protrusion in the wall. Thorough questioning revealed that the patient had undergone a larynx operation more than 20 years previously due to wall instability, with insertion of an autologous bone implant.

4.5.3 Malignant Tumours

Most malignant primary tumours of the lung (66%) are bronchogenic carcinomas, which represent the most frequent cause of cancer death in males (35%)

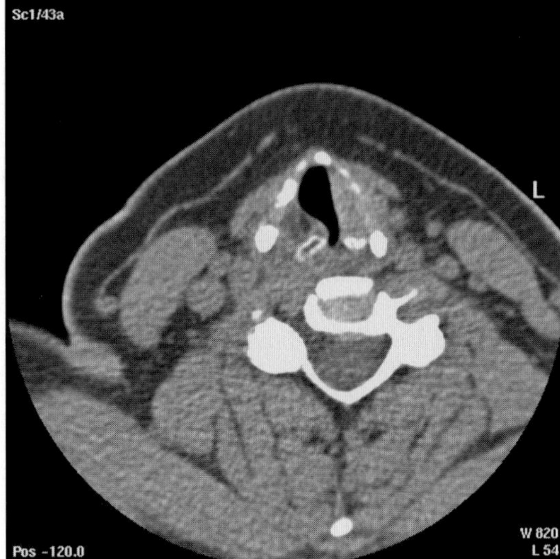

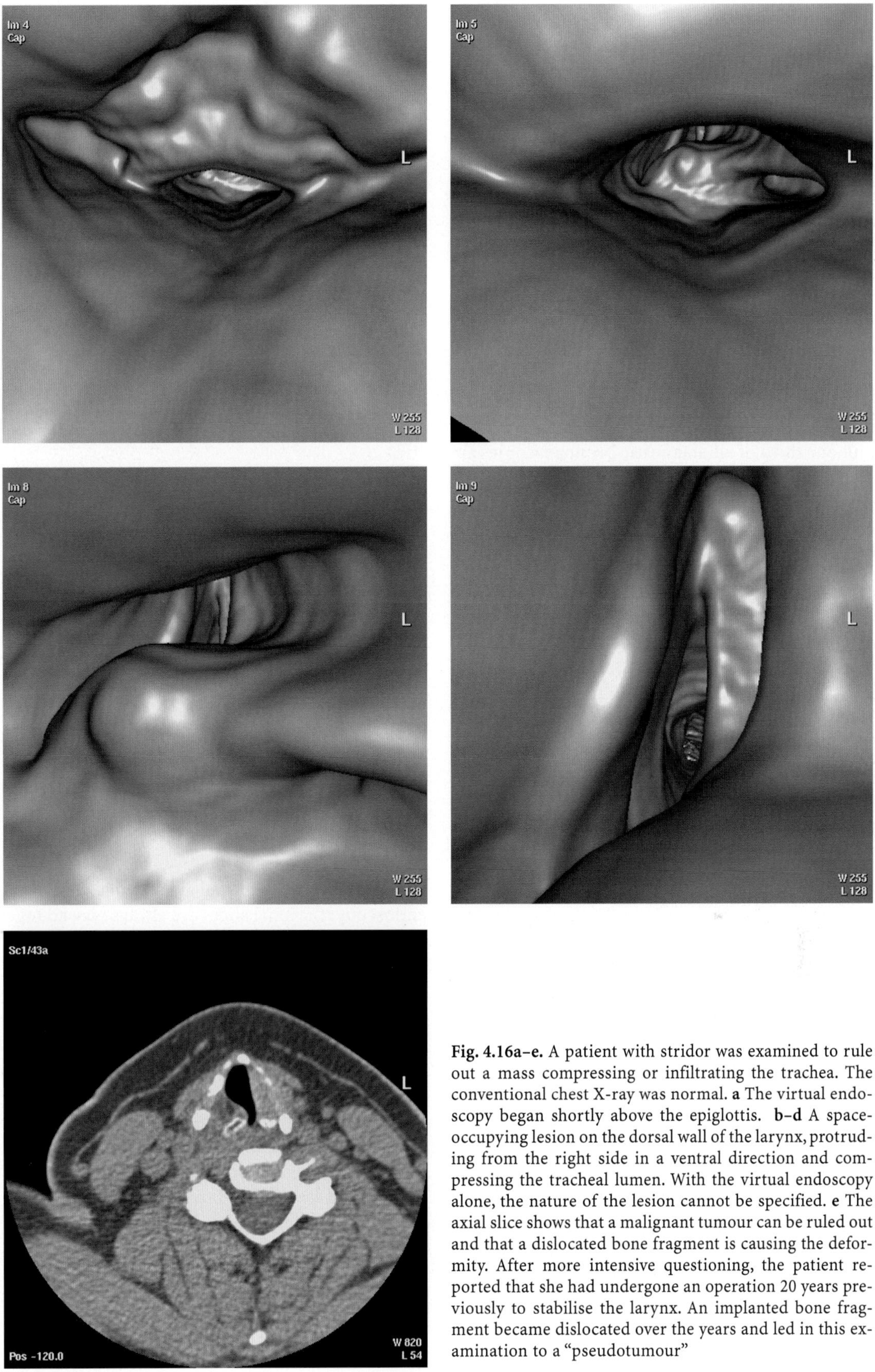

Fig. 4.16a–e. A patient with stridor was examined to rule out a mass compressing or infiltrating the trachea. The conventional chest X-ray was normal. **a** The virtual endoscopy began shortly above the epiglottis. **b–d** A space-occupying lesion on the dorsal wall of the larynx, protruding from the right side in a ventral direction and compressing the tracheal lumen. With the virtual endoscopy alone, the nature of the lesion cannot be specified. **e** The axial slice shows that a malignant tumour can be ruled out and that a dislocated bone fragment is causing the deformity. After more intensive questioning, the patient reported that she had undergone an operation 20 years previously to stabilise the larynx. An implanted bone fragment became dislocated over the years and led in this examination to a "pseudotumour"

and females (18%). Falling within the group of the bronchogenic carcinomas are squamous cell carcinoma (30–35%), adenocarcinoma (25–35%), small-cell undifferentiated carcinoma (20–25%) and large-cell undifferentiated carcinoma (10–15%). Bronchogenic carcinoma represents the second most common mass in the lung following benign granuloma. Further malignant tumours are alveolar cell carcinoma, lymphoma, primary sarcoma of the lung, plasmocytoma (primary or secondary), clear cell carcinoma, carcinoid, giant cell carcinoma and finally metastases (Fig. 4.17). Flexible bronchoscopy has become firmly established specifically for diagnosing and obtaining histological evidence of a malignant tumour (Arroliga and Matthay 1993; Lam and Shibuya 1999). It is also eminently suited for staging bronchial carcinomas (Ferguson 1990). About one third of all diagnostic bronchoscopies are intended to clarify a pulmonary lesion detected by conventional chest X-ray or CT. Table 4.4 shows the average diagnostic yield of flexible bronchoscopy with the currently available means for tissue removal as reported by Arroliga and Matthey (1993).

Table 4.4. Diagnostic yield of flexible bronchoscopy (data from Arroliga and Matthey 1993)

Technique	Number of patients	Average diagnostic yield (%)
Brushing	273	39 (29–50)
Forceps biopsy	190	27 (15–46)
Washing	176	43 (42–46)
Bronchoalveolar lavage	154	37 (24–64)
Double-hinged curette	131	89 (82–97)

CT, especially with the long-existing possibility to acquire thin sections, plays a principal role not only in the detection of primary lung malignancies, but also in the characterisation and staging of pulmonary lesions. Multiple signs have been defined in thin-section CT such as cut-off, bronchus compression, irregular or smooth narrowing (Gaeta et al. 1993) (Fig. 4.18). CT possesses a decisive advantage: it attains diagnostic information regarding the pulmonary parenchyma that methodically cannot be gained with true bronchoscopy. A tumour that does not visibly alter the surface of the bronchi escapes detection in flexible bronchoscopy. The tumour signs that generally apply for bronchoscopy (Table 4.5) (Ikeda 1974) can be categorised into direct and indirect signs.

Table 4.5. Signs of tumour on true and virtual bronchoscopy

Signs of tumour	Visibility on flexible bronchoscopy	Visibility on virtual bronchoscopy
Indirect signs		
Stenosis	++	++
Compression	++	++
Swelling	++	+
Direct signs		
Tumour		
Intraluminal mass	++	++
Extraluminal mass	–	–
Necrosis	++	–
Infiltration		
Vascular dilatation	++	–
Mucosal irregularity	++	–
Loss of cartilage structure	+	–
Obstruction	++	++

After considering the information in Table 4.5, it becomes obvious that the virtual bronchoscopy is inferior to flexible bronchoscopy with respect to endoluminal tumour diagnosis if criteria are evaluated that depend upon natural pigmentation. Mucosal infiltrations are not visible on virtual endoscopy if the only indication is a change in mucosal colour. The spatial resolution in virtual endoscopy also does not compare to that of flexible bronchoscopy. Thus, evaluation of virtual bronchoscopy should be restricted to the gross morphology of the bronchi and direct visualisation of intraluminal masses. However, as the virtual endoscopy is calculated from cross-sectional image data, all information surrounding the tracheobronchial tree is additionally available. The greatest handicap of true endoscopy – its inability to see through the bronchial wall – does not exist in virtual endoscopy: the axial slices are always viewed together with the endoluminal reconstruction, filling in any diagnostic gaps.

Naidich et al. (1997) summarised the situations where virtual bronchoscopy is desirable:

- Follow-up examination after radiotherapy or laser treatment in patients with malignant lesions in the airways
- Identification of lesions in the airways (in particular, in peripheral branches or in areas beyond a stenotic or obstructed segment which cannot be observed by flexible bronchoscopy)
- Preliminary evaluation before flexible bronchoscopy

A further indication for virtual endoscopy is the rare case when a flexible bronchoscopy is contraindicated. An example is shown in Fig. 4.19. In the initial bronchoscopy, a tracheal perforation occurred

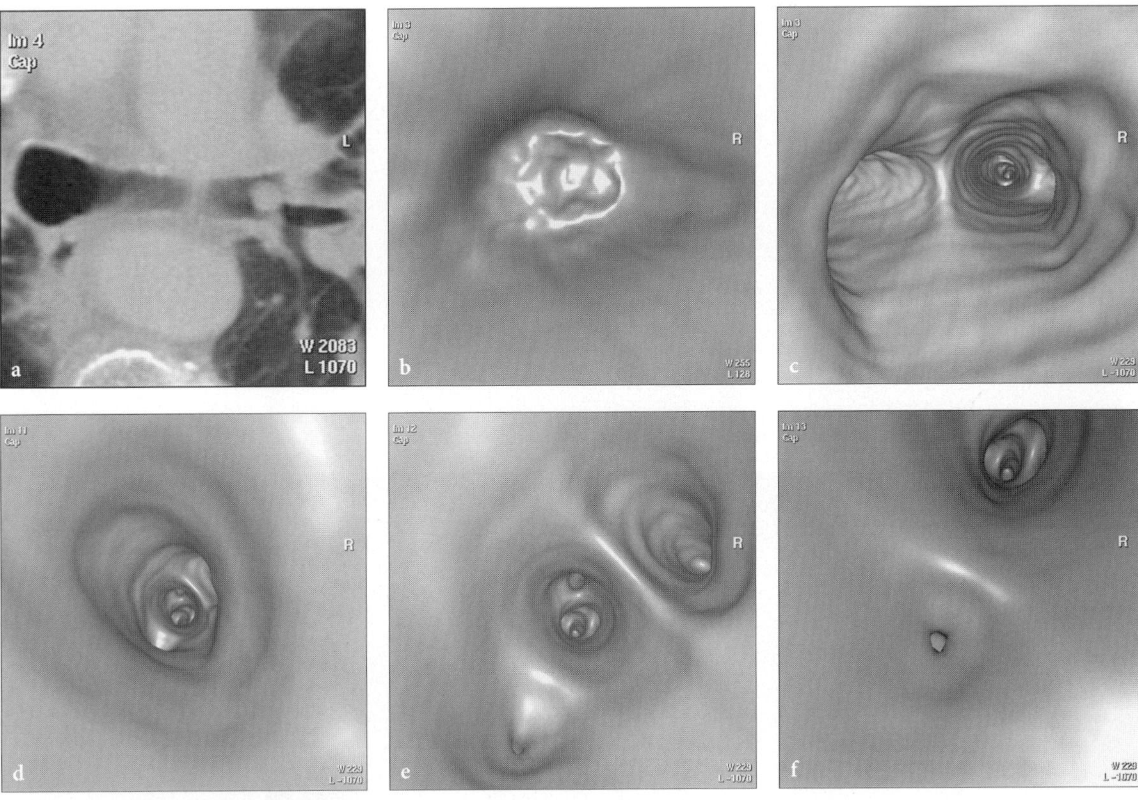

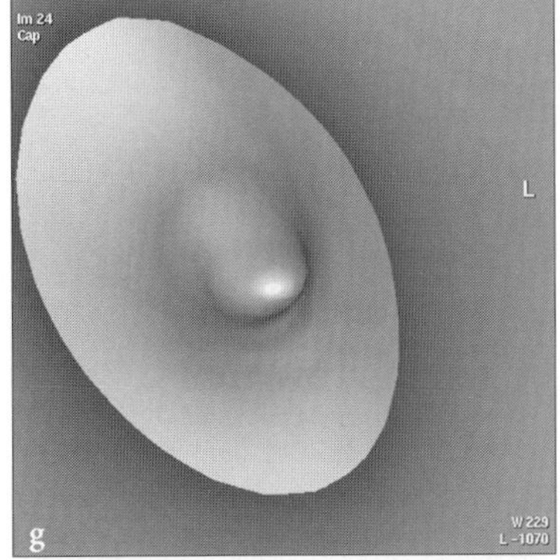

Fig. 4.17a–j. Examples of bronchial metastases in various forms. **a,b** Images from a patient with round metastases of a renal cell carcinoma. The round form and the location of the lesion are characteristic for metastatic disease. **c–j** Metastases from breast cancer behave differently: they can completely obstruct a bronchus (**g**); they can also lead to a circular stenosis (**f**). In such a case, clear demarcation of the finding from, for example, bronchial carcinoma is not possible. Images **h** and **i** demonstrate how a combination image is created: Surface extraction of the tracheobronchial tree (surface or volume rendered) is followed by a TTP reconstruction with the classification of air. The two images can be superimposed, thus creating a combined visualisation of the bronchi and the air-containing lung tissue. Note that the middle lobe is not inflated due to the metastatic occlusion

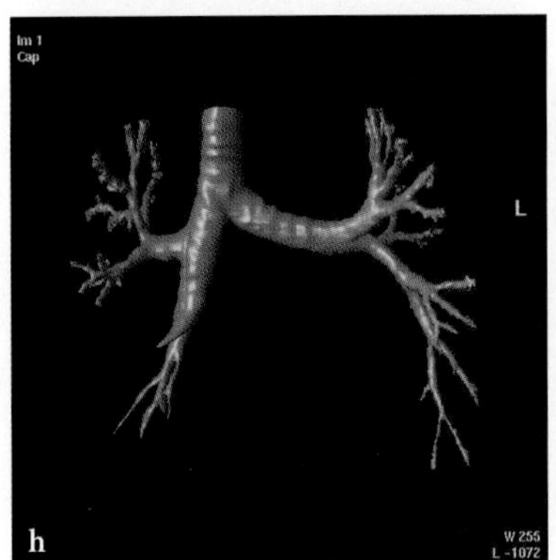

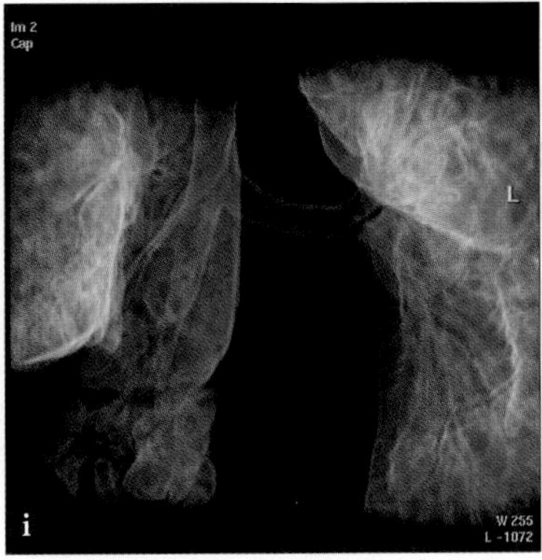

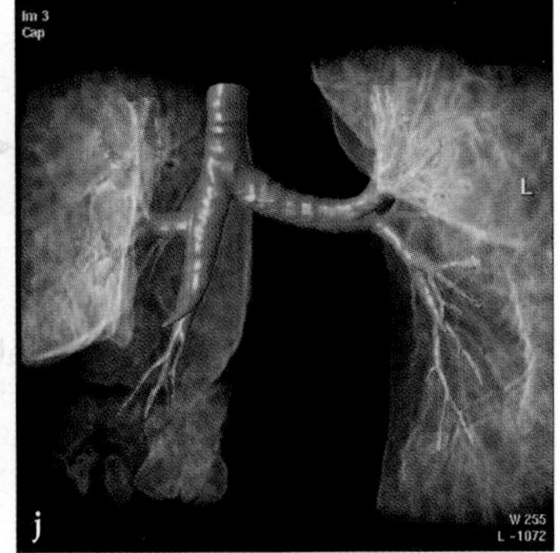

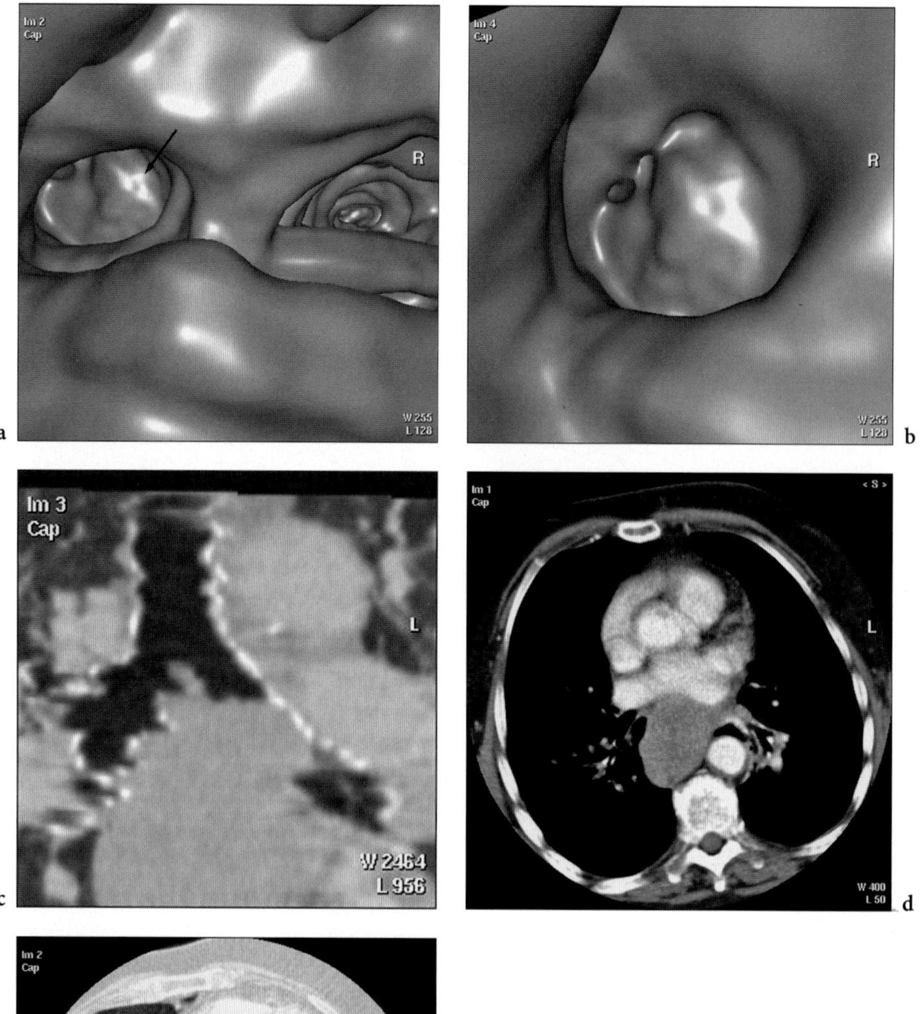

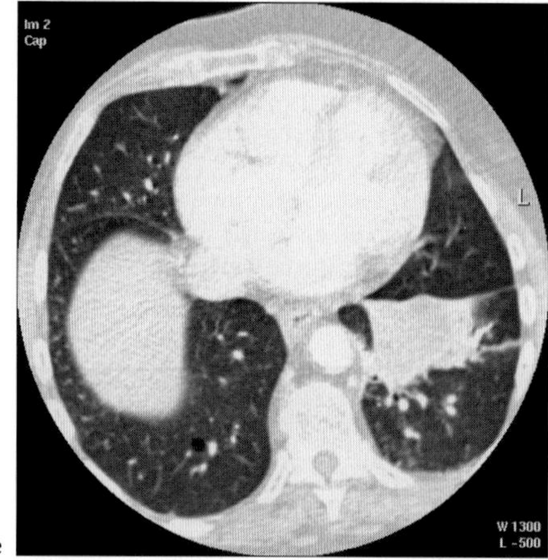

Fig. 4.18a–e. A 79-year-old patient who was examined by means of spiral CT with 7 mm slice thickness and intravenous injection of contrast material (**d**). The second, dedicated spiral acquisition was obtained with 1.5 mm slice thickness without repeated injection of contrast material. From these data, the virtual bronchoscopy was calculated. **a** A view onto the carina. Already, the nearly complete stenosis of the left main bronchus is seen (*arrow*). **b** A close-up shows the stenosis with a filiform remaining lumen. Due to dyspnoea, the patient could not hold her breath very long, explaining the strong breathing artefacts. **c** Especially the coronal reconstructions display not only the artefacts, but also the tumour on the left side. **e** The stenoses (*left*) lead to partial lower lobe atelectasis

due to the extensive tumour manifestation and the resulting infiltration of the tracheal wall. Repeated bronchoscopy was clinically judged to be too dangerous. Virtual bronchoscopy involves no mechanical irritation or air insufflation and was thus the method of choice for imaging the perforation. The non-invasiveness of virtual endoscopy was the decisive criterion in this case.

4.5.4 Bronchiectasis

The diagnostic presentation of bronchiectases can be difficult with flexible endoscopy. The diagnosis is usually based upon indirect indications, e.g. the detection of extensively inflamed and vulnerable or thickened, atrophic mucosa or the evidence of pu-

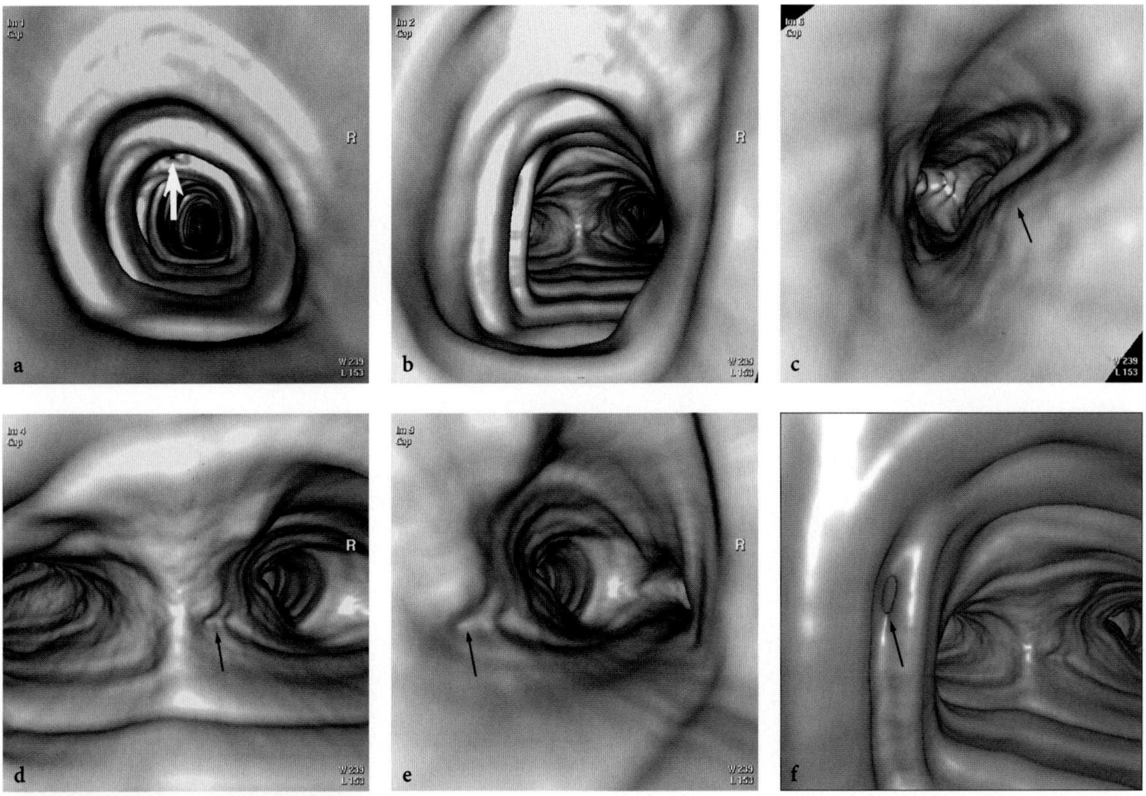

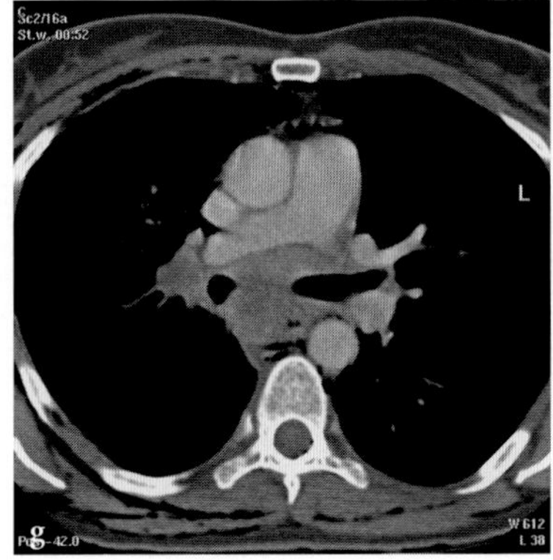

Fig. 4.19. Virtual endoscopy from a spiral CT (1.5 mm slice thickness) in a patient with histologically proven bronchial carcinoma. **a,b** The approach towards the carina, whose coarse surface already hints at tumour invasion. **c** View into the left main bronchus; **d** view of the infiltrated carina; **e** view into the right main bronchus. In all three images, the tumour infiltration can be visualised (*arrows*). **f** Careful inspection revealed a small hole in the tracheal wall on the left side (*arrow*). During the bronchoscopy performed to obtain histological material, the fragile tracheal wall was perforated in at least two places (*arrows* in **a** and **f**). **g** Axial CT shows both the extensive tumour mass and the pneumomediastinum and soft tissue emphysema that resulted from the perforations

trid, infectious secretions. An accurate projection of the morphology is seldom possible due to the perspective distortion.

In such cases, virtual endoscopy has a critical advantage: the diagnosis can be reached with the axial images alone. Since the position of the viewing direction is unlimited, bronchiectases can even be viewed from within in the direction of the proximal bronchus (Fig. 4.20); panorama images or 360° turnarounds are also possible. A very impressive presentation form is the TTP, and also the combined presentation from TTP of the lung together with the surface representation of the bronchi (Fig. 4.21).

4.5.5 Intervention

The main disadvantage of flexible bronchoscopy, already mentioned, is the absence of a view through the bronchus. For example, if a transbronchial biopsy of a mediastinal lymph node is planned (Dasgupta and Mehta 1999), the pulmonologist must estimate from the customary chest CT the biopsy location through which the externally lying lymph node can be reached (Ewert et al. 1997). This may explain why transbronchial biopsies do not have high sensitivity. By generating a virtual bronchoscopy the optimal

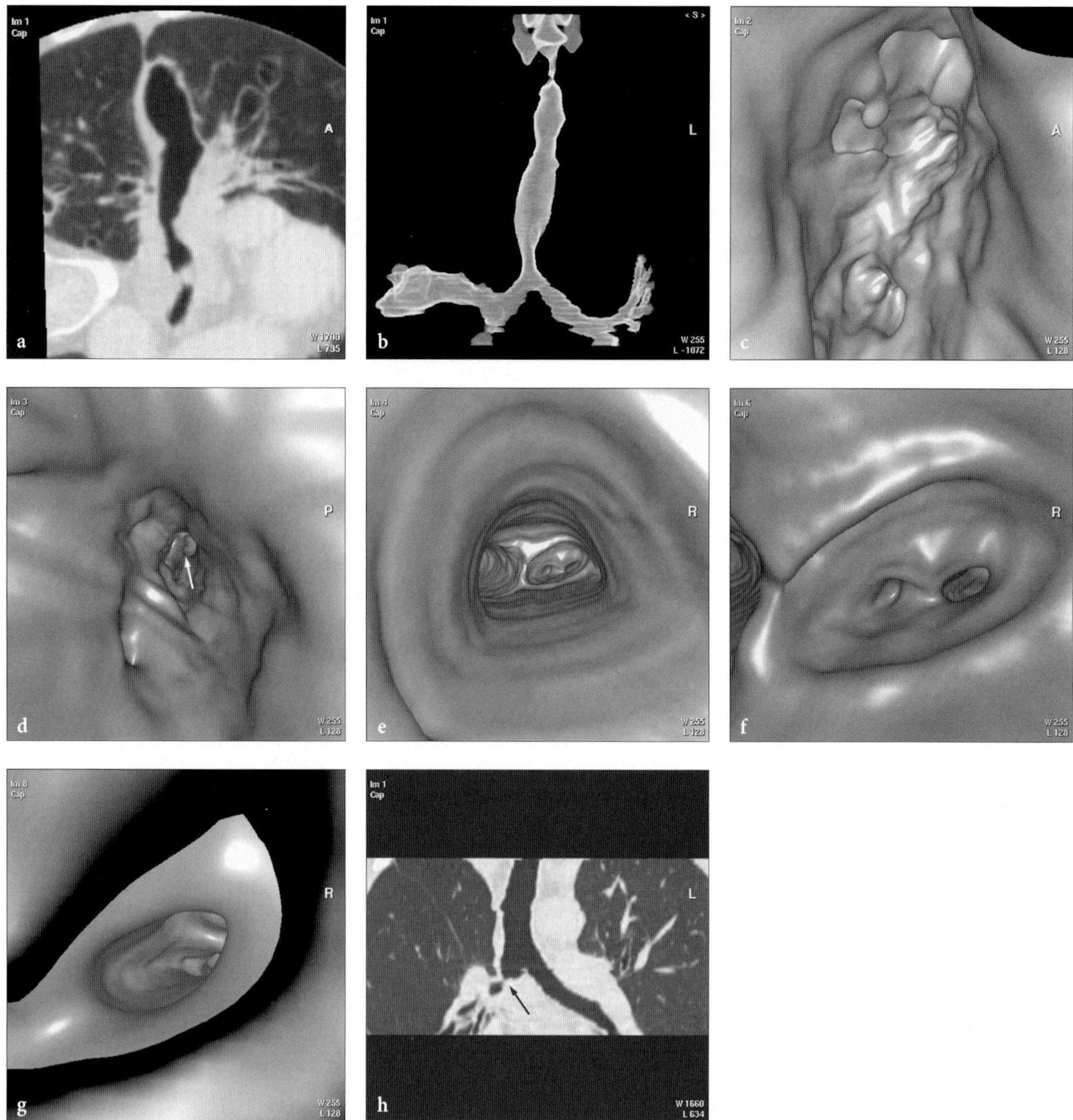

Fig. 4.20a–h. A 57-year-old patient with chronic recurring bronchitis. The massive bronchiectases can be detected in the spiral CT (**a**) and are also well distinguished in the TTP presentation (**b**). **c** A virtual view within the largest bronchiectasis. **d** A retrograde view of the "feeding" bronchus (*arrow*). Owing to the extensive disease manifestation, the patient underwent a lobectomy. Postoperatively, true bronchoscopy revealed a substantial stenosis of the main right bronchus that could not be passed endoscopically. **e–g** Virtual bronchoscopy, on the other hand, can evaluate the bronchi distal to the stenosis unhindered. **h** In the coronal MPR the postoperative ring stenosis is clearly discernible as well

access point for the biopsy procedure can be determined in advance (Hopper 1999). Some initial experiences have been reported (Bricault et al. 1998), but no larger studies that confirm an increase in sensitivity by using virtual planning assistance have been published to date.

A further, often postulated implementation is the measuring of stenoses to optimise stent fitting and implantation (Kim 1998). However, one must take into consideration the perspective distortion inherent to virtual endoscopy that is intentionally computed to create an image similar to a flexible bronchoscopy (Fleiter et al. 1997). Precisely the same distortion prevents exact measurement on true bronchoscopy as well. There is thus no rationale for the use of virtual presentations as the basis for mea-

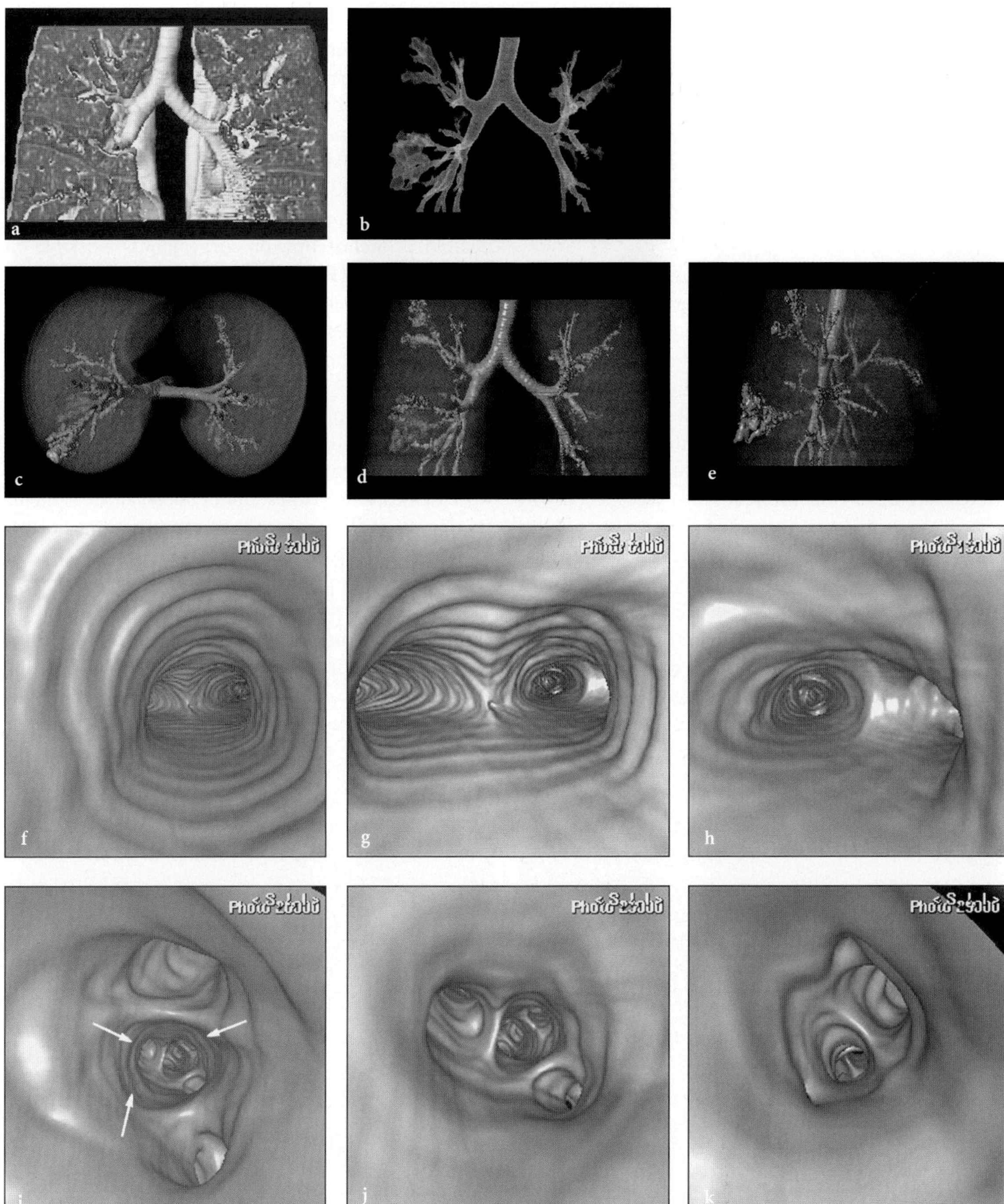

Fig. 4.21a–k. A 21-year-old patient with diffuse bronchiectasis. On true endoscopy, the extent of the disease was very difficult to appreciate because absolute diameters cannot be obtained with certainty due to the perspective distortion. Similarly, in virtual endoscopy (**f-k**) one could not give the diagnosis immediately. Particularly in image **i**, the *arrows* point at the ectatic bronchus, from which further branching into segmental bronchi follow. The ectatic bronchus is scarcely detectable. On the other hand, the other images (**a-e**) impressively show the extent of the bronchiectasis. For such cases, hybrid presentations from surface reconstructions of the tracheobronchial tree and TTP presentations of the lung tissue are very illustrative (**c-e**)

suring structures. For accurate measurements, distortion-free MPRs or mIPs are the methods of choice.

4.6 Application in Paediatrics

Applying ionising radiation in the paediatric population requires painstaking consideration. Thus, the indication for a CT examination must be clearly and individually defined. A modern low-dose spiral CT, e.g. with 10–25 mAs, corresponds to an average skin dose of 1–5 mGy (Rogalla et al. 1999). If CT is indicated, high-quality virtual endoscopies can be computed with an appropriate protocol. Likewise the indication for flexible bronchoscopy is, especially in very young children, restricted. Not only is it an invasive procedure, but also the inevitable sedation along with its risks need to be considered, special endoscopes must be used and also the examining physician should hold a high degree of experience.

In an initial study (Rogalla et al. 1997), 13 children with an average age of 5.3 years were examined with a low-dose spiral CT using 100 kV and 15–50 mAs. The slice thickness was 1.5 mm, and the pitch factor ranged from 1:1 to 1.3:1. The indications for virtual endoscopy included suspected aberrant bronchus, recurrent infiltrates, tracheal stenosis, middle lobe syndrome, etc. Using a viewing angle of 80–120°, a virtual endoscopy could be generated along a path in all patients. No sedation was necessary, and all children were breathing throughout the examination. Correlation with the findings from flexible bronchoscopy or surgery was possible in seven children (Fig. 4.22). The diagnostic information was, as expected, primarily present in the axial slices. Nonetheless, the virtual endoscopies were of surprisingly high quality, as noted by other authors (Konen et al. 1998; Lam et al. 2000); in particular, the documentation of findings is easier with the 3D than with axial slices.

With the introduction of EBT and multislice CT, which attains an 8 times higher speed at the same or even lower radiation exposure, examinations in children can be shortened. The result is not only increased acceptance by the children, but also decreased artefact susceptibility: fewer respiratory cycles occur during the examination period (Schoepf et al. 1998). Figure 4.23 shows a virtual endoscopy calculated from a multislice CT. As the entire examination period was 4 s, breathing artefacts are hardly present.

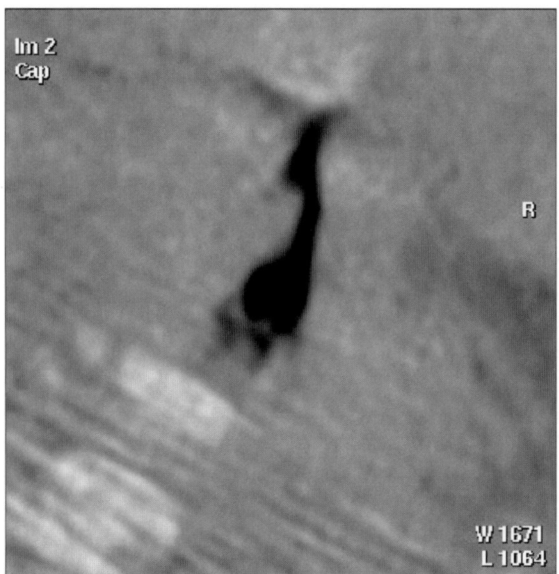

a

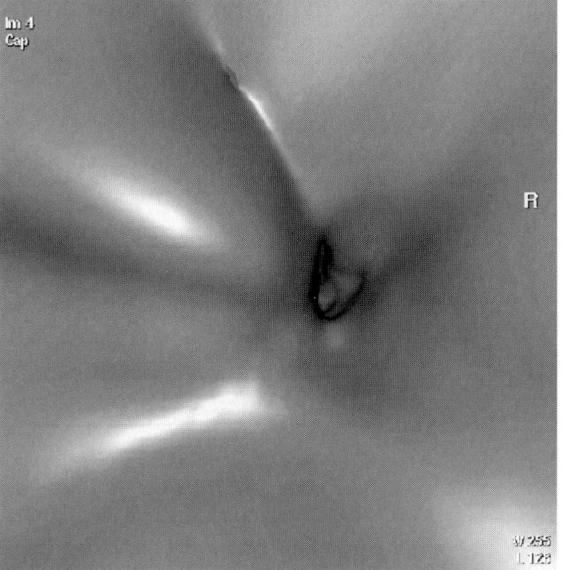

b

Fig. 4.22a,b. A 6-month-old child with clinically relevant stridor. The child had large cutaneous haemangiomas. A protrusion in the trachea in the low-dose CT (10 mAs; **a**), is easily recognised as a stenosis in the virtual bronchoscopy (**b**). The distal segment of the trachea and the bronchi were unremarkable. Since no intravenous contrast material was applied, characterisation of the lesion is not possible, but clinically haemangioma was considered probable. At a subsequent surgical intervention a haemangioma was confirmed and removed

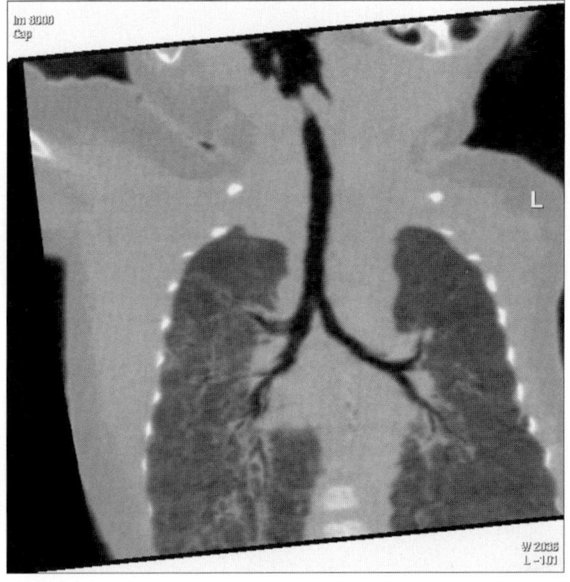

a

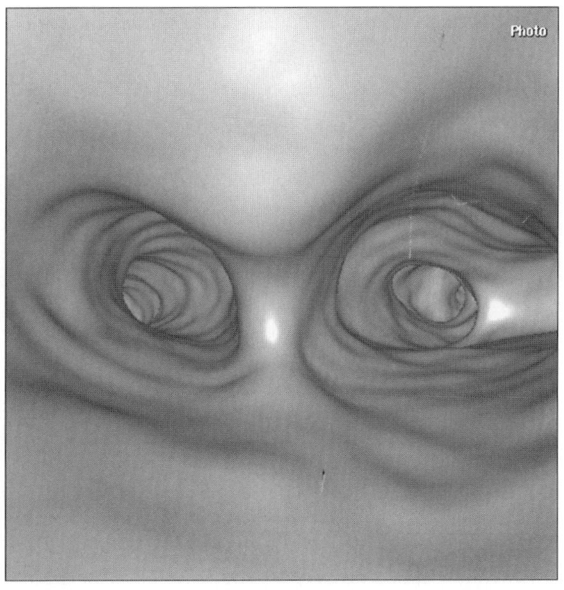

b

Fig. 4.23. Example of a multislice CT in a 6-week-old child. Owing to the rapid examination the axial slices and coronal reconstructions (3-mm average, **a**) are hardly influenced by breathing artefacts. Therefore, the virtual images are of excellent quality (**b**).

4.7 The Clinical Role

Defining the clinical role of virtual endoscopy is not so simple (Blezek and Robb 1997). The tracheobronchial tree is well suited for virtual presentation because the naturally high contrast independent of contrast agent is amenable to postprocessing. The following limitations are, however inherent to the method:

- Virtual bronchoscopy is a static examination technique; motion cannot be shown.
- Natural colour is absent. Changes such as surface infiltration or putrid secretion layers cannot be recognised as such (Fig. 4.24).
- The spatial resolution is limited. Depending on the CT technique used, it ranges between 1 and 5 mm, which is still approximately one order of magnitude less than the flexible bronchoscopy.
- Concurrent interventions are not possible; thus, the tumour diagnostic is made solely based upon the morphology.
- Radiation exposure is involved since the virtual image is based upon a CT examination.

On the other hand, there are various advantages, mostly founded in the underlying CT technique. The radiologist has access to the original slice images, which are especially indispensable for detecting extraluminal pathology. From this basis, the following benefits can be derived:

- Virtual bronchoscopy is non-invasive. Thus, it is indicated when flexible bronchoscopy cannot be performed.
- Stenoses, obstructions or endoscopically inaccessible areas are no obstacle for virtual endoscopy.
- Extraluminal information is always available (Fig. 4.25) and provides guidance for ensuing interventions.
- Through distortion-free presentation modes (MPR, mIP, etc.) exact measurements can be achieved, e.g. prior to stent implantation.

In order to be able to judge the clinical effectiveness, the advantages must be weighed against the disadvantages. No generalised statement can be offered because the individual methods and their disadvantages must be considered in light of the clinical situation. Without doubt, flexible bronchoscopy in the hands of an experienced pulmonologist will re-

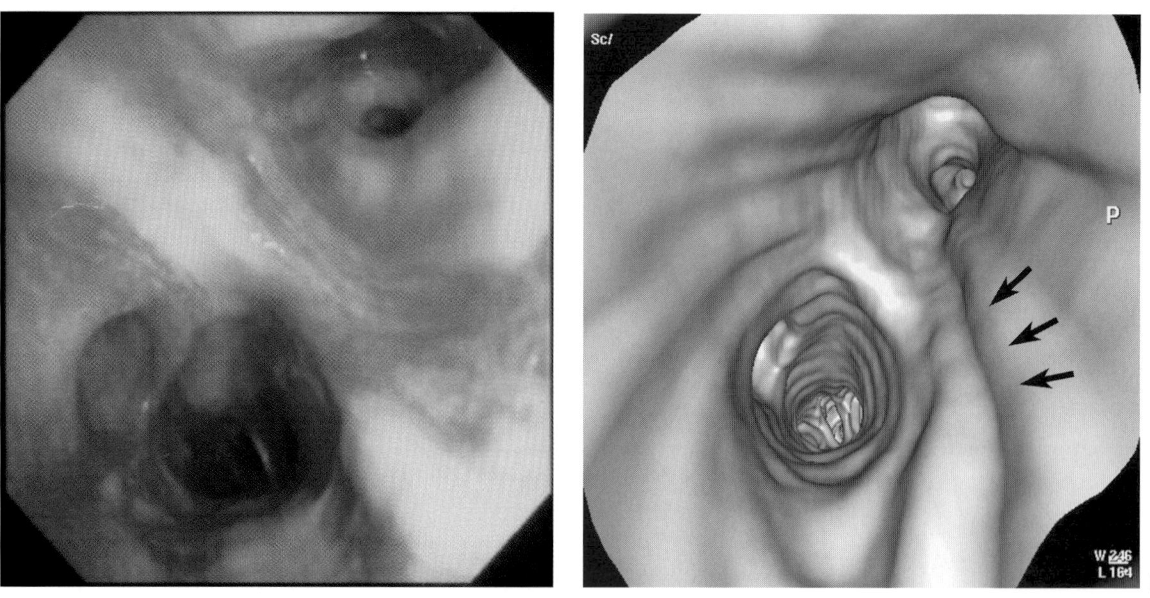

Fig. 4.24a,b. Example of a patient with tracheobronchitis. In the true endoscopy the putrid secretion layer on the carinae (*whitish colour*) is immediately detected. Since the surface of the virtual bronchoscopy is artificially reconstructed from tissues with various radiodensities, no true colour information is included, even if a colour may be programmed in the computer. Differentiation between pus and normal secretion is not possible on CT. Note also the stairway artefacts in the virtual endoscopy (*arrows*), caused by cardiac pulsations imprinted upon the tracheobronchial system. The artefacts always run parallel to the scanning plane (axial) and are therefore clearly differentiated from cartilage rings on the virtual endoscopy

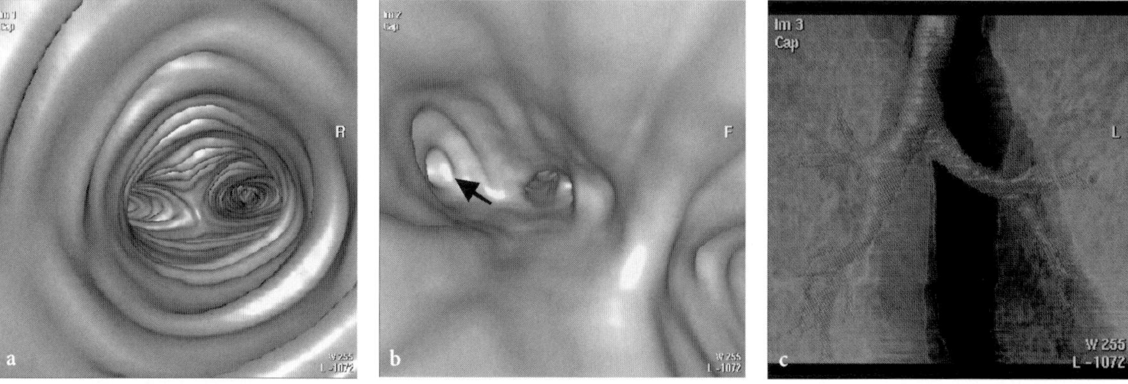

Fig. 4.25a–c. A 16-year-old female with serious left thoracic trauma after falling from a horse. In the initial bronchoscopy, the upper lobe bronchus could not be reached for inspection and further clarification of the post-traumatic anatomic relations was indicated, also in order to rule out congenital anomalies. **a,b** The low-dose CT (25 mAs) with virtual bronchoscopy demonstrates an occlusion of the upper lobe ostium (**b**, *arrow*). **c** In the combined presentation of the tracheobronchial tree and lung parenchyma (TTP), the occlusion with respect to its anatomical relations can be clearly located. Since no anomalies of the bronchi could be found (no accessory bronchi), the inflation of the parenchyma remained unclear. Obviously, in addition to the injury of the bronchus, a fistula formed in the upper lobe; however, this was not detectable on the thin-slice CT. Bronchiectases were not present on the axial CT

main the gold standard in the near future (Ahmad and Dweik 1999). However, along with the rapid advances in computing speed and the further expansion of multislice CT technology, virtual bronchoscopy will find its place in the daily routine and will continue to exist as one of many presentation forms to choose from for chest imaging. Once virtual images are available from standard CT examinations essentially without delay (Englmeier et al. 1999), eliminating extensive computing time or even the need for a second examination, clinical acceptance can be expected to increase dramatically. As a clinical teaching device (Buthiau et al. 1996; Krapichler et al. 1998), virtual endoscopy can greatly contribute to continuing education and to the qualification of operating personnel, which ultimately benefits the patient.

References

Ahmad M, Dweik RA (1999) Future of flexible bronchoscopy. Clin Chest Med 20:1–17

Arroliga AC, Matthay RA (1993) The role of bronchoscopy in lung cancer. Clin Chest Med 14:87–98

Blezek DJ, Robb RA (1997) Evaluating virtual endoscopy for clinical use. J Digit Imaging 10:51–55

Bricault I, Ferretti G, Cinquin P (1998) Registration of real and CT-derived virtual bronchoscopic images to assist transbronchial biopsy. IEEE Trans Med Imaging 17:703–714

Burke AJ, Vining DJ, McGuirt WF, Jr., Postma G, Browne JD (2000) Evaluation of airway obstruction using virtual endoscopy. Laryngoscope 110:23–29

Buthiau D, Antoine E, Piette JC, Nizri D, Baldeyrou P, Khayat D (1996) Virtual tracheo-bronchial endoscopy: educational and diagnostic value. Surg Radiol Anat 18:125–131

Dasgupta A, Mehta AC (1999) Transbronchial needle aspiration. An underused diagnostic technique. Clin Chest Med 20:39–51

Dorffel WV, Fietze I, Hentschel D, et al (1999) A new bronchoscopic method to measure airway size. Eur Respir J 14:783–788

Englmeier KH, Haubner M, Krapichler C, Reiser M (1999) A new hybrid renderer for virtual bronchoscopy. Stud Health Technol Inform 62:109–115

Ewert R, Dorffel W, Rogalla P, Mutze S (1997) Computed tomography-guided transtracheal needle aspiration of paratracheal lymphadenopathy in endoscopically normal patients. Invest Radiol 32:667–670

Ferguson MK (1990) Diagnosing and staging of non-small cell lung cancer. Hematol Oncol Clin North Am 4:1053–1068

Fleiter T, Merkle EM, Aschoff AJ, et al (1997) Comparison of real-time virtual and fiberoptic bronchoscopy in patients with bronchial carcinoma: opportunities and limitations. AJR Am J Roentgenol 169:1591–1595

Gaeta M, Barone M, Russi EG, et al (1993) Carcinomatous solitary pulmonary nodules: evaluation of the tumor-bronchi relationship with thin-section CT. Radiology 187:535–539

Guidelines for competency and training in fiberoptic bronchoscopy (1982) Section on Bronchoscopy, American College of Chest Physicians. Chest 81:739

Hopper KD (1999) CT bronchoscopy. Semin Ultrasound CT MR 20:10–15

Hopper KD, Iyriboz AT, Wise SW, Neuman JD, Mauger DT, Kasales CJ (2000) Mucosal detail at CT virtual reality: surface versus volume rendering. Radiology 214:517–522

Ikeda S (1974): Atlas of flexible bronchofiberscopy: Thieme, Stuttgart, Germany

Jover A, Garbarini A, Krempf M, Bonifassy R, Migueres J (1978) [Bronchial fibroscopy. Indications and results]. Poumon Coeur 34:283–290

Kim H (1998) Stenting therapy for stenosing airway disease. Respirology 3:221–228

Klingenbeck-Regn K, Schaller S, Flohr T, Ohnesorge B, Kopp AF, Baum U (1999) Subsecond multi-slice computed tomography: basics and applications. Eur J Radiol 31:110–124

Konen E, Katz M, Rozenman J, Ben-Shlush A, Itzchak Y, Szeinberg A (1998) Virtual bronchoscopy in children: early clinical experience. AJR Am J Roentgenol 171:1699–1702

Krapichler C, Haubner M, Engelbrecht R, Englmeier KH (1998) VR interaction techniques for medical imaging applications. Comput Methods Programs Biomed 56:65–74

Lacrosse M, Trigaux JP, Van Beers BE, Weynants P (1995) 3D spiral CT of the tracheobronchial tree. J Comput Assist Tomogr 19:341–347

Lam S, Shibuya H (1999) Early diagnosis of lung cancer. Clin Chest Med 20:53–61

Lam WW, Tam PK, Chan FL, Chan KL, Cheng W (2000) Esophageal atresia and tracheal stenosis: use of three-dimensional CT and virtual bronchoscopy in neonates, infants, and children. AJR Am J Roentgenol 174:1009–1012

Liebler JM, Markin CJ (2000) Fiberoptic bronchoscopy for diagnosis and treatment. Crit Care Clin 16:83–100

Mitchell DM, Emerson CJ, Collyer J, Collins JV (1980) Fibreoptic bronchoscopy: ten years on. Br Med J 281:360–363

Mori I (1986) Computerized tomographic apparatus utilizing a radiation source. U.S. Patent No. 4,630,202

Naidich DP, Gruden JF, McGuinness G, McCauley DI, Bhalla M (1997) Volumetric (helical/spiral) CT (VCT) of the airways. J Thorac Imaging 12:11–28

Neumann K, Winterer J, Kimmig M, et al (2000) Real-time interactive virtual endoscopy of the tracheo-bronchial system: influence of CT imaging protocols and observer ability. Eur J Radiol 33:50–54

Remy J, Remy Jardin M, Artaud D, Fribourg M (1998) Multiplanar and three-dimensional reconstruction techniques in CT: impact on chest diseases. Eur Radiol 8:335–351

Rodenwaldt J, Kopka L, Roedel R, Margas A, Grabbe E (1997) 3D virtual endoscopy of the upper airway: optimization of the scan parameters in a cadaver phantom and clinical assessment. J Comput Assist Tomogr 21:405–411

Rogalla P, Enzweiler C, Schmidt E, Taupitz M, Bender A, Hamm B (1998) [Thoracic diagnostics with electron beam tomography]. Radiologe 38:1029–1035

Rogalla P, Scheer I, Stöver B, Hamm B (1997) Virtual endoscopy of the tracheo-bronchial tree in children. Radiology 205(P):297

Rogalla P, Stöver B, Scheer I, Juran R, Gaedicke G, Hamm B (1999) Low-dose spiral CT: applicability to paediatric chest imaging. Pediatr Radiol 29:565–569

Sackner MA (1975) Bronchofiberscopy. Am Rev Respir Dis 111:62–88

Schoepf UJ, Seemann M, Schuhmann D, et al (1998) [Virtual and three-dimensional bronchoscopy with spiral and electron beam computed tomography]. Radiologe 38:816–823

Standards for training in endoscopy (1976) Statement of the Committee on Bronchoesophagology, American College of Chest Physicians. Chest 69:665–666

Summers RM (1997) Navigational aids for real-time virtual bronchoscopy. AJR Am J Roentgenol 168:1165–1170

Wang G, Vannier MW (1999) The effect of pitch in multislice spiral/helical CT. Med Phys 26:2648–2653

5 Virtual Endoscopy of the Small Intestine

P. Rogalla

CONTENTS

5.1 Introduction

Despite the development of a so-called intestinoscope, with a calibre as thin as a fibreoptic or electric endoscope (endoscope with a CCD camera at the tip), the small intestine has remained generally inaccessible to complete endoscopic evaluation (Van Dam and Brugge 1999). For a long time, at least since the introduction of the fractionated passage by Pansdorf (1937), radiological diagnostic procedures of the small intestine have played a central role in patient care. Due to the length and position of the small bowel, comprehensive intestinal imaging has posed a difficult challenge. Further complicating this task are the considerable variation in intestinal transit time from person to person, the unforeseeable enteral distribution patterns of contrast medium, and the superimposition of contrast-filled bowel loops upon more posterior segments. Partly due to the difficulties associated with examining the small intestine and partly because the entities that involve the small intestine, with the exception of Crohn's disease, are very rare, few radiologists have ventured into diagnostics of the small bowel.

The fractionated passage according to Pansdorf (1937) is a method still used today to display the small intestine in its entirety. The examination technique makes it possible to exclude larger pathological conditions; however, a definitive diagnostic statement about the organ is seldom feasible. During the initial days of radiological diagnosis, many researchers invested much energy into improving small intestine imaging using concepts that were, for the most part, based on various techniques (Pribram and Kleiber 1927). In practically all of these trials, the authors recognised that a continuous presentation of the organ was much more successful following duodenal intubation than after fractionated oral contrast medium administration. Even the initial reports on single and double contrast imaging of the small bowel confirmed that improved diagnostic accuracy was only possible after duodenal intubation (Gershon-Cohen and Shay 1939). Likewise, subsequent reports recommended an infusion of a larger amount of diluted contrast medium. However, at that time (1943), the lack of adequate materials and difficulties with duodenal intubation were the primary problems preventing a successful enteroclysma (Schatzki 1988). One of the first large series was published in 1951 and reported on the experience following 300 successful examinations of the small intestine (Lura 1951).

Sellink helped initiate a worldwide breakthrough with his work on the enteroclysma procedure (Sell-

P. Rogalla, MD
Department of Radiology, Charité Hospital, Humboldt-Universität zu Berlin, Schumannstrasse 20/21, 10117 Berlin, Germany

INK 1974, 1976). Whether this technique, which is less pleasant for the patient and technically more difficult for the physician than fractionated contrast medium administration, is actually diagnostically necessary has never been resolved (MAGLINTE et al. 1982; NOLAN et al. 1985; OTT et al. 1985 a,b). However, multiple studies have revealed that enteroclysma subsequent to duodenal intubation provides better diagnostic information than other techniques (EKBERG 1977; FLECKENSTEIN and PEDERSEN 1975). To create a double contrast, Sellink had initially recommended air or water for negative contrast. GMÜNDER and WIRTH (1970) followed by the use of methylcellulose as a negative contrast agent. More than 20 years of experience have now been accumulated worldwide with this technique, that is, first infusion of approximately 300 ml barium suspension followed immediately by infusion of methylcellulose. Despite many, sometimes local, modifications to this procedure, enteroclysma has become a firmly established standard procedure in radiological diagnostic imaging.

5.1.1 Why Introduce a New Examination Technique for the Small Intestine?

Despite the various diagnostic revelations, enteroclysma has some limitations. Enteroclysma allows limited information or no information at all regarding the extraintestinal anatomy or pathology. Although especially the motility of the organ can be analysed due to the dynamic character of this examination technique (which can be very useful for differential diagnoses), the surrounding pathology remains only indirectly interpretable, for example through compression or displacement of bowel loops. The investigation of extraluminal conditions is a domain of cross-sectional imaging techniques, including ultrasound, computed tomography and magnetic resonance imaging.

5.2 Cross-sectional Examination Modalities

5.2.1 Sonography

Ultrasound is customarily used as the first examination modality. It is very widespread and easily available, does not involve ionising radiation and is relatively affordable (MACCIONI et al. 1997; POZNIAK et al. 1990). The principal disadvantage in ultrasonography is the barrier created by meteorism of the abdomen. Air-filled loops prevent evaluation of regions behind them; as a result, continuous and comprehensive evaluation is rarely achieved. Nonetheless, ultrasonography has proved a worthwhile diagnostic imaging tool for evaluation of chronic inflammatory bowel diseases.

5.2.2 Computed Tomography

The value of CT for the assessment of the entire abdomen including the small intestine has been recognised for quite some time (DUVOISIN and SCHNYDER 1990; JAMES et al. 1987). This applies to chronic inflammatory conditions (HORTON et al. 1999), as well as to acute situations (GAYER et al. 1999; MAKITA et al. 1999). The reason for the preferred implementation of CT lies not only in the ability to examine patients independent of their clinical condition, but also in the rapidity achieved with spiral or multislice CT, the implementation in other regions beyond the abdomen if pathology is suspected, and also the widespread availability (THOENI and ROGALLA 1994). The depiction of anatomical detail on CT is excellent; the susceptibility to motion artefacts, when using spiral or multislice CT, is minimal. In the light of these strengths, CT has also become established in paediatric care (SIEGEL et al. 1988).

Alterations in the intestinal wall thickness, one of the key findings in the evaluation of the small bowel, can be assessed with great accuracy by CT (LOW 1998) and can play a fundamental role in the differential diagnosis. CT is ordinarily conducted during the administration of i.v. contrast medium or shortly thereafter, leading to strong enhancement of vital tissue, including the well-vascularised intestinal mucosa. It is common to mark the gastrointestinal tract with oral contrast medium before initiating the CT examination (ROGALLA et al. 1996; SILVERMAN 1994). Unfortunately complete enhancement of the small intestine is rarely achieved, and various attempts have been made to improve the contrast quality with medications (THOENI and FILSON 1988). However, the discontinuous enhancement of the small intestine has remained a problem because segments of collapsed bowel loops persist and prevent the aetiological differentiation of the thickened mucosa. The radiation exposure that goes hand-in-hand with CT represents the most important disadvantage of this technique in relation to other cross-sectional imaging modalities.

5.2.3 Magnetic Resonance Imaging

Magnetic resonance imaging has enjoyed increasing recognition in recent years. Its most significant advantage over CT is the absence of ionising radiation. Additionally, MRI currently surpasses all other techniques in soft tissue differentiation (DEBATIN and PATAK 1999). Increasing attention has been recently paid to MRI due to its diagnostic potential in evaluating the small intestine (HA et al. 1998). Previous limitations such as poor spatial resolution and artefacts caused by peristalsis and breathing motions have been resolved through rapid breathhold sequences, which allow excellent evaluation of the abdominal cavity (LEE et al. 1998). Not only for the detection of neoplastic processes (SEMELKA et al. 1996), but especially in diagnosing and evaluating inflammatory bowel diseases (MADSEN et al. 1997, 1999), MRI has gained a stable footing among the cross-sectional techniques (THOENI and ROGALLA 1994). The manner and method by which the small intestine should be contrasted is still undefined. MRI contrast agents for T1- and T2-weighted imaging are being implemented and compared for their diagnostic utility in various clinical conditions (GRUBNIC et al. 1999).

However, MRI is encumbered by the same problem as CT: complete contrast of the small intestine is difficult to attain. In other words, collapsed bowel segments often hinder adequate clinical evaluation.

5.3 Contrast Options

Despite the theoretical plausibility, it is practically impossible to implement ultrasound for virtual endoscopy due to the absence of a definitive slice orientation. Furthermore, it would also be necessary to obtain complete water filling of bowel loops for continuous evaluation of the entire small intestine, precisely the same problem encountered for oral contrast administration in CT and MRI (ROGALLA et al. 1998).

The intestinal distension achieved with sufficient contrast material administration induces a hypoperistalsis that has proven useful in both CT and MRI. Alternatively, an attempt can be made to fill the small intestine with air or carbon dioxide through the duodenal tube following intravenous spasmolysis. Although this perspective does not seem logical, since the viscosity of methylcellulose plays a central role in distending the bowel wall, optimal preparation of the patient with air produces surprisingly extensive distension of the bowel (Fig. 5.1).

5.4 Patient Preparation

To obtain an optimal small bowel examination, even in standard cross-sectional imaging, the gastrointestinal tract should be emptied (SELLINK and ROSENBUSCH 1981). When examining patients with chronic obstipation, ample preparation is especially important. Furthermore, a full caecum impedes the passage of contrast medium to the distal ileum and can result in failure to enhance this region. Generally, the same preparation procedures apply as for conventional radiological examination of the small intestine (BINSWANGER and SELLINK 1980; MOREWOOD and WHITEHOUSE 1986).

First, the duodenal intubation is carried out under conventional fluoroscopic control with the goal of placing the tip of the applicator behind the ligament of Treitz (Fig. 5.2). The mixture, containing 180 ml of oral contrast material for CT and 1820 ml of methylcellulose, is administered through the positioned tube. The mixture may be injected with a flow rate of 140 ml/min; if the patient has clinical complaints, the rate can be reduced to a minimum of 50 ml/min. Administration of 1500–1600 ml usually fills the entire small intestine.

If an MRI examination is anticipated instead of CT, the oral iodine-containing contrast media can be replaced with oral MRI contrast media (e.g. Magnevist enteral, Schering, Germany). In the event that a combined CT and MRI examination is planned, oral MRI contrast agent can be mixed with the oral CT solution.

5.5 Examination Procedures

5.5.1 Computed Tomography

The injection of the oral contrast combination should generally begin immediately the patient has

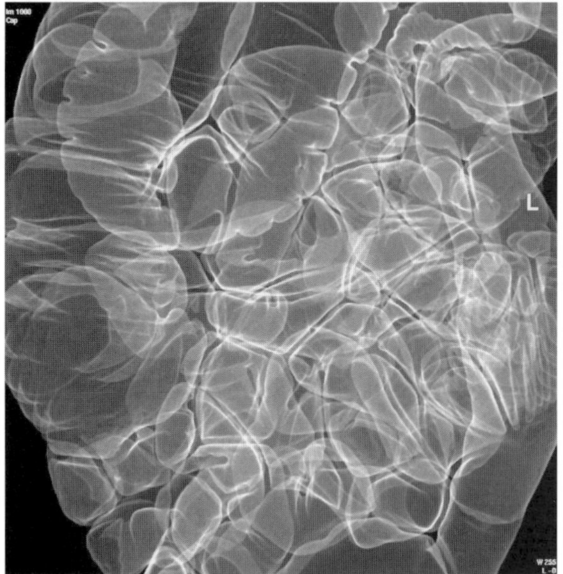

a

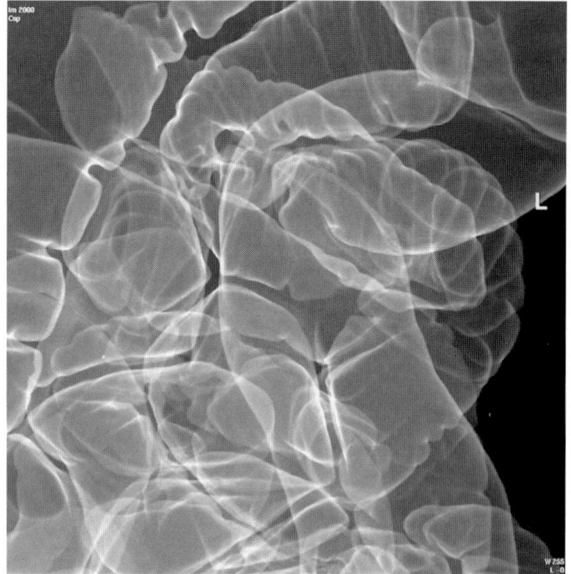

b

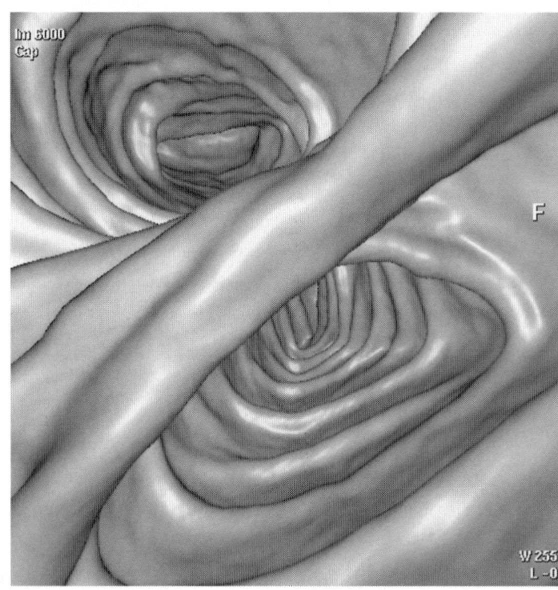

c

Fig. 5.1a–c. Images obtained after small bowel insufflation of CO_2 gas following duodenal intubation. **a** A TTP reconstruction of the small intestine (see text for detailed explanation of this technique). Only those interfaces that contain a density gradient of air against soft tissue are displayed. **b** An enlargement of **a**. Note the enormous detail resolution that is achieved, permitting observation of the individual intestinal folds. **c** Virtual endoscopy of a normal section of the jejunum. Morphological details of the jejunum are also well depicted in virtual endoscopy. Imaging parameters: multislice CT with 1 mm primary slice thickness, 0.6 mm reconstruction interval. Reconstruction matrix of TTP 1024×1024, of the virtual endoscopy 512×512

been positioned on the CT table. In accordance with the standard hospital protocol, the addition of a spasmolytic agent (e.g. Buscopan or glucagon) can be administered intramuscularly in order to reduce peristalsis and the resultant artefacts. It should be kept in mind, however, that the speed of a peristaltic wave is much lower than that of spiral CT; thus, even without spasmolysis movement artefacts are not necessarily present.

Between 1500 and 1800 ml are sufficient to fill the small bowel. Depending on the technical specifications of the available CT unit, single low-dose slices (e.g. 10-mm scans with 10 mAs) can serve to monitor the intestinal distension in the terminal ileum during contrast agent administration. Finally, continuous spiral CT of the abdomen should be performed. In this case, choice of the smallest possible slice thickness in combination with a pitch factor not larger than 2:1 (for spiral CT) permits examination of the entire abdomen during a single breathhold. In the latest generation of spiral CT devices, a slice thickness between 2.5 and 4 mm can be programmed together with a pitch factor of 1.5–2:1, resulting in a complete abdominal examination after 50–60 rotations. Most patients are capable of holding their breath for about 30 s after supervised, preparatory hyperventilation exercises. Shallow ex- and inspiration at the end of the spiral CT examination is of

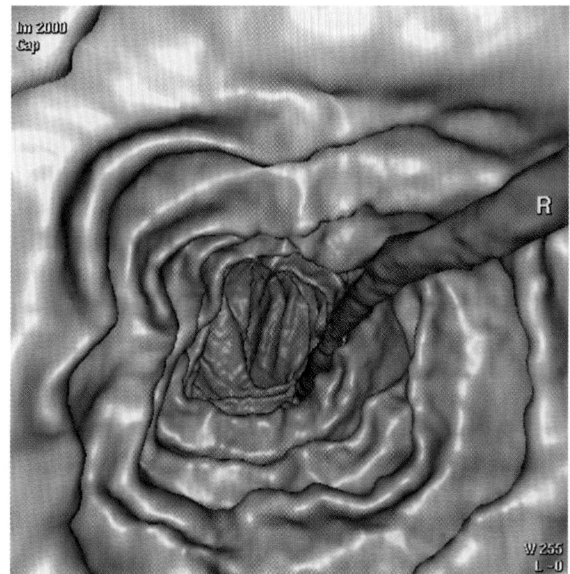

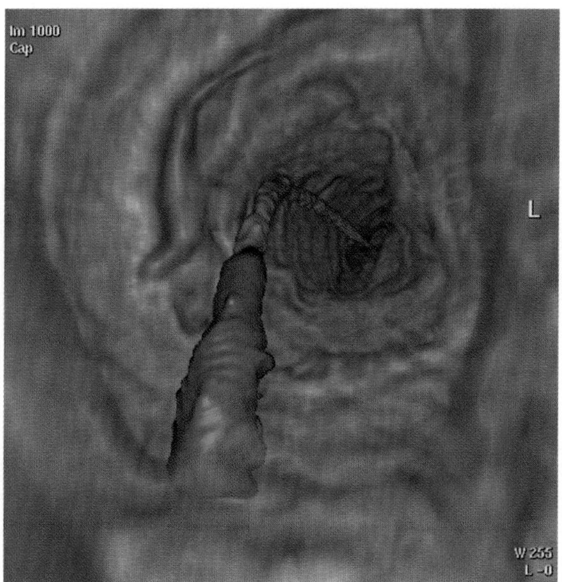

a b

Fig. 5.2a,b. Virtual endoscopic view into the jejunum. **a** A view along the tube. The metal olive is coded with another colour in order to allow improved demonstration. Display of the bowel wall as well as the tube is achieved with volume rendering technique, but with nontransparent presentation of the surface. **b** A view towards the tube. The tip of the tube (olive) was directly behind an intestinal fold. By using a transparent presentation of the intestinal wall (possible at any time in volume rendering), the olive tip can also be seen through the intestinal fold

no further consequence for image quality since the region being imaged at this point is at an ample distance from the diaphragm and hardly affected by breathing motions. This presupposes an examination direction from cranial to caudal. With the innovation of multislice CT, a speed 8 times that of spiral CT can be attained, supporting the use of a lower slice thickness. The currently available multislice CT procedures allow slice thicknesses of as little as 0.5 mm and are still rapid enough to examine the entire abdomen in one breathhold. An important consideration is that as long as the radiation exposure is not simultaneously increased, a thinner slice coincides with increased noise, and in this respect, sets the lower limit for slice thickness.

Analogous to all three-dimensional reconstructions from spiral data, the reconstruction interval should represent at least one third of the effective slice thickness. Thinner reconstruction intervals increase the number of reconstructed images, but do not improve three-dimensional image quality. An initial study on the optimal choice of slice parameters showed, as might be expected, that the smallest lesion detectable on virtual endoscopy of the small intestine must be slightly larger than the primary slice thickness of the CT (Rogalla et al. 1998). With a slice thickness of 1.5 mm and an overlapping slice reconstruction of about 50% (every 0.5–1 mm), round lesions with a diameter of 2–3 mm can still be recognised (Fig. 5.3). Although a small bowel model was used to maximise similarity to the natural situation, a limitation of the phantom study was that the plastic tube was surrounded by air and not by the physiological resorbing environment of the human body, so that the CT reconstructions were minimally influenced by image noise. In a sense, the model represents an ideal situation that is hardly achievable in a patient. Furthermore, the contrast between air and "soft tissue" was very strong; with lower contrast, the image noise plays a greater role (see also Sect. 5.5.2). In other words, the study represents a spatial resolution investigation that also demonstrates the maximal potential resolution of virtual endoscopy.

The diagnostic value of intravenous contrast agent administration for CT is well established and generally accepted, especially in diagnosis of the abdomen and pelvis. Since the CT images that are used to establish a virtual endoscopy of the small intestine can (and should) also be viewed as "normal" images, the use of i.v. contrast material is well justified. It must, however, be emphasised that for the calculation of virtual endoscopy, bowel wall enhancement is not only necessary, but also leads to a slight reduction of the contrast between the intestinal lumen and

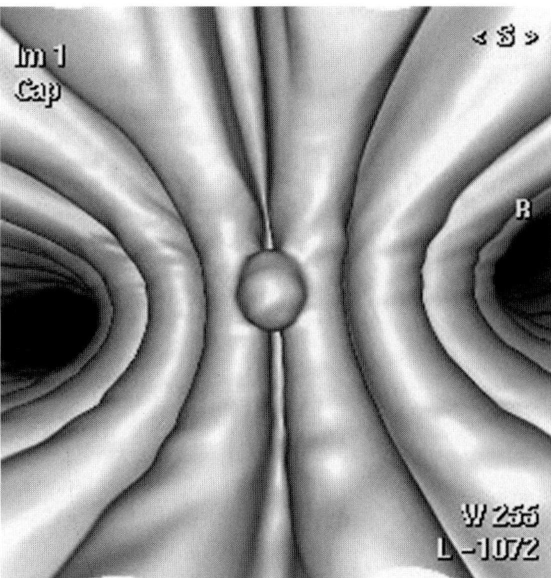

Fig. 5.3. Figure of a bowel phantom with an artificial 2-mm polypous lesion. The primary slice thickness was 1.5 mm, the reconstruction interval 1 mm. The round form of the lesion is still distinguishable. However, the phantom represents ideal intestinal conditions in which the walls are perfectly smooth and no confusion results from stool remnants or artefacts

the mucosa. Sufficiently high radiodensity of the intestinal contrast mixture (as previously described) can counterbalance this effect.

5.5.2 Multislice CT

The multislice CT technique that has been available since 1999 requires the same patient preparation for intestinal contrast as is necessary for spiral CT; the prerequisites for complete distension of all bowel loops and avoidance of spastic contractions are also similar.

The currently available devices for multislice CT, also known as multidetector CT or multirow CT, are generally 8 times quicker than a spiral CT with a revolution time of 1 s. The gantry rotates twice per second, and four slices are simultaneously obtained during one 360° rotation. It is possible to take advantage of the increased speed of multislice CT in two ways: by maintaining the same slice thickness, the examination is completed in one eighth of the time, or the slice thickness can be reduced to one eighth and the examination duration remains the same. A combination of both can naturally also be programmed. Slice thicknesses of 1–2.5 mm are implementable for abdomen and pelvic examinations and correspond to a breathhold of approximately 30 s or less.

A fundamental physical problem is encountered when choosing very low slice thicknesses: because very few photons can be received per detector, the image noise with, for example, slices 1 mm wide is very strong and can hinder image interpretation. A further problem is created by the large number of images produced. Up to 700–800 images per patient examination are easily reached (approx. 400–500 MB) and this is very demanding on the storage capacity, network and viewing stations. Currently, there are only few workstations that can handle such a huge amount of image data at once. A minimal prerequisite is a storage capacity of more than 500 MB RAM; in order to guarantee an acceptable processing speed even 1000 MB (1 GB) RAM is required.

Multislice CT exerts an important impact on virtual endoscopy: thin slices correspond to higher resolution in the longitudinal axis of the patient (*z*-axis). With an examination protocol of 1-mm contiguous slices and a reconstruction interval of 0.5 mm, the resulting image voxels ("voxel" is the standard abbreviation for volume element) have an isotropic geometry. As a result, secondary reconstructions in any arbitrary plane have practically the same spatial resolution as the originally acquired axial scans (Fig. 5.4). As discussed in Chap. 1 (Technical Background) and Chap. 6 (Virtual Endoscopy of the Colon), image noise can become a significant problem if the density difference between the two tissue types that are to be differentiated is too small. The gain in spatial resolution through the choice of a very thin slice thickness is offset by the correspondingly increasing image noise (Fig. 5.5). To date, experience with multislice CT is not extensive enough to permit a general recommendation for the choice of slice thickness. However, it is probable that also for standard examinations of the abdomen and pelvis, a slice thickness of 1 mm will prevail.

5.5.3 Magnetic Resonance Imaging

The MRI examination can be conducted alone (Aschoff et al. 1997; Rieber et al. 1998) or immediately following a CT examination. The application rate for the contrast agent is chosen in the same manner as for CT, and the bowel filling can be simi-

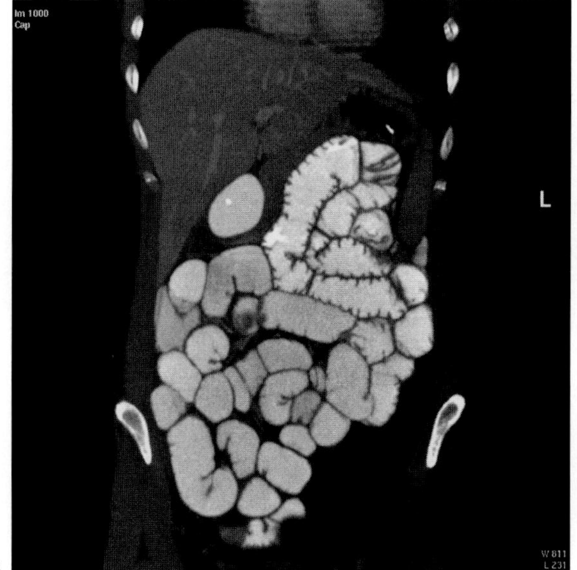

a

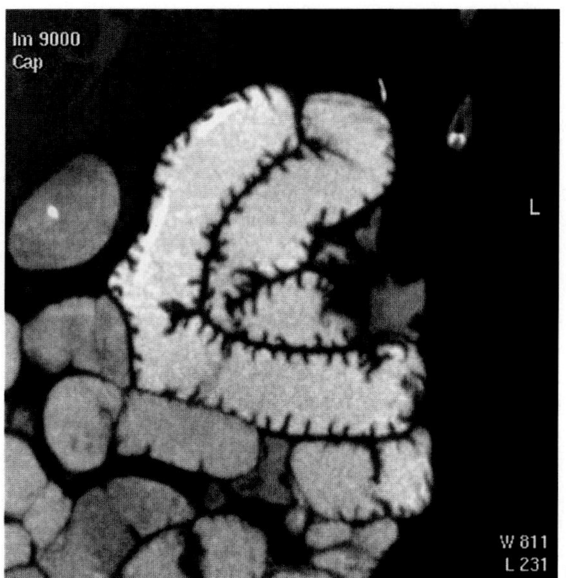

b

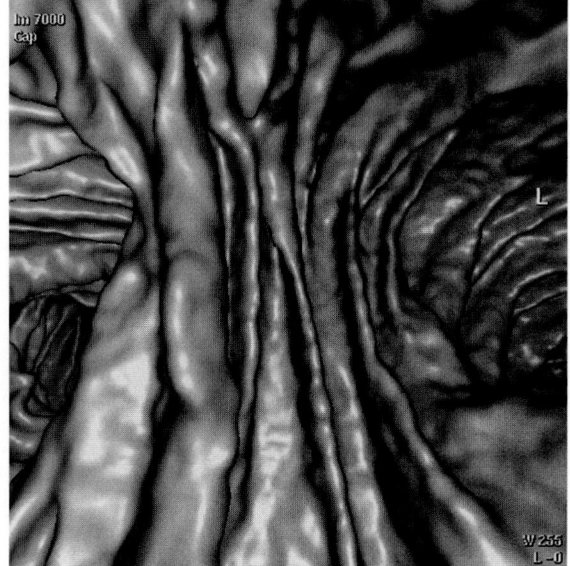

c

Fig. 5.4a–c. Secondary reformations in the coronal plane of a multislice CT. The primary slice thickness was 1 mm with a reconstruction interval of 0.5 mm. The resulting voxels are isotropic, explaining why the reformations have a spatial resolution practically identical to that of the original axially acquired scans. Note the clear demonstration of the jejunal folds (**a**), also seen in detail in the enlargement (**b**). The view is directed towards a "flexure", allowing sight of the approaching and departing loops in one image. Note the enormous detail resolution of the fold surface

larly monitored with single-shot images or with real-time imaging sequences. Once the entire small bowel until the terminal ileum is adequately distended, images are obtained, depending on contrast agent, using T1-weighted (e.g. FLASH) or T2-weighted (e.g. HASTE) sequences. Suppression of peristalsis is generally more relevant in MRI than CT, implying that use of an intramuscularly applied spasmolytic agent is advisable in most cases.

In MRI, just as in CT, the slice thickness should be set as low as possible. Coronary slices are advantageous for postprocessing, considering that in axial orientation two partitions are generally necessary in order to image the entire abdomen. Most of the postprocessing programs for three-dimensional reconstructions have difficulty interpreting two partitions as one data block, even if a gapless transition is obtained between the consecutive slice positions.

Finally, in MRI, as in CT, the decision of whether to additionally administer an i.v. contrast agent (Faber et al. 1997) should depend upon whether it is indicated and whether the costs are offset by the expected diagnostic gain. Experience has revealed that an i.v. injection of gadolinium-DTPA often does not improve the diagnostic strength of a small bowel image; however, no comparative studies exist.

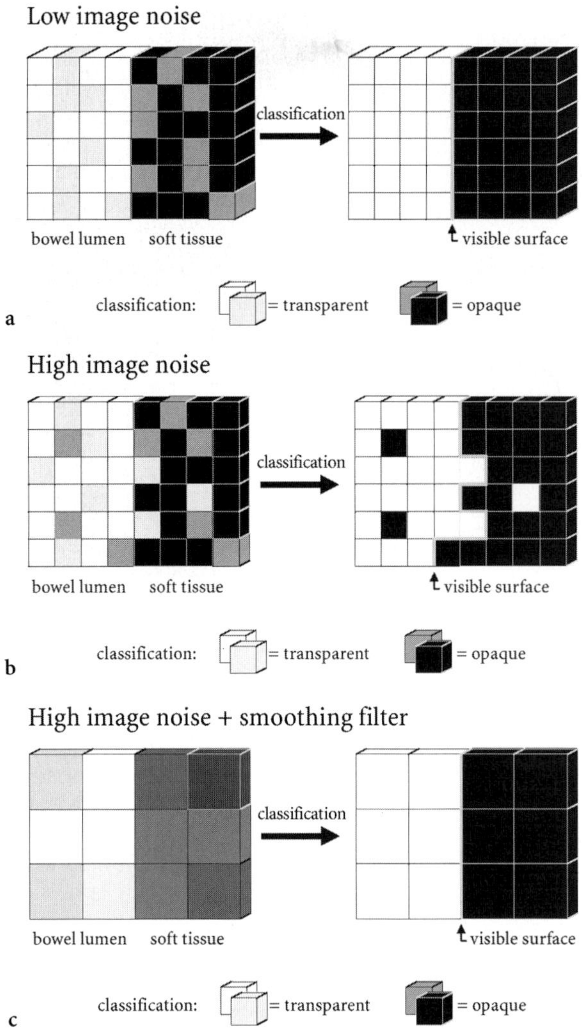

Low image noise

classification

bowel lumen soft tissue

visible surface

classification: = transparent = opaque

a

High image noise

classification

bowel lumen soft tissue

visible surface

classification: = transparent = opaque

b

High image noise + smoothing filter

classification

bowel lumen soft tissue

visible surface

classification: = transparent = opaque

c

Fig. 5.5a–c. Basic sketch describing the influence of image noise on a virtual surface reconstruction: **a** A grey value distribution of single voxels in a thick slice with limited image noise. The classification for the volume rendering technique was chosen in such a manner that all white and light-grey image points (representing the tissue type of contrast-filled intestinal lumen) are perceived as transparent and all other image points appear opaque in the reconstructed image. The image noise (some pixels deviate from the average brightness) has no influence on the reconstructed picture; the virtual wall viewable in the endoscopy has a smooth appearance. **b** A grey value distribution of the voxels by thinner slices with greater image noise. Now there are pixels in the tissue that would be classified as bowel lumen which have the grey value of soft tissue and are thus visible as flying objects in the reconstruction. Furthermore, pixels that are classified as another tissue type due to the image noise and that lie directly on the virtual surface lead to a depiction of holes or lumps on the visible virtual surface. These examples demonstrate that although the choice of a thinner primary slice thickness increases the spatial resolution, the virtual reconstruction is not necessarily improved. Two solutions are available for CT: the amperage (mAs) can be increased, in which case the image noise is reduced but the radiation exposure increases proportionally; alternatively, either a softer convolution filter (reconstruction kernel) can be chosen (selection during primary image reconstruction on the CT console) or an image filter, which reduces the image noise at the cost of spatial resolution (smoothing filter; **c**). However, as a consequence, the positive effect of a thinner slice (high *z*-axis resolution) is partly negated (low *x*/*y*-axis resolution). Thus, an unlimited reduction of slice thickness is confined by physical boundaries

5.6 Postprocessing and Visualization Techniques

5.6.1 Three-dimensional Reconstruction

The small bowel is a very complex, convoluted organ. Although a classical three-dimensional reconstruction is technically feasible, multiple superimposition of anterior bowel loops on posterior segments essentially hinders visualization, such that only the parts "facing" the viewer are well discernible. The more posterior segments are hardly assessable. Consequently, unless a significant alteration in the intestinal distribution is demonstrated, diagnostic value is often minimal.

5.6.2 Tissue Transition Projection

The reconstruction principles and the technical background of tissue transition projection (TTP) are comprehensively covered in Chap. 1. This technique produces a transparent demonstration of the imaged area (Fig. 5.6). A prerequisite for this display method is the existence of density differences, so-called gradients, between the neighbouring surfaces to be imaged, distinguishing opaque from transparent qualities. The resulting image is a display of the mucosal surface that strongly resembles the demonstration in conventional enteroclysma (Fig. 5.7). The TTP technique offers the viewer an opportunity to observe three-dimensional objects from all sides. Brightness and contrast can be adjusted to create optimal diag-

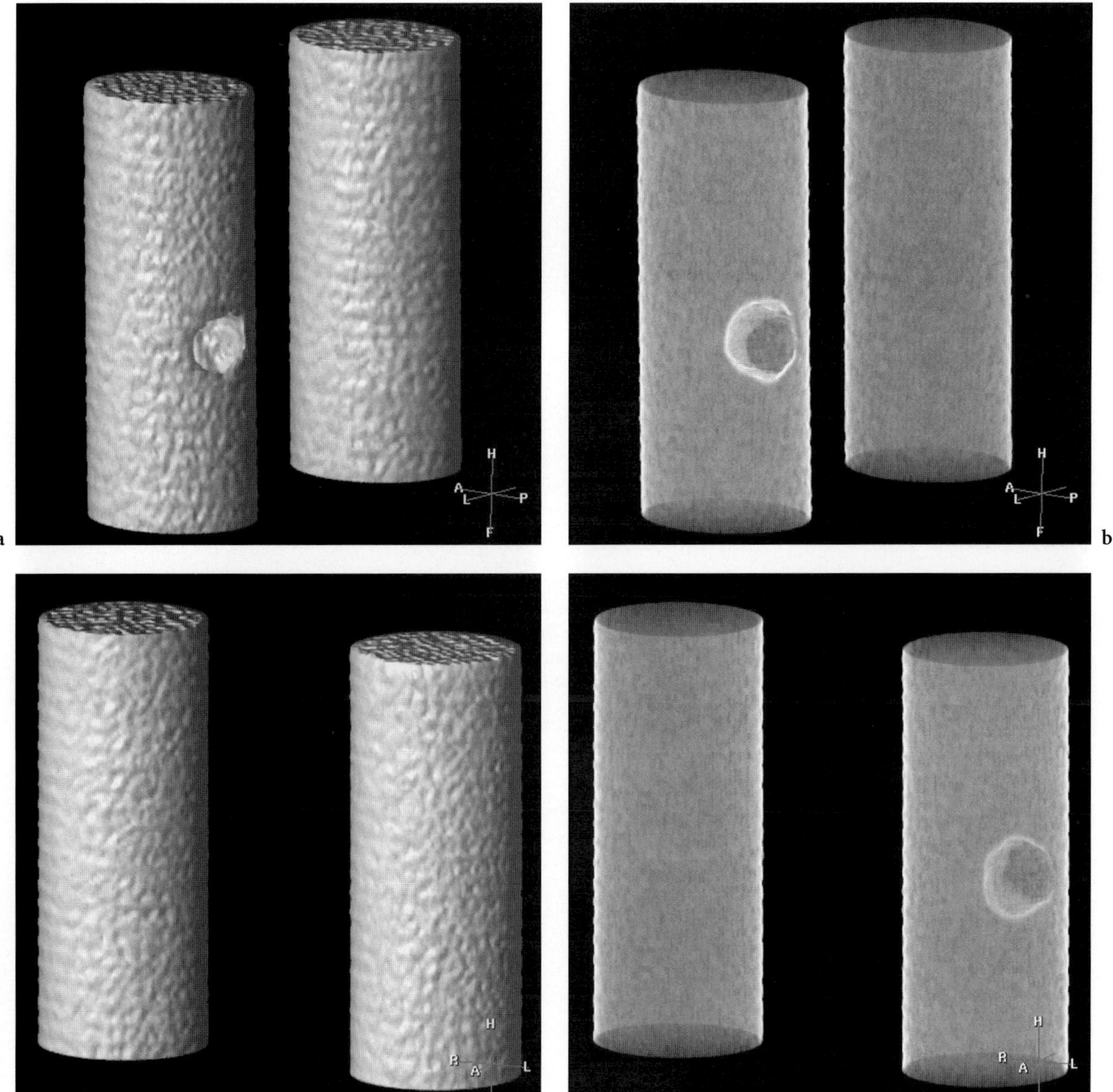

Fig. 5.6a–d. Principal image characteristics of tissue transition projections (TTP): A phantom consisting of two empty air-filled pipes was examined. A small polyp was inserted into one pipe. **a** A surface reconstruction (surface shaded display), in which the polyp is visible as an indentation due to its contact with the wall. **b** The TTP reconstruction also shows the polyp. **c** The three-dimensional object has been rotated so that the polyp is on the farthest surface from the observer. In other words, the polyp is covered by the pipe wall and no longer visible. **d** In the TTP reconstruction, however, the polyp and its morphology remain visible due to the transparent projection of the pipe wall. Due to the similarity between TTP images and conventional double-contrast studies under X-ray fluoroscopy, TTP images have also been referred to as virtual double-contrast reconstructions

nostic image quality. By adding a depth-encoding function, all portions of the intestine that are farther away from the viewer appear somewhat darker, enhancing the spatial resolution or three-dimensional impression. Additionally, a perspective distortion can be incorporated. For example, an image calculated with a 30° distortion resembles the distortion of a conventional X-ray. The extent to which the TTP technique is capable of displaying relevant clinical details must still be investigated.

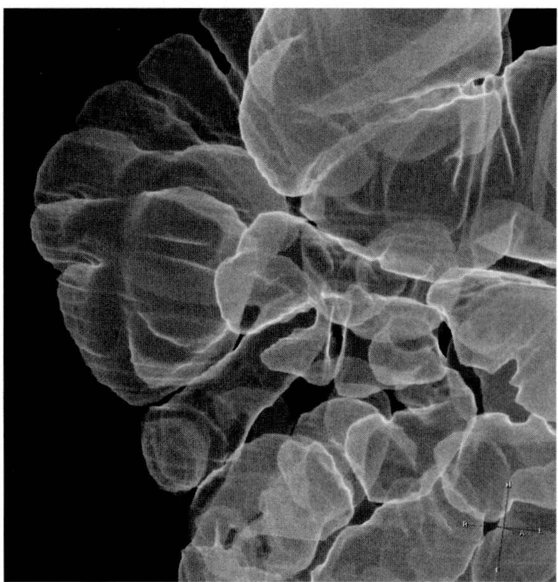

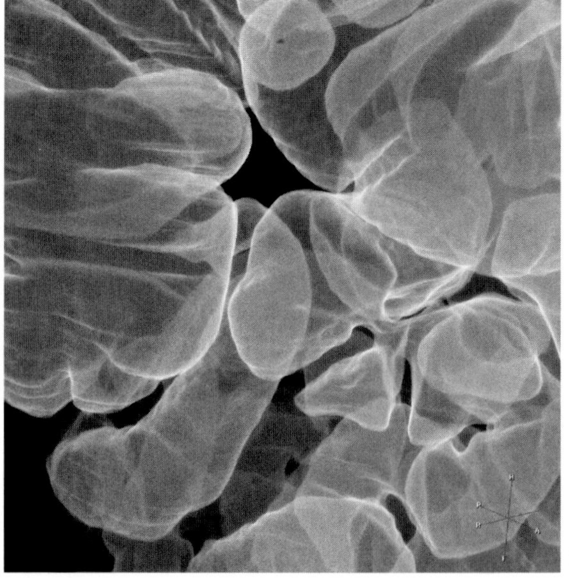

Fig. 5.7a,b. TTP of a patient who underwent a CT enteroclysma in order to rule out ileitis terminalis (Crohn's disease). **a** An overview in which overlapping bowel loops complicate a distinct evaluation of the terminal and preterminal ileum. **b** By rotating the object on the computer it is possible to bring the ileum forth in an enlarged reconstruction and attain an unobstructed view. Imaging parameters: spiral CT with 3 mm slice thickness, 5 mm/s table feed and 2 mm reconstruction interval. TTP was calculated with 2% depth encoding and 320 HU gradient threshold

5.6.3 Virtual Endoscopic Reconstruction

The fundamental reconstruction techniques for virtual endoscopy of the small intestine are similar to those for the large intestine. These techniques are extensively discussed in Chap. 6; the reader is referred there for more detailed information. The following is a short summary of the most important points. Two different reconstruction principles exist: surface rendering and volume rendering.

5.6.3.1 Surface Rendering

In the surface rendering technique, a threshold value determines which pixels will or will not be visible in an ensuing calculated model. The resulting model contains, in effect, much less information than the original image, namely only that on the object of interest. With relatively limited computer power this object can then be turned and viewed from all sides; after calculating a perspective distortion, a view from within is also possible. The advantages of this technique are the relatively low demand on hardware and software and the rapid processing speed while viewing, once the model has been calculated.

5.6.3.2 Volume Rendering

The volume rendering technique retains each pixel from all slices at all times, and through a classification system the investigator can determine which points should be transparent, which semi-transparent and which should appear opaque. A smooth transition is also possible. For each selected viewing angle, the computer must recalculate all pixels for that image. A model calculation does not exist. This technique has the significant disadvantage that the hardware demands are enormous; therefore, implementation of this technique has experienced much delay. The most notable advantages of the volume rendering technique are that, in contrast to the surface rendering technique, no data are lost and that in addition to the opportunity to select any viewing angle, the classification can be interactively altered during image viewing. Semi-transparent tissue presentation is possible only with the volume rendering technique.

In opposition to virtual endoscopy of organs that are filled with air, on the reconstruction from contrast medium-filled vessels or the small intestine (if not filled with air) the density differences on CT between contrast medium and surrounding tissues are not as intense as between air and soft tissue. The less the contrast, the more meaningful the influence of image noise for the reconstruction. Figure 5.8 shows the difference between the virtual reconstruction of a small intestine filled with air and one filled with contrast agent. In the volume rendering technique, it is possible, by means of a smooth transition function, to display the surfaces of interest as surfaces with depth, rather than as hard surfaces as in the surface rendering technique. The image noise can thus be displayed in a less disturbing fashion. Saving a preselected baseline setting by which reconstruction parameters might then be adjusted according to examination quality has proved to be very useful.

It has been shown that for a virtual endoscopic reconstruction, a polypous lesion must be at least as large as the predefined slice thickness in order to be demonstrated (Rogalla et al. 1998). Consequently, it can be expected that in virtual endoscopy, a lesion with a diameter of 4–5 mm will be easily recognised if the primary slice thickness of a spiral CT was 3 mm. A respective examination protocol through the entire abdomen with a 3-mm slice thickness is currently possible with a 1 s spiral CT. With the introduction of multislice CT that permits complete examination of the abdomen with a particularly low slice thickness, e.g. 1 mm, the potential to detect lesions as small as 1–2 mm in diameter is created. The full extent to which such a low slice thickness will negatively influence image noise in the virtual endoscopy must still be clinically investigated.

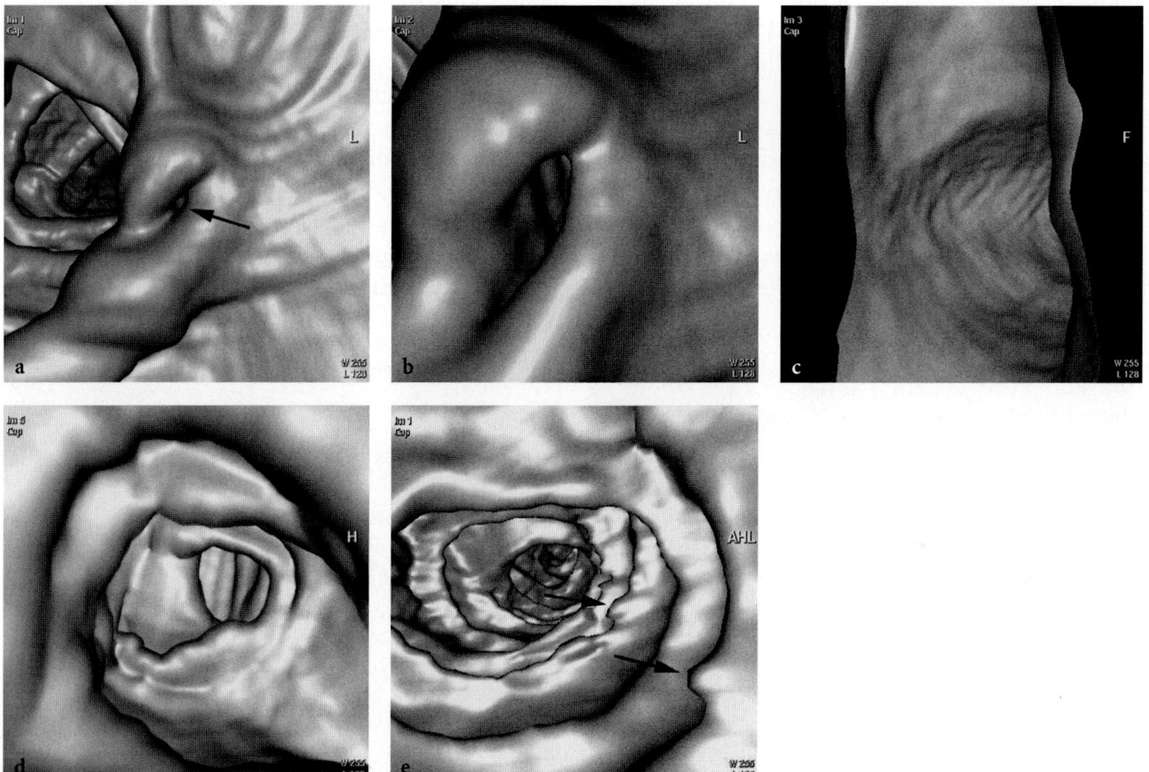

Fig. 5.8a–e. Comparison of two techniques to distend the small bowel. **a–d** The virtual reconstruction of an intestinal study in which the colon was filled with CO_2 gas through a rectal tube after spasmolytic i.v. medication. **a** A virtual view from the caecum onto the ileocaecal valve, which is slightly open (*arrow*). **b** A close-up of the ileocaecal valve. **c** The view through the valve into the terminal ileum. **d** The image represents a virtual view of the middle ileum, which was well distended and also filled with gas. Due to the high density difference between air (or CO_2 gas) and soft tissue on CT, the virtual reconstruction produces soft and natural looking surfaces, similar to the virtual images within the colon. Image noise has very little influence. **e** The virtual reconstruction of the small bowel (ileum) in a patient with similar body weight and circumference. The small intestine was filled with a mixture of methylcellulose and oral contrast medium that had a density of 350–450 HU. Therefore, the maximum density difference between the lumen filled with the contrast material and the bowel wall reached 250–350 HU, about one third of the difference between air and soft tissue. As a consequence, the image noise starts to become influential and can be appreciated in the virtual reconstruction as a somewhat irregular surface with polyp-like figures (*arrows*)

5.6.4 Hybrid Technique

Depending upon the monitor adjustments in CT, the intestinal contents will appear for the most part homogeneously white or, when filled with air, homogeneously dark. These image components do not contain any diagnostic information and can be colour coded with three-dimensional intestinal information. As a result, two images – the multiplanar axial slice and the virtual reconstruction – are practically presented on top of one another (Fig. 5.9). This so-called hybrid technique has the advantage that without using sophisticated navigational tools, essentially the complete small bowel can be presented as a hollow organ while simultaneously imaging extraintestinal conditions or pathology. The disadvantage is that in order to obtain an adequately detailed presentation of the small intestine, an image matrix of 512×512 pixels is too coarse and hence not sufficient for displaying fine endoluminal processes. A more desirable alternative is the reconstruction of the hybrid images with a 1024×1024 point matrix. In this case, however, the processing time and the memory capacity of the computer increase fourfold for each image. In addition, the colour information contained in each image further increases the memory requirements (dependent upon the internal computer image format) relative to a purely black-and-white CT image. The investigator must calculate with 2–4 MB per image.

Printing and distribution of images in the hybrid technique is also somewhat cumbersome because the representation in black and white on a standard X-ray film only complicates image interpretation. Colour documentation seems to be a prerequisite if hybrid images are to be distributed.

5.6.5 Navigation, Pathfinding

As already mentioned, the small intestine, attaining a length of 3–5 m, is highly convoluted and comprehensive navigation is technically difficult and extraordinarily time consuming. Without automatic pathfinding by the computer, approximately 1–2 h would be required for a manual navigation on current workstations. Despite the recommended contrast medium filling of the small intestine through enteroclysma, in most cases intermittent bowel segments that are not well distended remain. Although the less distended segments of the small bowel can also be interpreted well in axial or multiplanar slices, the remaining lumen in these segments can be so small that navigation through them is no longer pos-

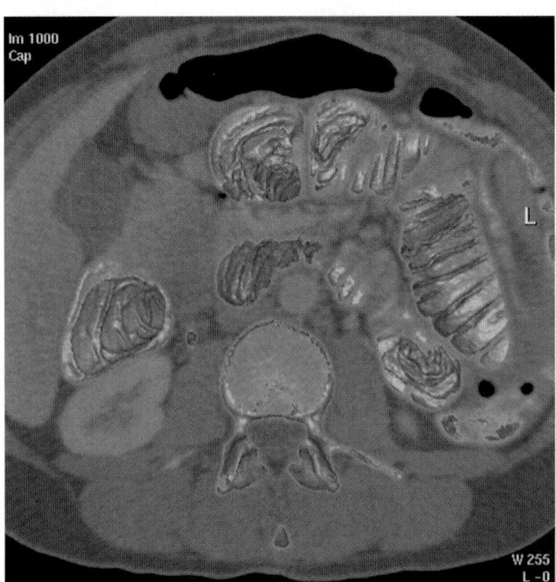

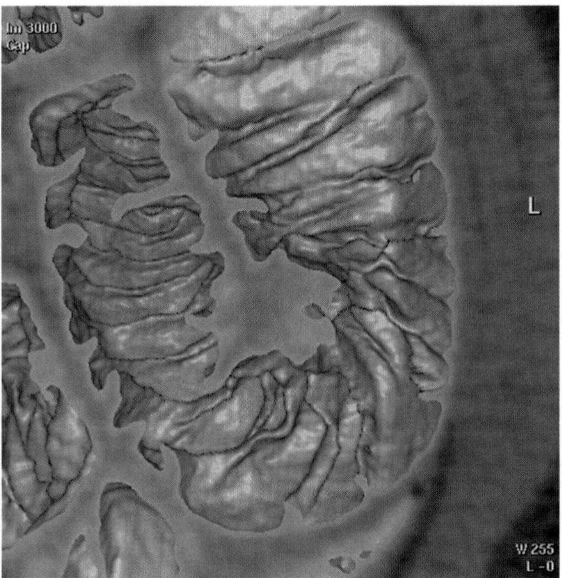

Fig. 5.9a,b. Principle of the hybrid technique: the areas in the presented CT slice that, in the case of small-intestine diagnostics, are filled with radiodense contrast material and therefore would appear to be homogeneously white are replaced with virtual depth information. **a** An axial slice; **b** an enlargement of a slice from a region further caudal. Note the enormously detailed depiction of the bowel anatomy in the hybrid technique. The axial slice information is not lost with this form of presentation. The calculation of the images can in principle run automatically on a workstation since no manual interaction (e.g. tracing a path) is necessary

sible. Therefore, even with maximal usage of the workstation's display of cross-sectional reference images, it is possible only with much effort, and sometimes not at all, to obtain a comprehensive endoscopic representation of the entire small intestine. Based on experience from the evaluation of more than 60 patients, it is sensible and time efficient to initially review the axial and coronal reconstructions, or in the MRI the axial and coronal primary images, and then to use the virtual endoscopy only in selected areas as an assisting procedure and for documentation of findings. It should nonetheless be emphasised that with advancing technical developments, most of all in the area of pathfinding, this situation may change and inspection of the endoluminal virtual images may become the first step when evaluating the small bowel.

Table 5.1. Overview of possible radiological manifestations of Crohn's disease and their visibility on cross-sections and virtual endoscopy

Pathological findings	CT/MRI cross-sections	Virtual endoscopy
Mucosal granularity	–	–
Aphthous lesions	–	–
Lymphoid hyperplasia	–	±
Cobblestoning	–	±
Deep ulcerations	+	±
Fistulae	++	±
String sign	++	+
Wall thickening	++	–
Fibrofatty proliferation	++	–
Mesenteric involvement	++	–
Phlegmon/abscess	++	–

–, Not visible; ±, rarely visible; +, visible; ++, clearly visible

5.8 Imaging Findings

5.8.1 Inflammatory Diseases

5.8.1.1 Crohn's Disease

Crohn's disease is generally seen as a disease of the entire gastrointestinal tract with a tendency toward segmental spreading (Wills et al. 1997). Most frequently affected, in up to 95% of cases, is the terminal ileum, with or without the caecum. The proximal jejunum and duodenum are more seldom affected (up to 10%). Crohn's disease is a chronic granulomatous process that causes transmural inflammation of the gastrointestinal tract, commonly with extension into the serosa and the mesenteric lymph nodes (Brzezinski and Lashner 1997).

One must differentiate between features that can be seen alone with virtual endoscopy and those that require additional assistance from axial or multiplanar cross-sectional images. In many instances, only the all-inclusive viewing of the various images makes the diagnosis of Crohn's disease possible, especially when the condition is neither clinically apparent nor strongly suspected. Table 5.1 gives an overview of discernible pathological characteristics in Crohn's disease:

The detection of initial changes, e.g. diffuse mucosal granularity (Glick and Teplick 1985) or aphthous lesions (Fujimura et al. 1996), is, as always, a domain of fibreoptic endoscopy or the conventional barium enema study. With fibreoptic endoscopy, all mucosal changes are excellently viewed (taking into consideration the use of magnifying endoscopic techniques), and biopsy specimens can be obtained in the same session, allowing pathological confirmation of the diagnosis. A prerequisite is naturally that the affected bowel segment can be reached, and this is generally the case only in the terminal or preterminal ileum. The relatively poor recognition of early mucosal changes with the cross-sectional imaging technique, and hence also with virtual endoscopy, is based on the fact that the spatial resolution, due to methodological differences, is substantially less than that of conventional fluoroscopy: the resolution on CT and MRI is approximately 10-fold inferior.

Lymphoid follicles are a normal occurrence in lymphatic tissue, which is also located in the intestinal wall (Kelvin et al. 1979). The lymphoid follicles can be spotted in approximately 50% of all barium studies performed in children and in about 13% of all air-contrast barium enemas performed in adults (Laufer and deSa 1978). They appear in a scale of about 1–3 mm, the lower limit of resolution of both CT and MRI. Even if single follicles can be detected, their appearance on CT and MRI is atypical and a specific classification is therefore practically impossible. Virtual endoscopy, with its improved spatial, three-dimensional display, displays round surfaces in a manner that is easier for the eye to perceive. Assuming the follicles are at least 3 mm in size, it is also possible to occasionally view single follicles in virtual endoscopy; however, they tend to take the form of an unspecific, irregular surface of the mucosa.

"Cobblestoning" occurs as a result of the accumulated, lined up ulcers which form a network crisscrossed by fissures. The mucosa between the fissures is oedematous and swollen, resulting in the characteristic cobblestone aspect (Goldblum and Petras 1997). This appearance is only one of numerous forms of inflammatory pseudopolyposis (Lichtenstein 1987). Although easily detected in the conventional barium study, the cobblestone pattern can be seen on cross-sections only if the difference in level between the base of the fissure and the mucosa is great enough and surface elevations of at least 1–2 mm are present. Virtual endoscopy also has a presentational advantage, because the widespread pattern is easier to display three-dimensionally than cross-sectionally.

Deep ulcerations and fistulas are always detectable in CT and MRI when, as described for the other changes, they are extensive enough to be recognised by the limited spatial resolution of these cross-sectional modalities. Especially when reconstruction enlargements from the raw data of spiral CT are attempted, CT is a step ahead of MRI concerning spatial resolution, so that with good contrast quality of the intestinal lumen, deep ulcerations are better recognised than on MRI. For fistulas, the trademark of Crohn's disease, CT is dependent upon filling of the fistula with contrast medium. Otherwise, differentiation between a fibrous layer or infectious infiltration and an actual fistula becomes extremely difficult or impossible. In this respect MRI has strategic advantages, since even a secretory filling of a fistula duct in comparison to the surrounding fat can be displayed excellently in T2-weighted sequences, making contrast filling unnecessary. Virtual endoscopy can display a fistula duct only if it stands in obvious continuity to the intestinal lumen, in other words when a contrast-filled, decipherable connection exists (Fig. 5.10). Otherwise, although an attempt to create a virtual endoscopy in the fistula duct could be made, the virtual endoscope must be manually focussed on the fistula. This requires a preliminary interpretation of the cross-sectionals. The resulting diagnostic gain is, however, no more than moderate.

The spastic contraction of the intestine by the so-called string sign is a functional stenosis without prestenotic dilation. Increasing fibrous changes of the intestinal wall often leads to a fixed stenosis with signs of obstruction. Both findings, the string sign without prestenotic dilation and the fixed stenosis, can be displayed very well with cross-sectional modalities. Stenoses are naturally easy to recognise on virtual endoscopy as well. However, the length and also the degree of the stenosis are not so clearly evident. All further pathological features of Crohn's disease, i.e. wall thickening, fibrofatty proliferation, mesenteric involvement and phlegmons or abscesses, are classical conditions that justify the diagnostic power of cross-sectional modalities. Obviously, these changes are undetectable in virtual endoscopy. Bowel loop displacements, which occur in the framework of fatty proliferation ("creeping fat"), can, for example, present similarly in the TTP technique as in the conventional barium study. Experience to date is too sparse to allow judgement of whether presentation forms such as TTP actually provide diagnostic support.

5.8.1.2
Infectious Diseases

Crohn's disease is often described as the most important chronic small intestinal inflammation. On the other hand, many other inflammatory bowel diseases occur rarely and therefore have allowed limited experience with virtual endoscopy. Next to bacterial pathogens, mostly *Salmonella*, *Shigella*, and *Escherichia coli*, viruses, such as rotavirus, can also cause enteritis. Most pathogens carry an enterotoxic effect and do not cause any morphologically detectable mucosal damage. Therefore, such enteritides are not (even indirectly) revealed using CT, MRI or virtual endoscopy.

5.8.1.3
Eosinophilic Enteritis

Eosinophilic enteritis is histologically characterised by extensive eosinophilic cell infiltration in all wall layers. The jejunum and stomach antrum are favoured locations. Radiologically detectable are irregularly thickened or formed folds, which also lead to shrinking of the lumen. Infiltration and damage to the muscle layers result in local dilations and wall thickening; findings that are only partially recognised on virtual endoscopy. Since the differential diagnoses of lymphoma, Crohn's disease or nonspecific infection (e.g. yersiniosis) are difficult to rule out, little diagnostic assistance is currently expected from virtual endoscopy.

5.8.1.4
Parasites and Worms

Due to the extremely infrequent occurrence of parasitic infections in industrialised countries, no experience has been collected to date with virtual endoscopy.

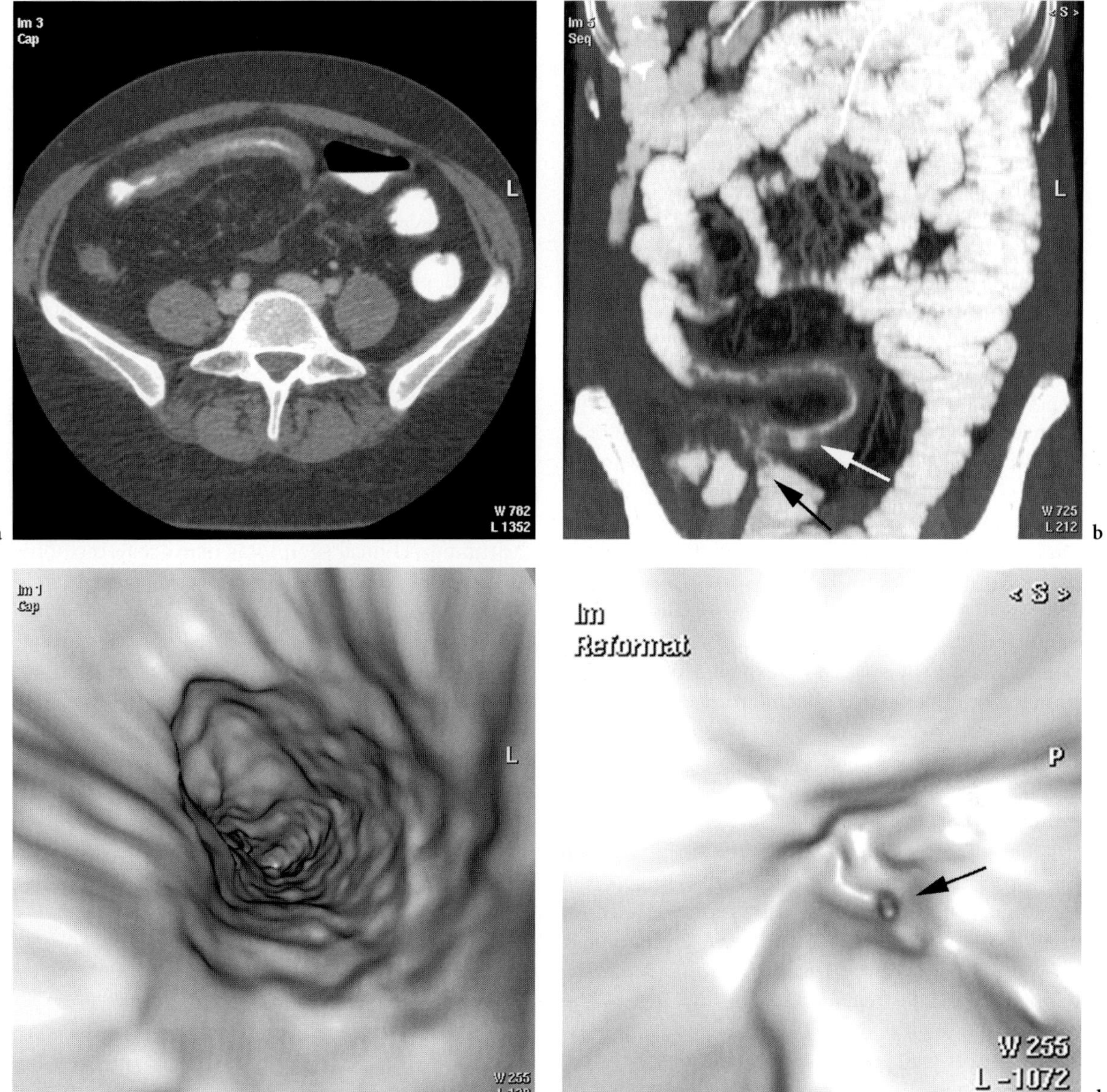

Fig. 5.10a–d. A young female patient with histologically proven Crohn's disease. **a** An axial slice already containing most of the features of Crohn's disease; a long segment of the preterminal ileum wall is thickened; additionally, the typical fatty proliferation in the immediate vicinity of the inflamed bowel loop (creeping fat) is depicted. **b** A coronal reconstruction showing that the ascending colon is barely filled with contrast agent, but the rectum does contain some. This contrast agent distribution pattern can only occur through an entero-enteral fistula, which is marked with an *black arrow*. The *white arrow* points at an ulceration referred to as a pseudodiverticulum in the diseased bowel segment. **c** A virtual view from the healthy part of the ileum onto the diseased portion. The lumen stenosis is conspicuous. **d** The ileo-rectal fistula is also observable from the rectum. The *arrow* points towards the ostium of the fistula. Imaging technique: spiral CT, 3 mm slice thickness, 2 mm reconstruction interval, oral contrast administration via a duodenal tube

5.8.1.5 Whipple's Disease

Whipple's disease, also termed intestinal lipodystrophy, stems most likely from an infection with an as yet unidentified pathogen. Next to changes in practically all organs (joints, heart, central nervous system, skin) intestinal wall thickening with a knotty constitution and mesenteric lymphadenopathy characteristically occur. Both of these findings are well demonstrated with cross-sectional modalities but elude virtual endoscopic detection. Only when knotty mucosal infiltration appears is it possible to see this in virtual endoscopy. Experience has not yet been obtained due to the rarity of this condition.

5.8.1.6 Tuberculosis

Since the introduction of pasteurised milk and the tuberculostatics, intestinal tuberculosis has become a rarity in industrialised countries. Nonetheless, the number of cases has risen in recent years, mostly due to the increase in immune-compromised patients, for example those with HIV infections or iatrogenic aetiology (e.g. bone marrow transplant). The terminal ileum and the ileocaecal region are favoured areas; the picture is, however, similar to the aphthous changes in Crohn's disease. Differentiation between the two entities is often not possible, and it is assumed that many infections of the terminal ileum wrongly attributed to tuberculosis before the discovery of Crohn's disease (Crohn et al. 1932) were actually Crohn's ileitis terminalis. The differential diagnosis must also include sarcoidosis and typhus. Also here, it is dubtful whether virtual endoscopy might be of use in the differential diagnostic procedure.

5.8.1.7 Radiation Enteritis

The small intestine is rather sensitive to ionising radiation. Acute radiation reactions are generally not an indication for a contrast medium examination. A dose of 45 Gy or more leads to chronic radiation damage. The intestine reacts with changes in the mucosa and the blood vessels and in connective tissue of deeper wall layers. Macroscopically, there are dense peritoneal adhesions and a thickened and shrunken mesentery with shrivelled and shortened intestinal loops. The intestinal wall is thickened and swollen. The lumen can be compressed into a high-grade stenosis. Ulcers can also appear. As already mentioned in the section on Crohn's disease, mucosal changes are first recognised in virtual endoscopy when they attain a size of at least 3 mm. Stenoses are easily recognised and the intestinal wall thickness is seen perfectly well in the cross-sectional images.

5.8.2 Neoplastic Diseases

Small intestinal tumours are rare (Howe et al. 1999; O'Riordan et al. 1996). The frequency of primary tumours is reported as 1:100,000 or 1.5–6% of all gastrointestinal tract tumours (Serour et al. 1992). About one half are malignant, and the malignant tumours are three times more frequently symptomatic. Overall, small bowel tumours are most frequently found in the ileum (41%), followed by the jejunum (36%), and the duodenum (18%). Due to their rarity and the inadequate diagnostic techniques, detection is often delayed. A very important examination is the so-called push endoscopy (Adrain and Krevsky 1996; O'Mahony et al. 1996; Zaman and Katon 1998). Despite the supreme advantage of being able to perform a biopsy in the same session, this procedure is very unpleasant for the patient. Since the introduction of enteroclysma, the radiological accuracy in diagnosing small intestinal tumours has substantially improved. Small and asymptomatic processes are also often detected. With increasing size of the tumour, clinical symptoms may occur, including an ileus, due to partial or complete displacement of the intestinal lumen. The often intermittent obstruction occurring in approximately 25% of the patients is also the most frequent manifestation of small intestinal tumours. In another 25%, gastrointestinal bleeding appears as a leading symptom (Morris 1999). In such patients, angiography and scintigraphy can be of indispensable assistance. Differential diagnostic categorisation of small bowel tumours is hardly feasible with conventional enteroclysma, and also for larger tumours, which are visualised on CT even without optimal intestinal enhancement, the classification can be very difficult.

5.8.2.1 Benign Tumours

Most benign small intestinal tumours (O'Riordan et al. 1996) originate from deeper layers of the bowel wall. In descending order of frequency, the following tumours may appear: leiomyomas (36%–49%), adenomas (15%–20%), lipomas (14%–16%), haemangiomas (13–16%), lymphangioma (5%) and neurogenic tumours (1%). The above-mentioned tumours usually lead to only mild stenosis of the lumen and therefore rarely cause an ileus, except as a result of an invagination (intussusception). Polyps occur in the framework of, for example, Gardner's syndrome or Peutz-Jeghers syndrome (Westerman and Wilson 1999). The latter arises from the muscularis mucosae and produces hamartomas that usually grow inwards in the intestinal lumen and can reach extreme sizes.

Polypous mucosal lesions in the small bowel can be well demonstrated as polyps on virtual endoscopy, assuming thorough and adequate oral administration of contrast medium, as outlined in Sect. 5.4, Patient Preparation. Although the small intestine does not present the same problem as the colon, i.e. that stool remnants are so solid and formed that they can be mistaken for polyps, residues of chyme that adhere to the intestinal wall can complicate the examination and create the impression of wall irregularities. In any case, such virtual-endoscopic findings should be compared with the respective axial or multiplanar slices in order to differentiate artefacts from enteral contents.

If, according to an applied rendering algorithm, only a gradient from highly enhanced bowel lumen to less dense bowel wall is used, air bubbles could be misinterpreted as polyps (Fig. 5.11). In such a case, however, the correlation with the original cross-sectional images can immediately clarify uncertainties.

5.8.2.2 Malignant Tumours

The most frequent among the malignant small intestine tumours (Howe et al. 1999) is carcinoid tumour (46–48%) (Ciccarelli et al. 1987). With decreasing frequency follow adenocarcinomas (25–26%), lymphoma (16–17%), leiomyosarcoma (9–10%), vascu-

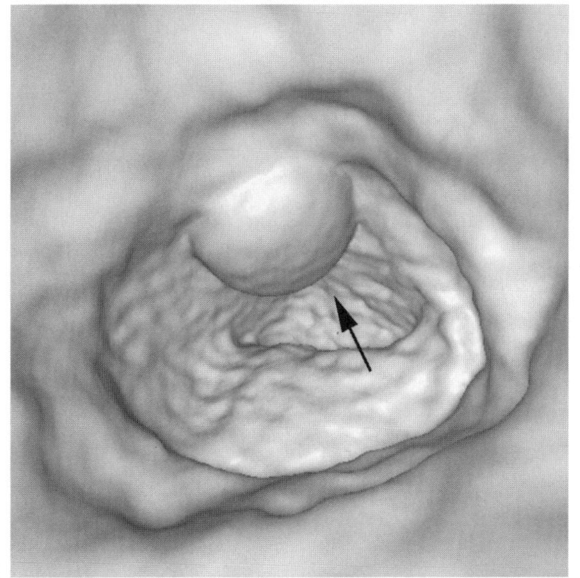
a

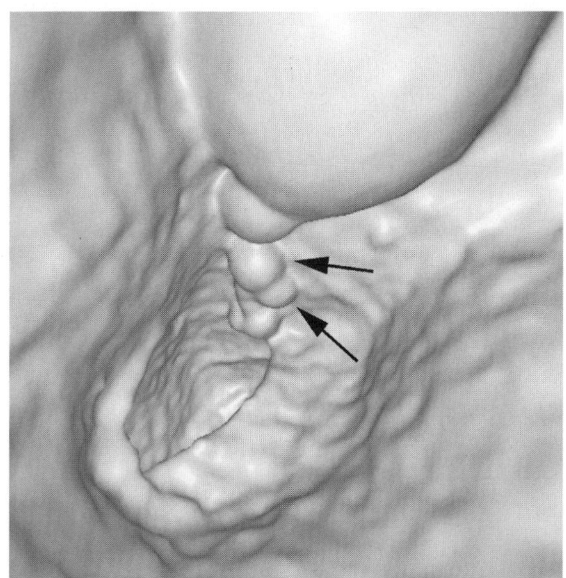
b

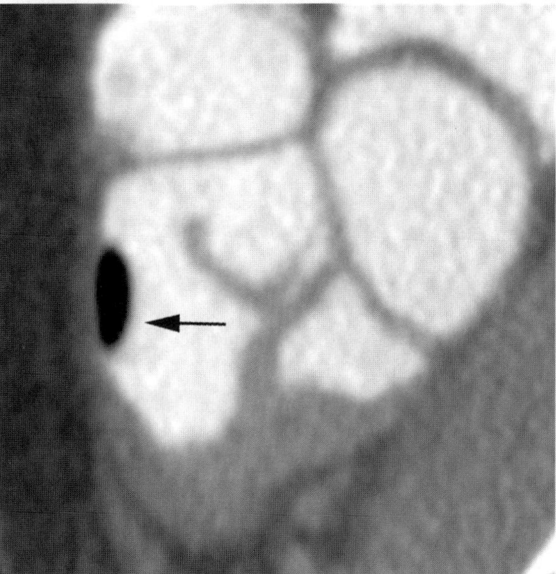
c

Fig. 5.11a–c. An example of air bubbles in the contrasted bowel. The bubbles take on the impression of a smoothly bordered polyp. This example reveals the importance of viewing the axial or multiplanar images when in doubt (**c**); in a cross-sectional image, it is not possible to confuse a polyp with an air bubble

lar malignancies (1%), fibrosarcoma (0.3%) and metastatic tumours (Fig. 5.12). The cardinal symptoms are pain due to intermittent obstruction, weight loss, gastrointestinal bleeding (DESCAMPS et al. 1999; MORRIS 1999) and occasionally also a palpable abdominal mass. However, 30% of the tumours are clinically asymptomatic.

Virtual endoscopy can visualise tumours well as long as they cause a morphological alteration of the luminal bowel wall (Fig. 5.13). Problems may arise if the tumour lies on a sharp bend in a bowel loop and is not coated by contrast agent. Under such circumstances, the tumour can only be suspected on virtual endoscopy based on the interruption of the pattern of intestinal

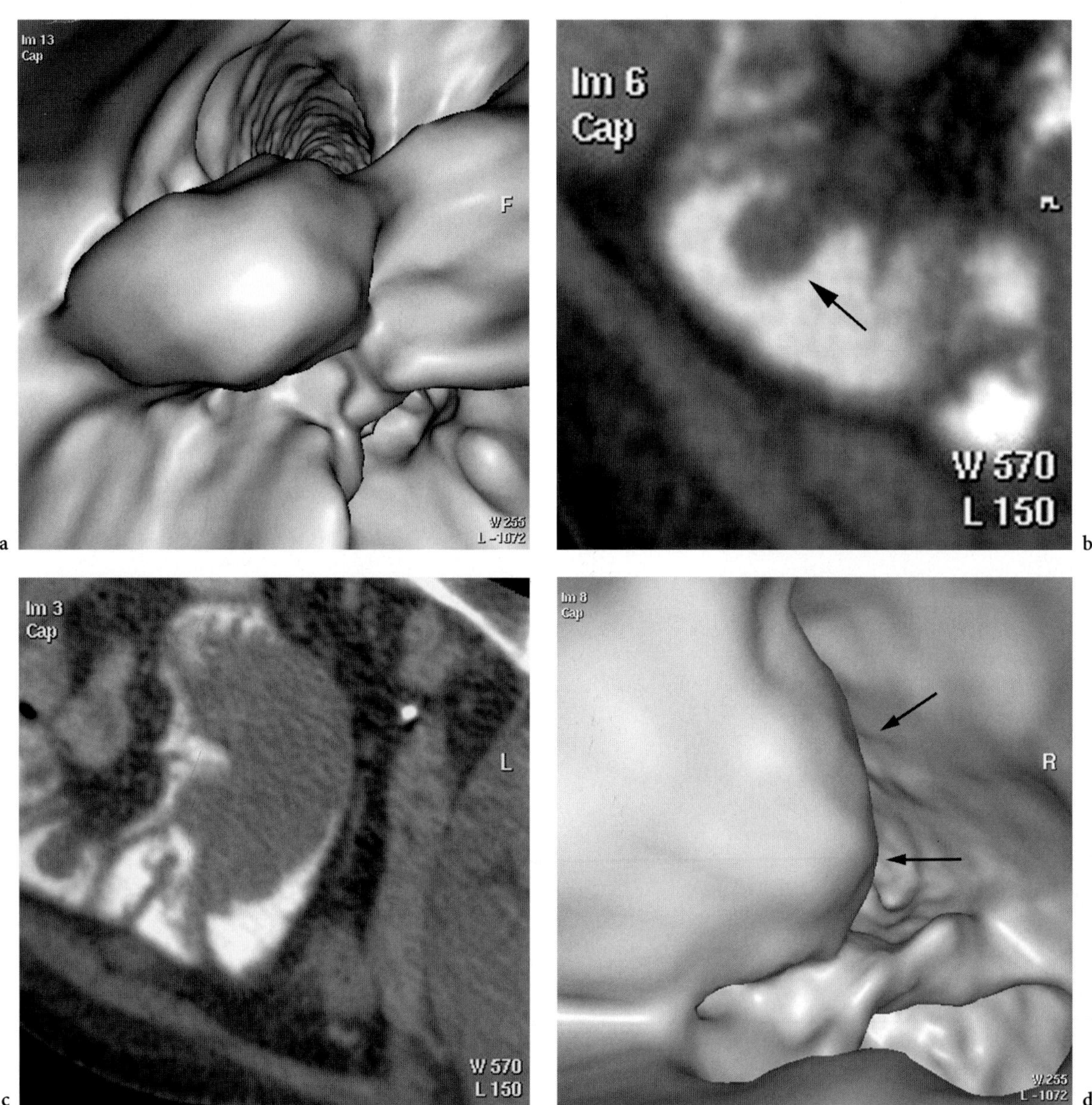

Fig. 5.12a–d. Virtual endoscopy with the corresponding multiplanar images of a female patient with melanoma metastases. In the intestinal lumen on the virtual image (**a**) a metastasis is depicted with a polyp-like figure, which can be confirmed in the MPR (*arrow;* **b**). Even when carefully scanning the original axial slices, this finding can easily escape detection. A neighbouring, larger metastasis caused marked narrowing of the lumen. This finding cannot be overlooked in the axial slice (**c**), and the virtual endoscopy can only provide clear confirmation of the findings (*arrows;* **d**). No knowledge of the metastases existed prior to the CT. The example further shows that without entire contrasting of the intestine, such findings can easily be overlooked. Imaging technique: spiral CT with 3 mm slice thickness, 5 mm/s table feed, 2 mm reconstruction interval

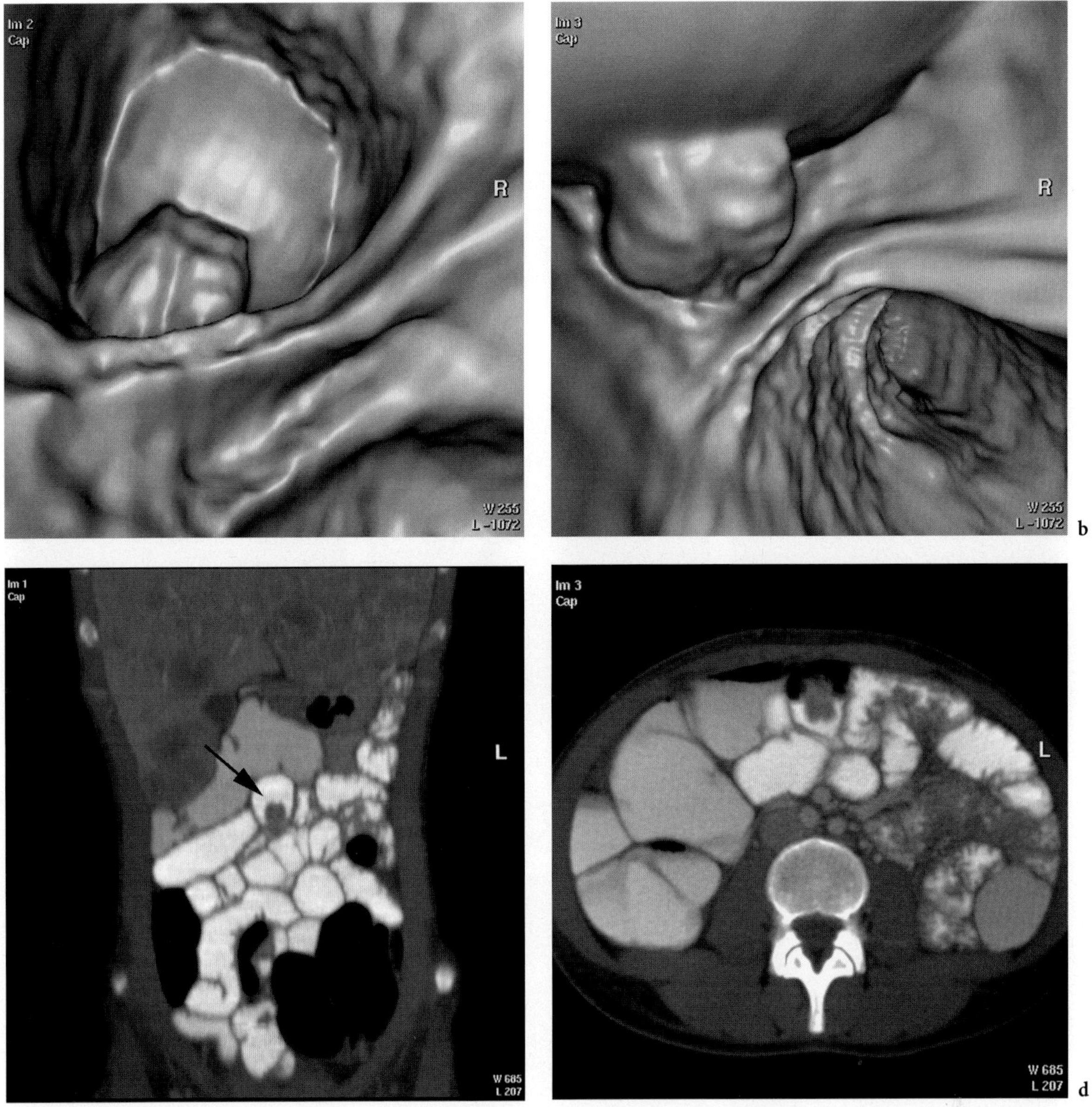

Fig. 5.13a–d. Virtual endoscopy of the small bowel in a young woman who presented with multiple focal liver lesions. The liver was biopsied, and the initial suspicion of a carcinoid based on laboratory values could be confirmed. The subsequent small bowel enteroclysma was indicated in order to find the primary tumour. **a,b** Virtual views in which the polypous tumour lies directly adjacent to a remaining air bubble which is signified by the smooth surface in the horizontal direction. **c** The tumour can also be demonstrated in the multiplanar reconstruction *(arrow)*; however, the disseminated liver metastases cannot be viewed on virtual endoscopy. Virtual endoscopy is naturally not suited for general evaluation of conditions outside the intestinal lumen. **d** Suboptimal contrast enhancement of the small intestine. Several loops of the jejunum are already empty and poorly distended, and subsequent filling of the large colon is seen. The contrast medium in the large colon shows a lower density than the mixture in the small bowel (dilution effect), indicating that the small intestine was not adequately prepared for the examination. Imaging technique: spiral CT with 3 mm slice thickness, 5 mm/s table feed, 2 mm reconstruction interval

folds. Once again, the axial or multiplanar images can then support or dismiss the virtual endoscopic findings.

Metastases need not always grow in polypous fashion(Blecker et al. 1999); rather, they sometimes cause widespread infiltration of the small intestine (Stenbygaard and Sorensen 1999). Although in these cases there is a pathological presentation of the wall on virtual endoscopy, here too a definitive diagnosis is first made when the axial images have been reviewed. Currently, virtual endoscopy cannot directly display the bowel wall thickness. With malignant tumours, the infiltration depth is also of ultimate importance and these factors can be optimally recognised on cross-sectional images (Fig. 5.14).

The TTP technique, which is very similar to conventional enteroclysma in its display format, allows an informative overview of the small intestine; tumour-related stenoses become very distinct. Current problematic areas in TTP are large segments of the small bowel that are not filled with contrast agent. This also might be misinterpreted as a stenosis or a luminal lesion.

5.8.3 Other Small Bowel Diseases

Numerous changes other than inflammatory bowel diseases must be considered in the spectrum of differential diagnoses: amyloidosis, lymphangiectasia, endometritis, diverticula and many more. Due to their rarity, there is limited experience of what findings are apparent on virtual endoscopy and what detection rates can be expected. For global configuration anomalies (malrotations, hernias) one can expect virtual endoscopy to have no great value. In contrast, three-dimensional presentations such as TTP may become very helpful because they depict the bowel in its entirety.

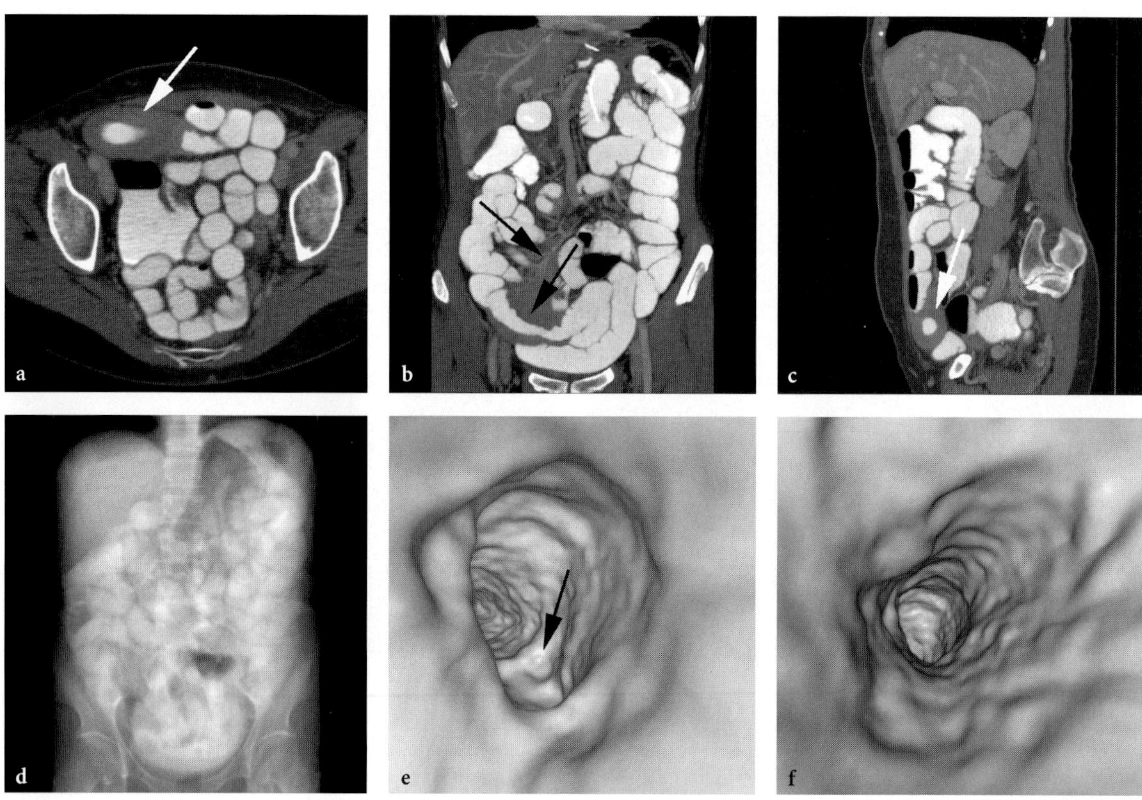

Fig. 5.14a–n. A middle-aged woman with histologically verified non-Hodgkin's lymphoma (status post cervical lymph node excision). Following conventional CT, lymphoma manifestation in the small bowel was suspected. Subsequent small bowel enteroclysma was technically of limited quality and diagnostically inconclusive, although suspicion of small intestine involvement was expressed. The patient was ultimately referred for combined CT/MRI enteroclysma. This example is perfectly suited to compare the visualization techniques described in the text. **a** Axial CT at the level of the hip joint. The circular thickening of the wall is clearly recognisable, representing a manifestation of the lymphoma (*arrow*). The coronal (**b**) and sagittal (**c**) multiplanar reformation of the conducted multislice CT (1 mm slice thickness, 0.5 mm reconstruction interval) also clearly show the findings in the ileum (*arrows*). The coronal view simultaneously demonstrates the extensive involvement of the mesenteric root in one image. **d** A thick slice reconstruction in the coronal plane, also termed computed volume projection (CVP). The image resembles a conventional radiograph. The small bowel finding is, however, hardly detectable, illustrating the diagnostic limitation of simple radiography. **e,f** The virtual endoscopic impression of the diseased part of the ileum. The natural intestinal folds of Kerckring are completely absent; instead, an unsettled, irregular surface texture with clearly discernible ulcers is depicted (*arrow*). The intestinal lumen is not notably stenotic

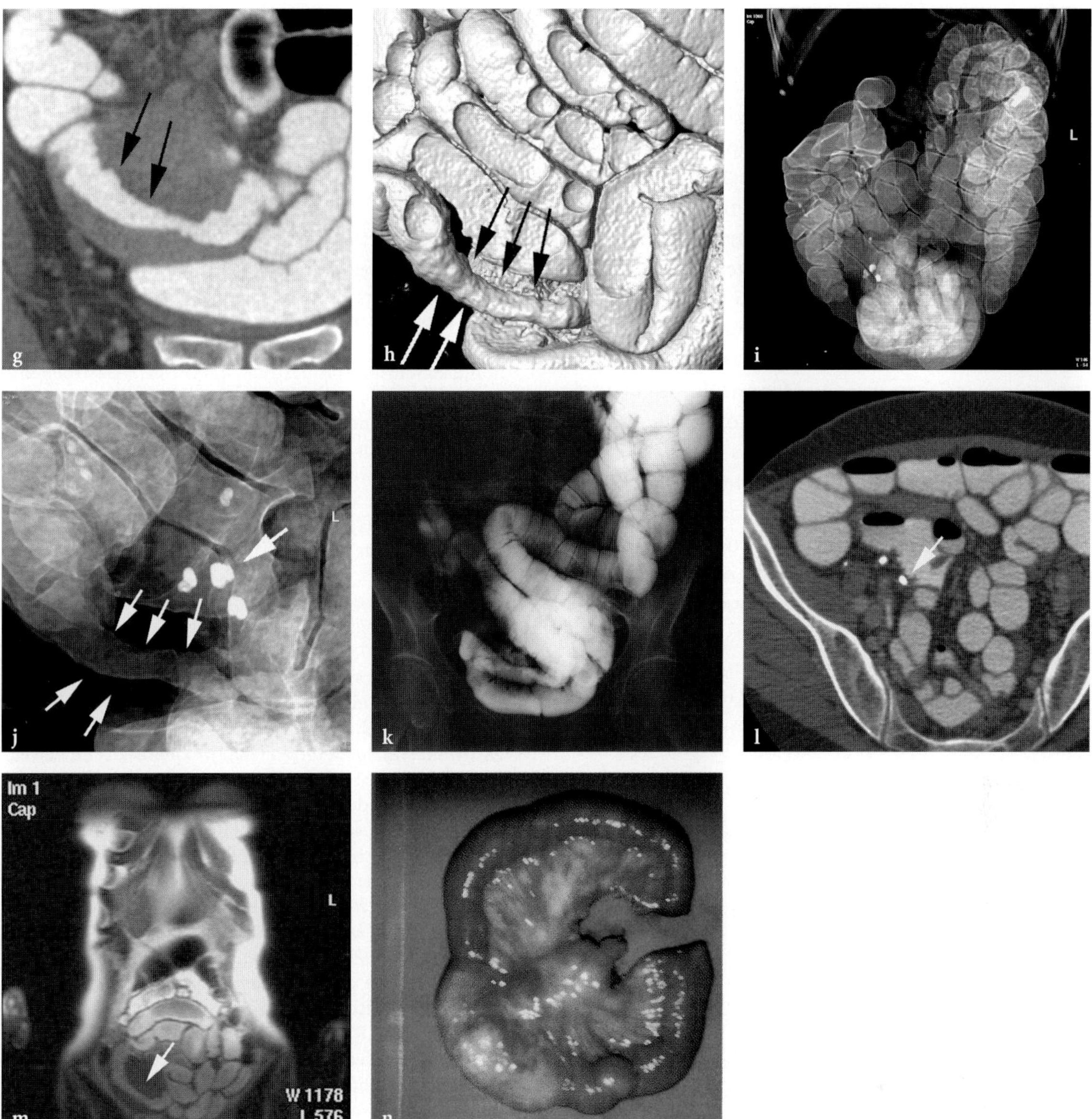

Fig. 5.14a–n. (Continued) **g** Virtual endoscopy does not permit observation of the wall thickening or, most of all, of the peri-intestinal involvement. Although the image is very indicative of tumour disease in the small intestine, a specific differential diagnostic classification, especially against chronic inflammatory bowel disease, may be difficult. **h** A three-dimensional surface reconstruction containing the perceivable finding (*arrows*). In addition, the remaining air bubbles create the appearance of indentation in the intestinal wall. However, this image demonstrates that only the intestinal loops that are not covered by other intestinal segments can be judged. The shaded surface display is therefore only diagnostically useful in certain instances. **i,j** TTP reconstructions, which have a similar appearance to the conventional enteroclysma (**k**). Although the transparency in the presentation makes viewing of the overlapping intestinal loops less pleasant, the findings are detectable in the deeper lying segments. The rounded figures marked with an *arrow* represent calcified lymph nodes, confirmed by the corresponding axial image (**l**). **m** The intestinal affection is also clearly observable on MRI immediately following CT. Due to the position of the finding (*arrow*) on the border of the imaging area (HASTE sequence, body phased array coil), the contrast is not optimal and is insufficient especially for virtual endoscopy. The surgical specimen of the resected bowel loop (**n**) confirmed the preoperative image findings

5.9 Summary

What is the diagnostic benefit of virtual endoscopy of the small intestine? The question can be posed with regard to all reconstruction techniques that use primary image data to create new, three-dimensional representations. Not only is all diagnostic information contained in the primary image data (otherwise it could not be incorporated into the reconstructions), but every further computing step bears the danger that diagnostic information will disappear in the course of processing. Meanwhile, algorithms bring the additional disadvantage of artefacts.

In conclusion, the original cross-sectional image remains a diagnostic tool that cannot be replaced.

The discrepancy between the material and time that have to be invested in virtual endoscopy and the maximal achievable diagnostic benefit is relatively large in small bowel diagnostics owing to the complexity of the organ, especially its length. Consequently, virtual endoscopy of the small bowel is to be seen as an additional presentation form, which cannot substitute consideration of the original axial slices.

Further technical developments in the field of primary imaging modalities, currently most of all in CT with multislice technology, have highlighted the problem of viewing image data: 500–1000 images per examination is no longer a rarity. The immense quantity of images must initially be transferred over a network and saved in archives. Beyond this technical challenge, the clinical radiologist is once again presented with the problem of managing the data flood. Of interest would be a way of compressing the image data without extensive information loss. Aside from image compression technologies that compress the pure image data in the computer, methods that carry out information compression and thus simplify diagnostic decisions have gained increasing interest. In this respect, virtual endoscopy is only one technique among many others that possesses the above-mentioned potential. The extent to which small bowel radiology will actually profit cannot yet be stated with certainty.

With further developments, particularly in the area of computing speed and as a result of the immediate availability of virtual endoscopic images following the examination, virtual endoscopy may gain in diagnostic value.

References

Adrain AL, Krevsky B (1996) Enteroscopy in patients with gastrointestinal bleeding of obscure origin. Dig Dis 14:345–355.

Aschoff AJ, Zeitler H, Merkle EM, Reinshagen M, Brambs HJ, Rieber A (1997) [MR enteroclysis for nuclear spin tomographic diagnosis of inflammatory bowel diseases with contrast enhancement]. Rofo Fortschr Geb Rontgenstr Neuen Bildgeb Verfahr 167:387–391.

Binswanger RO, Sellink JL (1980) [Enteroclysis: improved and simplified contract media imaging of the small intestine]. Schweiz Med Wochenschr 110:867–869.

Blecker D, Abraham S, Furth EE, Kochman ML (1999) Melanoma in the gastrointestinal tract. Am J Gastroenterol 94:3427–3433.

Brzezinski A, Lashner BA (1997): Natural history of Crohn´s disease. In Allan RNJ, Rhodes JM, Hanauer SB (eds), *Inflammatory bowel disease*, 3rd edn. New York: Churchill Livingstone, pp 475–486.

Ciccarelli O, Welch JP, Kent GG (1987) Primary malignant tumors of the small bowel. The Hartford Hospital experience, 1969–1983. Am J Surg 153:350–354.

Crohn BB, Ginzburg L, Oppenheimer GD (1932) Regional ileitis: a pathological-clinical entity. J Am Med Assoc 99:1323–1328.

Debatin JF, Patak MA (1999) MRI of the small and large bowel. Eur Radiol 9:1523–1534.

Descamps C, Schmit A, Van Gossum A (1999) "Missed" upper gastrointestinal tract lesions may explain "occult" bleeding. Endoscopy 31:452–455.

Duvoisin B, Schnyder P (1990) [Computerized tomography of the small bowel]. Radiologe 30:280–285.

Ekberg O (1977) Crohn's disease of the small bowel examined by double contrast technique: a comparison with oral technique. Gastrointest Radiol 1:355–359.

Faber SC, Stehling MK, Holzknecht N, Gauger J, Helmberger T, Reiser M (1997) Pathologic conditions in the small bowel: findings at fat-suppressed gadolinium-enhanced MR imaging with an optimized suspension of oral magnetic particles. Radiology 205:278–282.

Fleckenstein P, Pedersen G (1975) The value of the duodenal intubation method (sellink modification) for the radiological visualization of the small bowel. Scand J Gastroenterol 10:423–425.

Fujimura Y, Kamoi R, Iida M (1996) Pathogenesis of aphthoid ulcers in Crohn's disease: correlative findings by magnifying colonoscopy, electron microscopy, and immunohistochemistry. Gut 38:724–732.

Gayer G, Zissin R, Apter S, Shemesh E, Heldenberg E (1999) Acute diverticulitis of the small bowel: CT findings. Abdom Imaging 24:452–455.

Gershon-Cohen J, Shay H (1939) Barium enteroclysis. AJR Am J Roentgenol 42:456–458.

Glick SN, Teplick SK (1985) Crohn disease of the small intestine: diffuse mucosal granularity. Radiology 154:313–317.

Gmünder U, Wirth W (1970) Doppelkontrastdarstellung. Schweiz Med Wochenschr 100:1236.

Goldblum JR, Petras RE (1997): Histopathology of Crohn´s disease. In Allan RN, Rhodes JM, Hanauer SB (eds), *Inflammatory bowel disease*, 3rd edn. New York: Churchill Livingstone, pp 311–316.

Grubnic S, Padhani AR, Revell PB, Husband JE (1999) Comparative efficacy of and sequence choice for two oral contrast agents used during MR imaging. AJR Am J Roentgenol 173:173–178.

Ha HK, Lee EH, Lim CH, et al. (1998) Application of MRI for small intestinal diseases. J Magn Reson Imaging 8:375–383.

Horton KM, Corl FM, Fishman EK (1999) CT of nonneoplastic diseases of the small bowel: spectrum of disease. J Comput Assist Tomogr 23:417–428.

Howe JR, Karnell LH, Menck HR, Scott-Conner C (1999) The American College of Surgeons Commission on Cancer and the American Cancer Society. Adenocarcinoma of the small bowel: review of the National Cancer Data Base, 1985–1995. Cancer 86:2693–2706.

James S, Balfe DM, Lee JK, Picus D (1987) Small-bowel disease: categorization by CT examination. AJR Am J Roentgenol 148:863–868.

Kelvin FM, Max RJ, Norton GA, et al. (1979) Lymphoid follicular pattern of the colon in adults. AJR Am J Roentgenol 133:821–825.

Laufer I, deSa D (1978) Lymphoid follicular pattern: a normal feature of the pediatric colon. AJR Am J Roentgenol 130:51–55.

Lee JK, Marcos HB, Semelka RC (1998) MR imaging of the small bowel using the HASTE sequence. AJR Am J Roentgenol 170:1457–1463.

Lichtenstein JE (1987) Radiologic-pathologic correlation of inflammatory bowel disease. Radiol Clin North Am 25:3–24.

Low VHS (1998) The query corner. Bowel wall thickening on CT. Abdom Imaging 23:107–110.

Lura A (1951) Enema of the small intestine with special emphasis on the diagnosis of tumors. Br J Radiol 24:264–271.

Maccioni F, Rossi P, Gourtsoyiannis N, Bezzi M, Di Nardo R, Broglia L (1997) US and CT findings of small bowel neoplasms. Eur Radiol 7:1398–1409.

Madsen SM, Thomsen HS, Munkholm P, Schlichting P, Davidsen B (1997) Magnetic resonance imaging of Crohn disease: early recognition of treatment response and relapse. Abdom Imaging 22:164–166.

Madsen SM, Thomsen HS, Schlichting P, Dorph S, Munkholm P (1999) Evaluation of treatment response in active Crohn's disease by low-field magnetic resonance imaging. Abdom Imaging 24:232–239.

Maglinte DD, Burney BT, Miller RE (1982) Lesions missed on small-bowel follow-through: analysis and recommendations. Radiology 144:737–739.

Makita O, Ikushima I, Matsumoto N, Arikawa K, Yamashita Y, Takahashi M (1999) CT differentiation between necrotic and nonnecrotic small bowel in closed loop and strangulating obstruction. Abdom Imaging 24:120–124.

Morewood DJ, Whitehouse GH (1986) A comparison of three methods for performing barium follow-through studies of the small intestine. Br J Radiol 59:971–973.

Morris AJ (1999) Small-bowel investigation in occult gastrointestinal bleeding. Semin Gastrointest Dis 10:65–70.

Nolan DJ, Cadman PJ, Jeffree MA (1985) Re: Detailed per-oral small-bowel examination versus enteroclysis [letter]. Radiology 157:836–837.

O'Mahony S, Morris AJ, Straiton M, Murray L, MacKenzie JF (1996) Push enteroscopy in the investigation of small-intestinal disease. Qjm 89:685–690.

O'Riordan BG, Vilor M, Herrera L (1996) Small bowel tumors: an overview. Dig Dis 14:245–257.

Ott DJ, Chen YM, Gelfand DW, Van Swearingen F, Munitz HA (1985a) Detailed per-oral small bowel examination vs. enteroclysis. Part I: Expenditures and radiation exposure. Radiology 155:29–31.

Ott DJ, Chen YM, Gelfand DW, Van Swearingen F, Munitz HA (1985b) Detailed per-oral small bowel examination vs. enteroclysis. Part II: Radiographic accuracy. Radiology 155:31–34.

Pansdorf H (1937) Die fraktionierte Dünndarmfüllung und ihre klinische Bedeutung. Rofo Fortschr Geb Rontgenstr Neuen Bildgeb Verfahr 56:627–634.

Pozniak MA, Scanlan KA, Yandow D, Mulligan G (1990) [Current status of small-bowel ultrasound] [published erratum appears in Radiologe 1990 Dec;30(12):597]. Radiologe 30:254–265.

Pribram BO, Kleiber N (1927) Ein neuer Weg zur röntgenologischen Darstellung des Duodenums (Pneumoduodenum). Rofo Fortschr Geb Rontgenstr Neuen Bildgeb Verfahr 36:739.

Rieber A, Wruk D, Nussle K, et al. (1998) [MRI of the abdomen combined with enteroclysis in Crohn disease using oral and intravenous Gd-DTPA]. Radiologe 38:23–28.

Rogalla P, Mutze S, Hamm B (1996): Body CT: state-of-the-art. Munich: W. Zuckschwerdt.

Rogalla P, Werner Rustner M, Huitema A, van Est A, Meiri N, Hamm B (1998) Virtual endoscopy of the small bowel: phantom study and preliminary clinical results. Eur Radiol 8:563–567.

Schatzki R (1988) Small intestinal enema. By Richard Schatzki, 1942. AJR Am J Roentgenol 150:499–507.

Sellink JL (1974) Radiologic examination of the small intestine by duodenal intubation. Acta Radiol (Stockh) 15:318–332.

Sellink JL (1976) Proceedings: Why enteroclysis of the small intestine? Br J Radiol 49:288–289.

Sellink JL, Rosenbusch G (1981) ["The ten commandments" for enteroclysis or ten golden rules for proper enteroclysis technique]. Radiologe 21:366–376.

Semelka RC, John G, Kelekis NL, Burdeny DA, Ascher SM (1996) Small bowel neoplastic disease: demonstration by MRI. J Magn Reson Imaging 6:855–860.

Serour F, Dona G, Birkenfeld S, Balassiano M, Krispin M (1992) Primary neoplasms of the small bowel. J Surg Oncol 49:29–34.

Siegel MJ, Evans SJ, Balfe DM (1988) Small bowel disease in children: diagnosis with CT. Radiology 169:127–130.

Silverman PM (1994): Handbook of helical (spiral) computed tomography: techniques & protocols. Corona Del Mar, CA, USA: Mallinckrodt Medical, Inc. by Med Write, Inc.

Stenbygaard LE, Sorensen JB (1999) Small bowel metastases in non-small cell lung cancer. Lung Cancer 26:95–101.

Thoeni RF, Filson RG (1988) Abdominal and pelvic CT: use of oral metoclopramide to enhance bowel opacification. Radiology 169:391–393.

Thoeni RF, Rogalla P (1994) Current CT/MRI examination of the lower intestinal tract. Baillieres Clin Gastroenterol 8:765–796.

Van Dam J, Brugge WR (1999) Endoscopy of the upper gastrointestinal tract. N Engl J Med 341:1738–1748.

Westerman AM, Wilson JH (1999) Peutz-Jeghers syndrome: risks of a hereditary condition. Scand J Gastroenterol Suppl 230:64–70.

Wills JS, Lobis IF, Denstman FJ (1997) Crohn disease: state of the art. Radiology 202:597–610.

Zaman A, Katon RM (1998) Push enteroscopy for obscure gastrointestinal bleeding yields a high incidence of proximal lesions within reach of a standard endoscope. Gastrointest Endosc 47:372–376.

6 Virtual Endoscopy of the Colon

P. Rogalla, N. Meiri, and C.I. Bartram

CONTENTS

P. Rogalla, MD; N. Meiri, RD
Department of Radiology, Charité Hospital, Humboldt-Universität zu Berlin, Schumannstrasse 20/21, 10117 Berlin, Germany
C.I. Bartram, MD
St Mark's Hospital, Northwick Park, Harrow, HA1 3UJ, UK

6.1 The Investigation

P. Rogalla, N. Meiri

6.1.1 Background

Colorectal cancer represents the third most frequently diagnosed cancer world-wide, and the second most diagnosed cancer in industrialised Western countries (Eddy 1990; Landis et al. 1998; Silverberg et al. 1990). For the United States, it is estimated that 129,000 new cases were diagnosed in 1999 (Cancer Facts and Figures 1999); however, when malignant polyps are considered, the true yearly incidence of colorectal cancer probably approaches 160,000 (Landis et al. 1998). Enormous geographical differences exist among countries, in certain instances, with respect to the incidence of colorectal cancer. For example, it is higher in Scotland than in England, and the incidence in both northern Italy and the northern United States is higher than in the southern areas of these countries (Devesa and Chow 1993). With regard to the difference between the two sexes in the occurrence of colorectal cancer, there has been little apparent change in the past 70 years: reports exist from 1922 revealing a predominance in men in a ratio of 6:5 (Schmieden and Scheele 1922), with rectal carcinoma occurring twice as often in men as in women.
In an evaluation of more than 120,000 patients with colorectal cancer in the USA in 1993, men were affected more often than women in both the black (ratio 6:5) and the white (ratio 7:5) populations (Devesa and Chow 1993). An interesting aspect of this study was that in the proximal regions of the colon this relation between the sexes was practically unnoticeable, but the further distal the cancer, the higher the proportion of men affected by it.

The age at onset has appeared to increase over the last few decades. While in 1922 the age of 40–60 years was given as the time of onset, recent reports indicate a peak incidence between the 70th and 80th years of life (Baron et al. 1994; Chu et al. 1994; Crucitti et al. 1995). Early detection and preventive removal of premalignant adenomatous polyps are believed to be the most probable reasons for the gradual decrease in both incidence and mortality since 1985 (SEER 1995). For an asymptomatic individual without any known risk factors for developing colorectal cancer, the likelihood that a malignant tumour will develop in the large intestine is nevertheless estimated at 6%. According to statistical analyses, life expectancy decreases by 6–7 years for patients with colorectal cancer (Boring et al. 1993), and the 5-year survival rate decreases from 45% for patients with locally confined colorectal cancer to 5% for patients with metastatic disease at the time of diagnosis.

The value of primary prevention of colorectal cancer has been under discussion, especially since epidemiological studies have shown that various dietary components appear to play an influential role in its development. It is widely held that lack of fibre in the diet is an important factor in the high incidence of colorectal cancer in Western countries. Since the early 1970s it has been suggested that, by reducing intestinal transit time and by acting as a diluent, dietary fibre could reduce the exposure of the large intestinal mucosa to potential carcinogens (Burkitt 1971). This hypothesis has gained support from epidemiological studies (Modan et al. 1975) and from recent work on the effect of fibre on mucosal cell turnover (Rooney et al. 1994). It has been suggested that another dietary influence is animal fat: a diet rich in animal fats not only causes increased excretion of bile salts in the faeces, but also promotes the growth of bacteria that can degrade bile salts to carcinogens (Imray et al. 1992; Modan et al. 1975). Furthermore, epidemiological studies have shown that a diet lacking in vegetables is associated with colorectal cancer (Leitzmann 1998; Modan et al. 1975), and it is believed that vegetables may increase the activity of colonic enzymes which protect against carcinogens. In a meta-analysis conducted in 1998, the authors found coffee consumption of more than four cups per day to have a protective role against development of colorectal cancer, but this applied only to populations in northern and southern Europe and Asia, not to the United States (Giovannucci 1998).

Despite this strong evidence accumulated over the years, some researchers still question the protective role of fibre intake against the development of colorectal cancer, since these results were not reproducible in a large, longitudinal epidemiological study in an American female population who semi-quantitatively reported their fibre intake (Fuchs et al. 1999). Further, more precise studies may be necessary to elucidate this discrepancy.

In an effort to identify individuals at increased risk of developing a colorectal adenoma, a cohort study of 47,723 male health professionals polled by repeated questionnaires (Giovannucci et al. 1995a) identified elevated body mass index, waist circumference, and waist-to-hip ratio as risk factors for colon carcinoma. Obesity and physical inactivity were associated with adenomas larger than 1 cm. In a cohort of 644 people with a family history of colorectal carcinoma who were screened by colonoscopy (Gaglia et al. 1995), the risk of adenoma increased with advancing age, male gender, and family history of "hereditary non-polyposis colorectal cancer" (HNPCC). The most significant predictor was the presence of cancer or adenoma in two or more generations of a family (regardless of HNPCC history).

Nevertheless, the recommendation to maintain a desirable body weight, reduce the intake of fat, especially saturated fats, alcoholic drinks (particularly beer), salt and smoked or grilled meat, and to consume plenty of fresh fruits and vegetables which contain fibre, antioxidants and phytochemicals – components currently recognised to play a preventive role – remains (Shike et al. 1990). Nicotine promotes the development of colonic adenomas, whereas, as proven for rectal cancer, physical activity has a protective role (Leitzmann 1998). Noteworthy is also the fact that patients who take prostaglandin synthesis inhibitors, such as Aspirin, on a regular basis show a 50% reduced risk for the growth of a malignant tumour in the colon or rectum (Giovannucci et al. 1995b).

6.1.2 Screening for Colorectal Polyps: Is It Useful?

6.1.2.1 Adenomatous Polyps

Approximately one-half to two-thirds of all colorectal polyps are of the adenomatous type, and by the age of 50 years, these may be found in about 25% of the population. The incidence increases with age and the possibility of malignant transformation with size. It is now widely accepted that:

- The prevalence of premalignant adenomas correlates well with the prevalence of carcinomas, the average age of adenoma patients being approx. 5

years lower than that of patients with carcinomas (Muto et al. 1975; Winawer et al. 1987).

- Adenomatous tissue often accompanies cancerous tissue, and it is unusual to find small cancers with no contiguous adenomatous tissue (Morson 1966).
- Sporadic adenomas are identical histologically to the adenomas of familial adenomatous polyposis (FAP), and the latter condition is unequivocally premalignant (Debinski et al. 1996; Wyman and Shorthouse 1996).
- Premalignant adenomatous polyps larger than 1 cm are more likely to display cellular atypia and chromosomal abnormalities than are smaller polyps (Muto et al. 1975; Winawer et al. 1997).
- The distribution of adenomas over the various colon segments is similar to that of carcinomas (Granqvist 1981).
- Adenomas are found in up to one-third of all surgical specimens resected for colorectal cancer (Chu et al. 1986; Eide 1986) (Fig. 6.1).

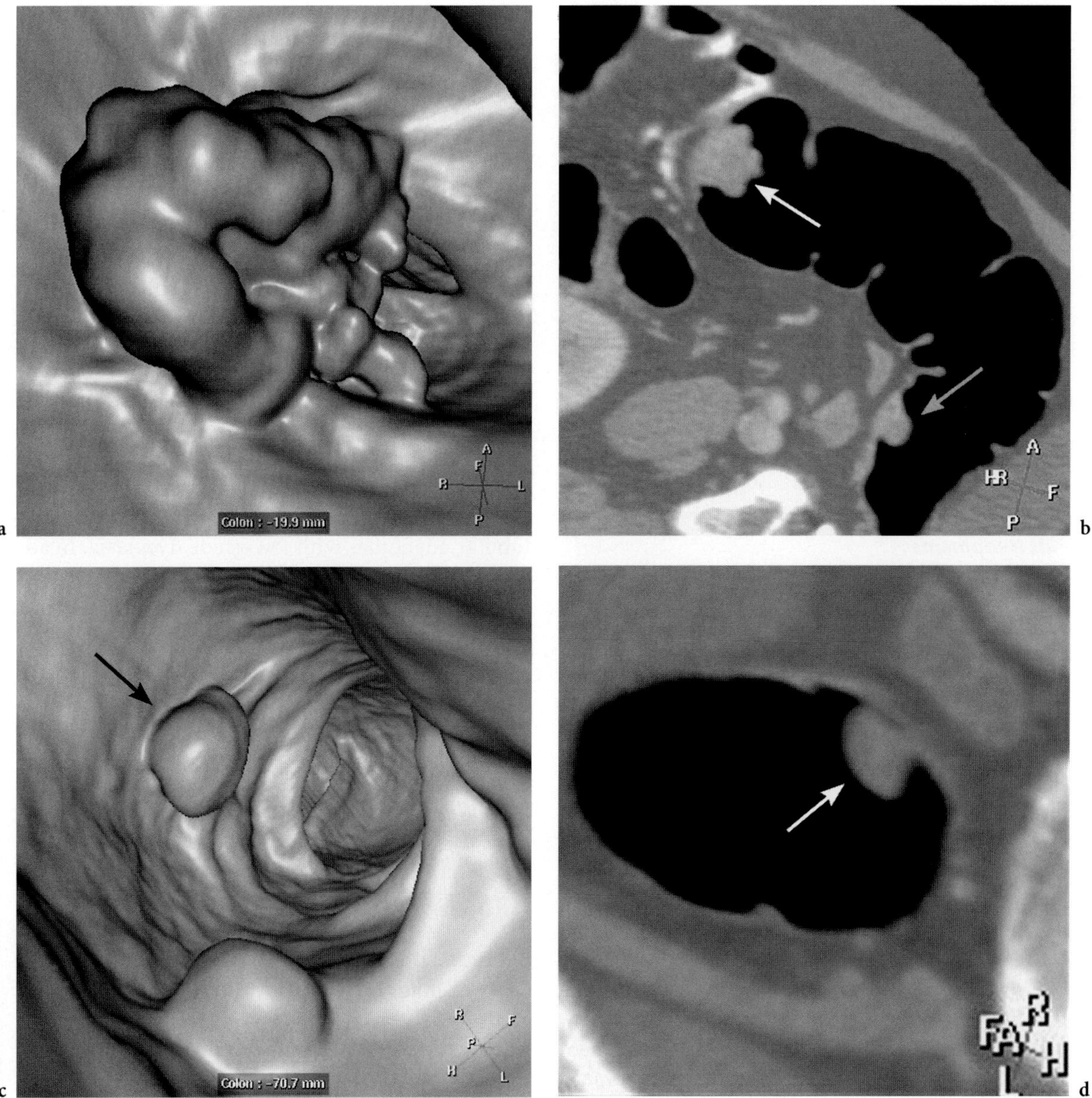

Fig. 6.1a–d. A 58-year-old man with multiple carcinoma manifestations. **a** The virtual endoscopy of a colon carcinoma in the descending colon. **b** A multiplanar reconstruction (MPR) through the bowel, showing the carcinoma (*white arrow*) in addition to a distally located polyp (*grey arrow*). **c** The virtual view of the polyp shows, however, a further smaller pedunculated polyp (*arrow*), displayed in an enlarged format as MPR in image **d.** In the framework of a total colectomy, a total of four carcinomas and at least nine adenomatous polyps were described

If the tumour is restricted to the bowel wall (WHO stages T1 and T2), it can be surgically resected with curative intent; however, individuals with T1 and T2 tumours are usually asymptomatic and therefore usually do not seek medical attention, so the tumour remains undetected. Moreover, 75% of colorectal cancers occur in individuals who do not belong to a risk group according to the current classification (Burt 1997). Bearing in mind that malignant transformation is found in approx. 1% of polyps less than 1 cm in size, compared to 10% of larger polyps (Muto et al. 1975; Winawer et al. 1997), early detection of colorectal polyps by screening asymptomatic individuals without any risk factors (and re-evaluating who should be in the target group) might be regarded as one of the leading goals in health care management.

6.1.2.2 Definition of Screening Technique

A screening technique is defined as the examination of individuals at risk of a disease prior to the development of symptoms. The disease for which the individuals are being screened must be common and severe, and the effectiveness of early detection for the prognosis must be proven. With colorectal cancer, both these conditions are unequivocally fulfilled.

6.1.2.3 Flat Neoplasms

Although the evidence that screening for colorectal cancer can reduce mortality (Byers et al. 1997; Winawer et al. 1997), individuals at risk of developing this disease remain largely under-screened. Although a considerable number of flat and depressed colorectal neoplasms have been reported in Japan (Kudo 1993), colorectal cancer mainly develops through precursors, and the "adenoma–dysplasia–carcinoma sequence" is still valid, giving rise to a need for an early preventive intervention such as endoscopic polyp removal, by which the subsequent development of colorectal cancer can be prevented (Murakami et al. 1995).

In contrast to adenomatous polyps, depressed, flat, diminutive neoplasms account for a very low percentage of the total number of colorectal neoplasms. Most reports describe small, flat, colorectal adenomas with an allegedly high malignant potential. These reports, most of which have come from Japan, assert that such lesions are common, that they may be missed during conventional colonoscopy, and that they frequently and rapidly degenerate into flat cancers. However, small, flat adenomas with a high malignant potential appear to be rare in Western countries (Bond 1995).

Early submucosal invasion (Fig. 6.2) is characteristic of the flat type of carcinoma (Kudo 1993), which is distinguished by rapid growth and the potential to arise de novo (Nakamura 1994). In a series of 3824 colorectal neoplasms, 2.7% (105), including 8 invasive carcinomas, with a size of 5 mm or less were classified as depressed, and only 1.5% (22) of 1475 neoplasms measuring 6–10 mm were classified as depressed, including 11 invasive carcinomas (Kudo et al. 1995). In another series, the proportion of depressed neoplasms was indicated as 5.7% (54/930) of those with a size of 5 mm or less and 1.3% (12/930) in the range of 6–10 mm. Altogether, 2 invasive carcinomas smaller than 5 mm and 4 carcinomas measuring 6–10 mm were found in the latter series (Fujiya and Maruyama 1997). Furthermore, large North American series of diminutive colorectal polyps reported a low incidence of high-grade dysplasia or invasive cancer (Waye et al. 1988); and even when experienced Western endoscopists searched for small flat adenomas, such lesions with the gross appearance of flat adenomas, as described by Japanese researchers, were occasionally found (Lanspa et al. 1992); however, the histopathological examination of these findings almost invariably indicated benign tubular adenomas with low-grade dysplasia. In addition, the finding of a small adenoma in Western countries does not necessarily identify patients with a premalignant mucosal defect. Long-term follow-up studies of patients who had only small tubular adenomas resected at proctosigmoidoscopy indicated no increased risk of subsequent cancer.

It can be generally stated that small flat adenomas exhibit minimal clinical importance in industrialised Western countries, (Bond 1995), although this topic continues to be debated heatedly in the literature (Jaramillo et al. 1995).

6.1.3 Current Investigation Techniques

There are several prerequisites for a screening technique. It must be:
- Accurate
- Acceptable
- Feasible
- Cost-effective

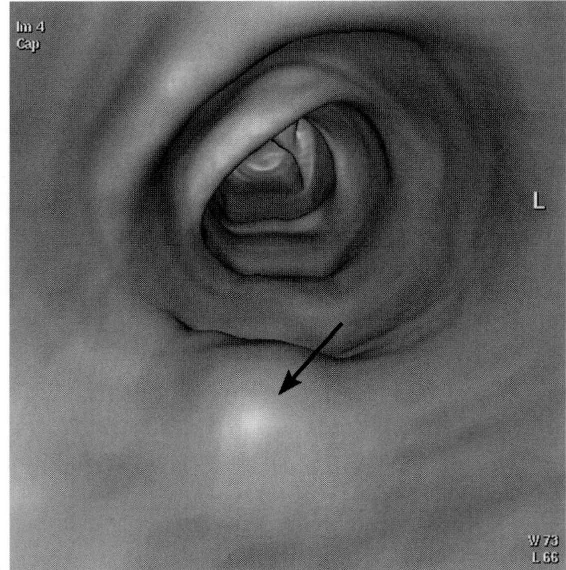

a

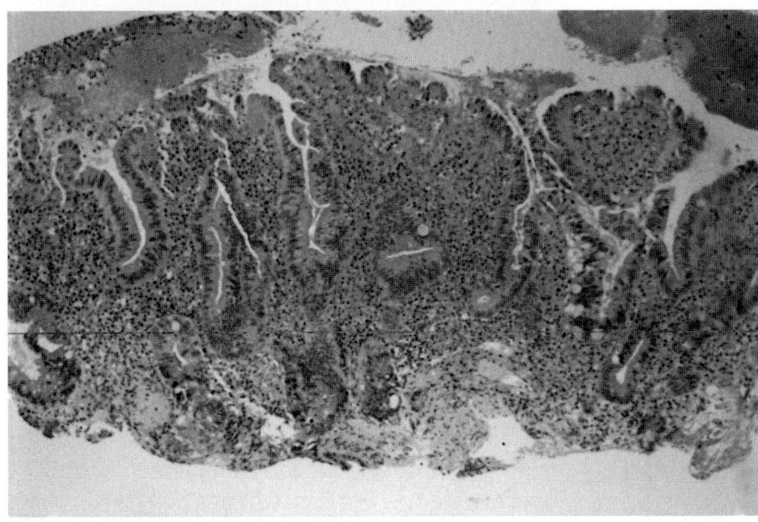

b

Fig. 6.2. a Virtual endoscopic view into the descending colon of a patient with longstanding history of ulcerative colitis. The slight bulge (*arrow*) represents a flat adenocarcinoma. **b** Histology from the flat colon carcinoma. The carcinoma grows within the mucosal layer and may not necessarily change the morphology of the mucosal surface

The American Cancer Society and the National Cancer Institute in the United States recommend for individuals at average risk a digital rectal examination and a faecal occult blood test annually, starting from the age of 45 years, and a sigmoidoscopy every 3–5 years, or a complete colonoscopy every 10 years, starting from the age of 50. As another example, health care providers in Germany reimburse physicians for an annual digital rectal examination and a faecal occult blood test, starting at the age of 45. Despite the non-invasiveness of both tests and continuing efforts of health care providers in public education, only 14% of the males in Germany take part in the screening programme. A similar poor response to screening programmes for colorectal cancer has been shown in the United States: for example, of 17,000 health care workers who had been invited to undergo a free colonoscopy, only 6% (959) responded. This reflects poor professional awareness as well as lack of acceptance of currently available tests. In one 1995 survey, respondents who had never been screened reported that they would rather sacrifice a month of life to avoid a flexible sigmoidoscopy and up to 3 months to avoid a colonoscopy (Bowdy 1998). Gender is another barrier, with women less likely (33%) than men (43%) to ever agree to a colorectal examination (Bowdy 1998). The major limitation to the widespread implementation of colorectal cancer screening has been the lack of a single test that meets all the requirements for screening.

6.1.3.1 Faecal Occult Blood Test (FOB, Haemoccult)

In the early 1970s, the FOB test was incorporated into screening programmes in most Western countries (Fig. 6.3). Its ineffectiveness can be judged from several studies: it has been shown that FOB testing results in the detection of only 30–40% of colorectal cancers and 10% of adenomatous polyps (ELLIOT et al. 1984; FROMMER et al. 1988; HOBBS et al. 1992; KRONBORG et al. 1987; REILLY et al. 1990). According to the results of the Minnesota study, the mortality due to colorectal cancer can be significantly reduced, by 33%, if the FOB test is used annually over a period of 13 years. This reduction is no longer significant (6%) if the FOB test is applied biennially (MANDEL et al. 1993). However, because the study was carried out on volunteers it was not a true randomised population study. In addition, the test used rehydrated Haemoccult, which is not very specific and resulted in a large proportion of healthy subjects (30%) undergoing subsequent negative colonoscopies.

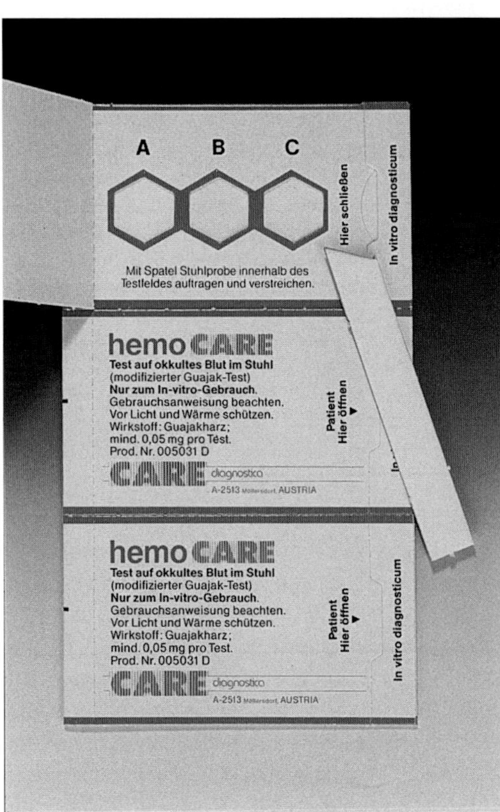

Fig. 6.3. Example of an FOB testing envelope

In a strictly population-based randomised study of 150,251 subjects aged 45–74 years (HARDCASTLE et al. 1996), a total of 893 cancers were diagnosed in the study group of which 26% were detected by screening, 28% presented as interval cancers, and 46% arose in patients who had refused the test. At a median follow-up of 7.8 years, 360 individuals had died of colorectal cancer in the study group, compared with 420 in the control group. This represents a significant reduction of 15% in cumulative mortality (95% confidence interval) in the study group. An almost identical study carried out in Denmark obtained analogous results, showing an 18% reduction in mortality (KRONBORG et al. 1996).

It can be stated that FOB screening can significantly reduce mortality from colorectal cancer, albeit modestly when applied to unselected populations. Thus, the challenge for the future should be to increase the compliance of individuals and to improve sensitivity and specificity of the screening test.

6.1.3.2 Flexible Sigmoidoscopy, Colonoscopy

Amidst the knowledge that about 70% of cancers and large adenomas are found in the distal 60 cm of the large bowel, flexible sigmoidoscopy has been proposed as a screening test (SELBY et al. 1992), and there is strong evidence that it is more sensitive than FOB testing (WHERRY and THOMAS 1994). As early as 25 years ago, it was shown that by means of repeated rectoscopy with subsequent removal of all visible polyps, the incidence of carcinomas could be decreased by 80%, and in consequent examinations, advanced cancers were not seen at all (GILBERTSEN 1974). These results have been confirmed in a case-control study: sigmoidoscopic screening can reduce the mortality rate of colorectal cancer by 70%. Furthermore, a single sigmoidoscopy has been reported to reduce the risk for a period of 10 years (SELBY et al. 1992).

Besides the fact that a colonoscopy is more expensive than a flexible sigmoidoscopy, the acceptance of colonoscopy is rather limited. Complications of diagnostic colonoscopies are mainly due to respiratory problems, and severe complications such as perforation occur predominantly in the sigmoid colon (overall rate: 0.1%). The mortality is reported to be below 0.015%, and if polyps are removed, the complication rate lies between 0.5 and 2% (FRÜHMORGEN and PFÄHLER 1990; ROGERS et al. 1975).

More important, particularly if different investigation techniques should be compared, are the miss rates for adenomatous polyps when the techniques are being used as a screening tool. In contrast to the common belief that fibreoptic endoscopy fulfils the indisputable role of the gold standard in colonic polyp screening, it has recently been confirmed that miss rates in fibreoptic colonoscopy are commonly underestimated. A total of 183 patients were endoscopically examined by an experienced endoscopist, closely followed by a second complete colonoscopy (REX et al. 1997): 27% of the polyps smaller than 5 mm, 13% of the polyps ranging from 5 to 9 mm in size, and 6% of polyps larger than 10 mm were missed upon the first colonoscopy, an overall miss rate of 24% (Table 6.1). Furthermore, in an analysis of 47 patients who had undergone complete colonoscopy within the past 3 years (HASEMAN et al. 1997), the authors could prove that in half of the patients the colon was not completely investigated, and the rest of the cancers were simply overlooked.

Table 6.1. Flexible colonoscopy: miss rates of polyps

Polyp size	Miss rate
<5 mm	27%
5–9 mm	13%
>10 mm	6%
All sizes	24%

Source: REX et al. 1997

Nevertheless, a cost-effectiveness study has shown that screening for colorectal polyps and cancer with sigmoidoscopy and faecal occult blood testing may not be cost-effective compared to screening with flexible colonoscopy of the entire colon (LIEBERMAN 1991). The author calculated the costs of preventing one death from colon cancer as $444,133 with sigmoidoscopy versus $347,214 with colonoscopy.

6.1.3.3 Double-Contrast Barium Enema

Numerous published results on the efficacy of double-contrast barium enema (DCBE) are available (BOLIN et al. 1988; BRADY et al. 1994; FORK 1981; FORK 1983). DCBE has been shown to be easier, cheaper and, in a more recent study, considerably safer than flexible endoscopy (BLAKEBOROUGH et al. 1997), with only one death in 56,786 DCBEs performed; safety is therefore five times greater than that of diagnostic total colonoscopy. In symptomatic patients, the sensitivity of barium enema for colorectal cancer is 65% to 75%, while its sensitivity for colorectal cancer in asymptomatic persons with a positive faecal occult blood test varies from 50% to 75% (JOHNSON et al. 1996; KEWENTER et al. 1995). Considerable energy has been devoted to the discussion of the relative merits of double-contrast enema and fibreoptic colonoscopy. Many of these studies have misleadingly compared examinations done by operators with widely varying degrees of experience and interest. In comparing results, it is essential that the examinations to be compared were both performed at a state-of-the-art level.

As already mentioned above, it is important to realise that there is an error rate inherent in flexible colonoscopy (GLICK et al. 1989). This is due in part to the fact that the caecum is not reached in a significant proportion of colonoscopies (HASEMAN et al. 1997; OBRECHT et al. 1984); additionally, there are significant endoscopic blind spots in the colon, resulting in overlooked polyps as demonstrated on double-contrast enema (LAUFER et al. 1976; MILLER and LEHMANN 1978). Vice versa, it must be stressed that false-positive and false-negative results in barium enema studies (FORK 1988) may occur in up to 1% and 7% of cases, respectively, and these errors usually occur in the sigmoid colon and caecum (ANDERSON et al. 1991; NORFLEET et al. 1991).

Discrepancies between radiological and endoscopic findings are not infrequent. In such instances, it should not automatically be assumed that the endoscopic findings are correct. It is clear that generally the results achieved with good quality colonoscopy and double-contrast enemas are comparable, especially when considering polyps greater than 1 cm in diameter (REX et al. 1986). Furthermore, little doubt exists that on barium enema studies, the precise position of a tumour can be determined (Fig. 6.4), a task which may prove difficult in flexible endoscopy considering that the only reliable landmarks are the anus and the terminal ileum (FRAGER et al. 1987). The combination of DCBE and flexible sigmoidoscopy has been shown to work well, with 100% sensitivity for detection of cancer and polyps larger than 5 mm in size (BLAKEBOROUGH et al. 1997).

6.1.3.4 Conventional CT, Spiral CT, and MRI

Although both endoscopic and double-contrast barium studies afford high accuracy, neither permits assessment of the depth of tumour infiltration or the spreading of the tumour to distant sites. Cross-sectional CT and MRI images of the abdomen and pelvis permit precise measurements of the thickness of the colonic wall, determination of the anatomical relationship of the colon to other abdominal and pelvic

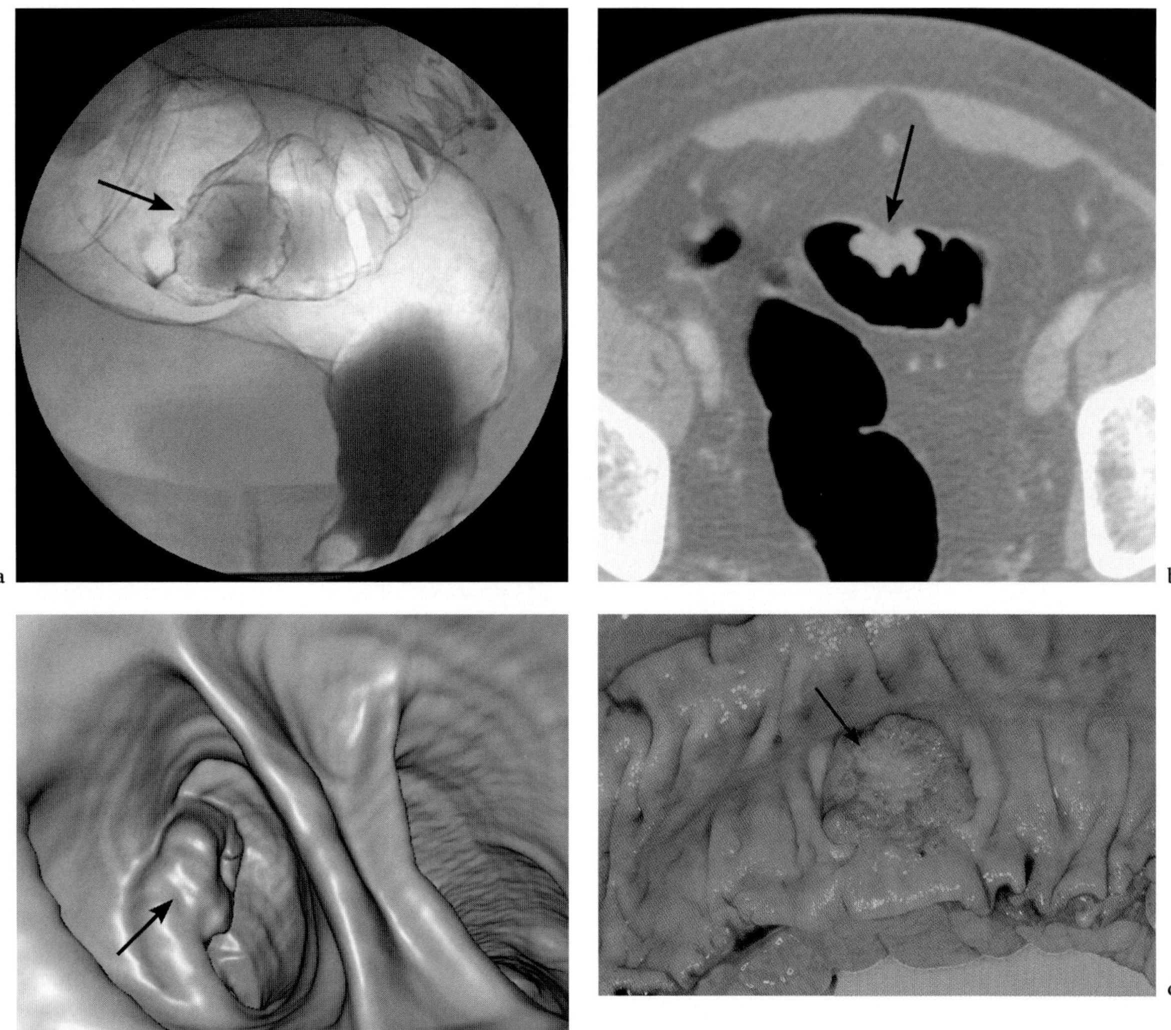

Fig. 6.4a–d. Double-contrast barium enema, axial CT slice, virtual endoscopy and histopathological specimen of the same tumour in the sigmoid colon. The central ulceration of the tumour is visible in all three images (**a–c**) as well as on the surgical specimen (**d**)

organs, and detection of the presence or absence of metastases to lymph nodes, adrenal glands, liver, bony structures or adjacent musculature (Thoeni and Rogalla 1994). Although CT and MRI offer many advantages for obtaining information on the extension of a tumour beyond the colonic wall (Husband et al. 1980), neither is a primary modality for evaluating patients with suspected tumours of the colon. Early and subtle changes of the mucosal surface and lesions less than 5 mm in diameter usually are not detected by conventional or spiral CT or MRI because often the rectum and colon are incompletely distended. Also, any retained and adherent faecal matter can result in an erroneous diagnosis of a colorectal neoplasm (Fig. 6.5). On cross sections, the rectum, the rectosigmoid and the ascending and descending colon are easily evaluated because of their fixed pelvic or retroperitoneal positions. Tumours in the hepatic and splenic flexures and transverse colon were previously less readily examined by cross-sectional imaging because colonic peristalsis and diaphragmatic excursions rendered these parts of the colon more difficult to evaluate (Thoeni and Rogalla 1995); however, with the use of spiral CT and fast pulse sequences in MRI, most of these problems have been eliminated.

CT results can be improved through the use of a relatively large and rapidly delivered bolus of intravenous contrast agent and rapid scanning. As CT

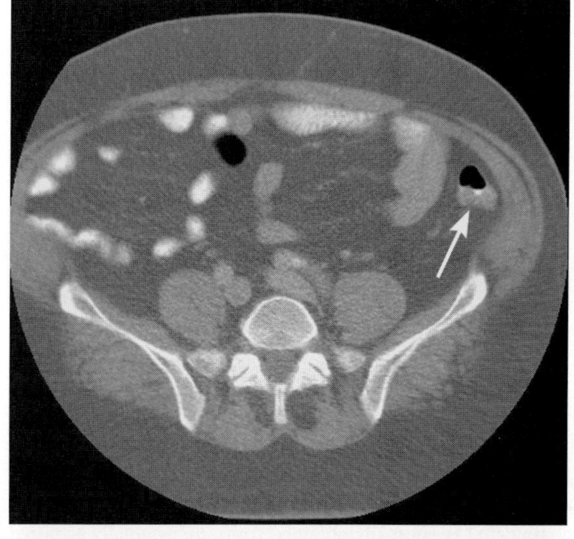

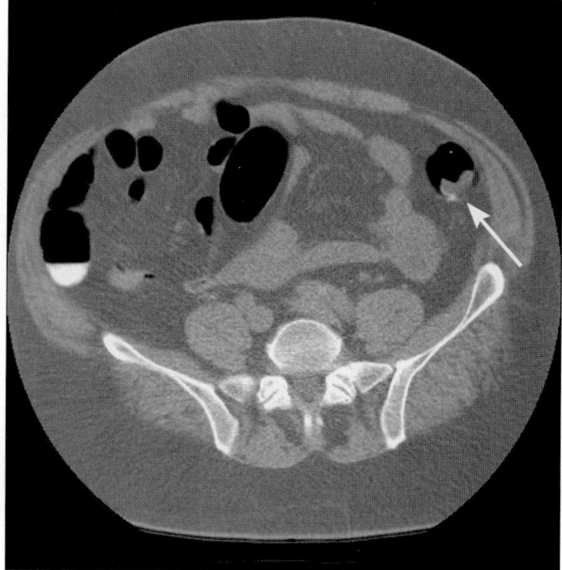

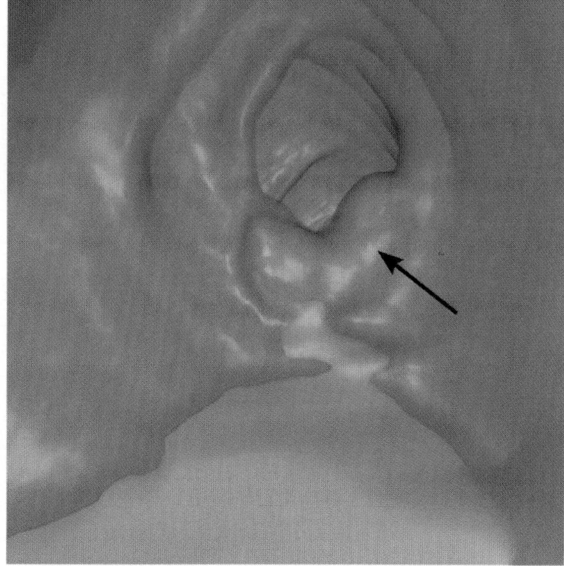

Fig. 6.5. a Abdominal CT scan after standard preparation with oral and rectal contrast material. A tumour (colorectal carcinoma) is hardly distinguishable (*arrow*) in the poorly dilated descending colon. **b, c** Re-examination of the same patient following the firm clinical suspicion of a colorectal carcinoma. Imaging in pneumocolon technique. The colorectal carcinoma is clearly demonstrated (*arrow*, **b**) in a well-dilated colon. Since staging was carried out during the initial examination, intravenous contrast agent was not used in the second session. The virtual endoscopy (**c**) displays the bowl-like carcinoma (*arrow*)

usually is used for staging and not for detecting of colonic lesions, thin sections of 3–5 mm width may facilitate demonstration of even small lesions. Nevertheless, it appears that CT rarely matches the resolution of density differences in the soft tissue which MRI can provide in the pelvis, with or without fat suppression and with or without gadolinium enhancement (Yee et al. 1994). In a recent study, the colon was filled with a water enema and subsequently examined in CT (Hundt et al. 1999). By means of a biphasic scanning protocol with a spiral run in the arterial and venous phase, the authors were able to attain sensitivity of 97.2% in the arterial phase and 89.1% in the venous phase for the detection of colonic carcinoma. Moreover, the accuracy of the staging results was a remarkable 81% for the arterial and 64.8% for the venous phase.

6.1.3.5 Ultrasonography

Due to the physical characteristics of acoustic waves, ultrasonography has played a rather limited role in the evaluation of the large bowel. However, some effort has been undertaken to strengthen the value of ultrasonography for the detection of colonic masses (Fig. 6.6) and even adenomatous polyps. Being relatively inexpensive, broadly available and free of radiation exposure, ultrasonography could represent an ideal screening technique, especially accom-

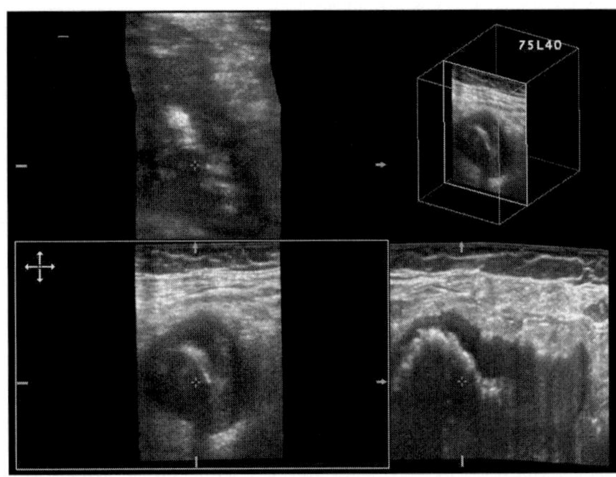

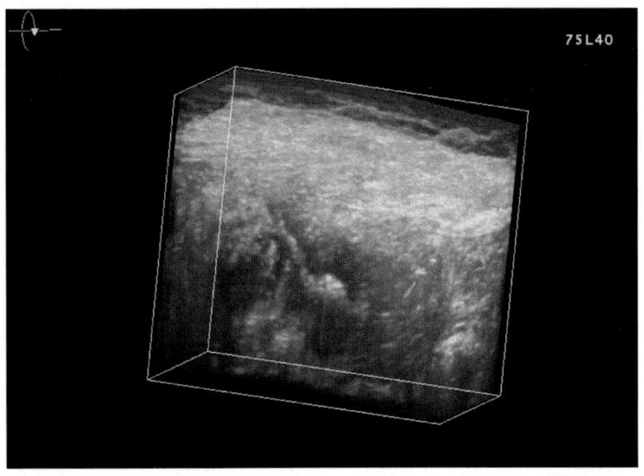

Fig. 6.6a, b. Ultrasound image of a colorectal carcinoma. With a location of the tumour relatively close to the abdominal wall, excellent demonstration of the tumour in US can be achieved (stage upon surgery: T3N1M0). By means of advanced software packages US images can also be processed into 3D displays. The real-time 3D image can be viewed from any perspective. The important diagnostic information (infiltration depth, lymphadenopathy etc.) is optimally obtained from the originally acquired cross-sectional images

modating applications in the paediatric population (Walter et al. 1992).

Despite highly promising results in a study conducted on 220 patients with colonoscopic correlation (Limberg 1990), where sensitivity of 91% for polyps larger than 7 mm and sensitivity of 94% along with specificity of 100% for colon cancers are reported, similar results have not been confirmed. Strikingly, the most recent study (Chui et al. 1994) revealed overall sensitivity of 6.9% for identifying polyps in the colon after filling the entire colon with water, and sensitivity of 12.5% for polyps equal to or more than 7 mm in diameter. In 52 subjects, the "hydrocolonic" ultrasound suggested the presence of five masses which could not be confirmed by colonoscopy. In addition, the ultrasound could not be completed due to complications related to the colonic filling with water. The authors concluded that ultrasound, even after colonic filling, is not suitable for polyp or cancer screening. In any case one must keep in mind that the results of sonographic examinations are strongly examiner-dependent.

6.1.4 The New Investigation Technique: Virtual Colonoscopy

6.1.4.1 Terminology

Although the new imaging technique – virtual colonoscopy – has been available to radiologists for more than 4 years, the terminology is still an unsettled issue. There are several suggestions, such as CT colography, CT colonography, CT pneumocolon or simply pneumocolon, all of which are more or less scientifically precise; however, while accurate, these terms are relatively uninformative to the broad medical and lay audience and a consensus as to the preferred version does not yet exist.

Alluding to the fact that the new imaging technique displays views into organs that have been purely calculated from cross-sectional data, alluding to the fact that surfaces, colours, shapes and light reflections are artificial and may have little to nothing in common with the reality imaged by CT or MRI, the less rigorous but more appealing and inclusive term "virtual colonoscopy" is preferred by many. This choice is not without precedence in the recent history of introducing new imaging modalities to the medical and lay public. More than 20 years ago, when computed tomography initially became available to radiologists as a new imaging technique, two radiologists published in the *New England Journal of Medicine*, using the term "CAT scanning" in their description of a then prevalent infectious disease, *cat* scratch fever. Professionals as well as patients and the lay public still understand and use the term "CAT scanning", regardless of the fact that the established and prevailing abbreviation is CT. Similarly, the term "virtual endoscopy" contains no information on the source data from which the images were calculated. Although in the recent past imaging parameters such as slice thicknesses, imaging speed, and imaging strategies have greatly converged between CT and MRI, some differences will remain between the two modalities, and it can be expected that the terms "CT colonography" and "MR colonography" will be perpetuated alongside "virtual colonography".

6.1.4.2
Source Data Requirements

In principle, any imaging modality delivering cross-sectional information is suitable for virtual colonoscopy. At present, CT and MRI represent the primary imaging sources. To avoid misregistration, the modality should provide continuous data information. For CT the use of spiral acquisition mode with overlapping reconstructions, and for MRI breathhold pulse sequences delivering gapless slice information, are mandatory. Similar to all other applications of virtual endoscopy, the basic, very simple rule is: *The thinner the slices, the better the spatial resolution,* and as a consequence of this, the smaller the polyps that can still be detected.

As discussed in the chapter covering the small intestine, the smallest polyp detectable has approximately the same size as the primary slice thickness. If spiral CT with 5-mm beam collimation has been used in the abdomen, it can be expected that the majority of polyps smaller than 5 mm will escape detection. By reconstructing overlapping slices at half the distance of the primary slice thickness, a 5-mm polyp will be imaged on two slices, being the minimum requirement to allow visualization on the reconstructed endoscopic view (Nyquist theorem).

Currently, most authors use spiral CT for virtual colonoscopy (Ahlquist et al. 1997; Beaulieu et al. 1998; Hara et al. 1996; Vining 1997). Further debate as to whether CT or MRI (Luboldt et al. 1998c) is superior for virtual endoscopy can certainly be expected. Magnetic resonance imaging has the undeniable advantages of not utilising ionising radiation and of providing better soft-tissue contrast resolution (Luboldt and Debatin 1998), but its disadvantages include limited availability, greater costs, longer examination time, and lower patient acceptance.

With the introduction of multislice CT scanners that are capable of scanning up to 8 times faster than the current spiral CT scanners, improving the *z*-axis resolution to the extent that there is no difference between the *x*-, *y*- and *z*-axis (isotropic voxel scanning), and reconstructing the images at more than twice the current rate, the debate as to which method is superior is far from settled. Thus, the following explanation refers principally to CT, and the potential for MRI in reference to specific aspects is mentioned.

In a phantom study (Beaulieu et al. 1998), the authors evaluated the influence of CT acquisition parameters on lesion detectability and sizing. Spherical lesions of 2.5, 4, 6, 8, and 10 mm in diameter were randomly placed in a bowel phantom, which was scanned with 3 mm slice thickness and pitch factors of 1:1 and 2:1, as well as with 5 mm slice thickness and pitch factor of 1:1. The 4-mm beads could be detected with 100% at 3 and 5 mm slice thickness, whereas 2.5-mm beads at 5 mm slice thickness or scans with a pitch of 2:1 were detected in only 78–94% of the cases. The authors concluded that 4-mm lesions require a slice width of at least 5 mm to be reliably detected.

6.1.4.3
Patient Preparation

The patient preparation for virtual endoscopy is more or less identical to the preparation established for DCBEs or flexible colonoscopy. The primary goal of the preparation is to empty the large bowel of its natural content. There are several medications on the market (Prepacol, Fleet, Klean-Prep, X-Prep, Picolax, Dulcolax, GoLytely, etc.), all of which consist of a mixture of salts and electrolytes. There have been numerous investigations evaluating the optimal bowel preparation technique for flexible colonoscopy (Drew et al. 1997; Sharma et al. 1997). In a recent study comparing oral sodium phosphate (NaP, Fleet) with polyethylene glycol electrolyte solution (PEG) the authors concluded that NaP cleans the colon as well as PEG but results in significant cost savings and improved patient compliance (O'Donovan et al. 1997). In our experience, the patients have tolerated NaP quite well, and the cleansing results are better than with any other preparation technique. However, the contraindications of NaP must be taken into consideration, most importantly, renal failure (Vukasin et al. 1997).

6.1.4.4
Spasmolytic Medication

It is recommendable to have the patient empty the bowels immediately before being placed onto the CT table to assure that the rectum contains as little remaining fluid as possible. After placing a rectal tube (Fig. 6.7), a spasmolytic agent should be administered either intravenously or intramuscularly. Both agents currently in clinical use (*N*-butylscopolamine and glucagon) can be chosen, depending on personal preference, availability, or official approval. However, there are several indications in the literature that the use of Buscopan (*N*-butylscopolamine) is preferable to glu-

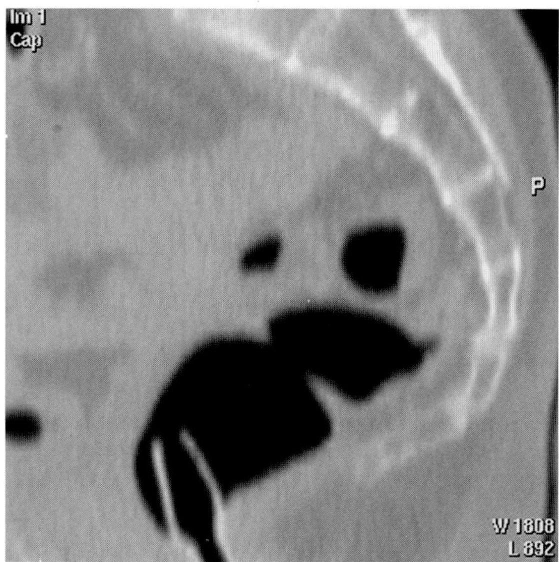

a

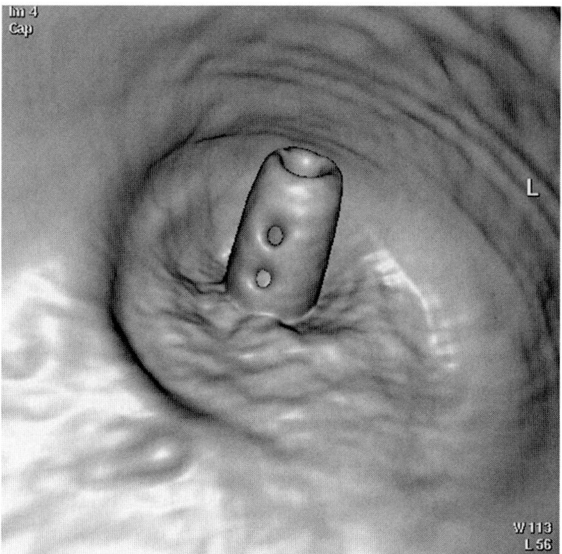

b

Fig. 6.7a, b. Sagittal and virtual reconstruction of the rectum with a rectal tube in place. The placement of the rectal tube should always proceed with maximal caution, possibly only after a digital exploration. The rectal digital examination should serve the diagnostic purpose of rectal carcinoma screening as well as prevent a perforation associated with forced placement of the rectal tube in the presence of a stenosis resulting from a carcinoma

cagon not only with respect to costs but also the improved distension of the colon. Recent investigations have even shown that the intravenous administration of glucagon has absolutely no influence on the colonic distension in virtual endoscopy (Morrin et al. 1999b; Yee et al. 1999), and considering the additional cost of approximately 50 Euros its use is therefore unjustifiable. Consequently, it was shown that glucagon also does not increase the polyp detection rate.

In a study on 124 patients, either 1 mg glucagon, 20 mg Buscopan or a placebo (physiological saline) was randomly injected intravenously. The authors reported that Buscopan led to better distension, especially of the rectosigmoid colon (Goei et al. 1995); however, the side effects of Buscopan, that is, the possibility of temporary visual impairment, should be considered, and patient consent must be obtained prior to the examination (Goei et al. 1995; Sissons et al. 1991). Furthermore, the contraindications for Buscopan must be regarded; they include glaucoma, prostatic hypertrophy, and heart disease (Cittadini et al. 1998; Fink and Aylward 1995).

6.1.4.5 Bowel Distension and Filling

6.1.4.5.1 Computed Tomography

Once the rectal tube has been placed, the colon can be insufflated either with room air by means of a balloon or with pressure-controlled carbon dioxide. In a study of ours, 40 patients were randomly separated into two groups: 19 received colon insufflation with carbon dioxide and 21 with room air assisted by a balloon-pump. The diameter of the colon was measured in four different positions in each patient and averaged per group. The results showed a trend towards superior distension with carbon dioxide (4.3 cm for CO_2 versus 3.5 cm for room air, p=0.07). This effect is most likely due to the fact that the intestinal mucosa passively resorbs the CO_2 via the lipid phase of the membranes, and the patient can then eliminate the gas through exhalation. This improves the patient's ability to tolerate the CO_2, and consequently discomfort is experienced at a later point in time than if room air were to be insufflated. As a result, the colon is better distended once insufflation is ended. In another series of 47 patients who were examined with a CO_2 insufflation followed by flexible colonoscopy, no complications arose, including during the consequent polypectomy with an electrical loop cutter.

6.1.4.5.2 Magnetic Resonance Imaging

MRI requires complete filling of the colon with fluid once a bowel cleansing procedure has been completed. This can be done with a mixture of water and gadolinium-DTPA in a 100:1 dilution (Luboldt and Debatin 1998). In addition, other contrast media, for example, manganese phosphate and iron glycerophosphate, have been evaluated with regard to providing contrast in the colonic lumen, acceptability to the patient and cost (LUBOLDT et al. 1998b). The addition of 0.8% cellulose as an enema additive increases the viscosity of the mixture and is reported to facilitate rectal filling. By applying ultrafast MRI sequences with fluoroscopic capabilities, the progress of the enema can be followed to assure optimal filling of the colon.

6.1.4.6 Scanning Techniques, Image Acquisition

6.1.4.6.1 Computed Tomography

Most authors perform the CT scanning direction from cranial to caudal (FENLON et al. 1998; HARA et al. 1997; JOHNSON et al. 1997; ROYSTER et al. 1997). This procedure is justified by the limited speed of the CT scanner and the goal of examining the whole abdomen with one spiral scan, during which the patients would be expected to hold their breath for more than 40–60 s. Although our experience is that most patients who have been adequately trained are capable of attaining a 30-s breathhold, it is not so problematic when scanning from top to bottom if the patient takes a shallow breath towards the end of the interval. At this point, the spiral has reached the pelvic area and breathing motion is hardly a disturbance.

Most of the current standard spiral CTs allow a scan duration of more than 50–60 s. Consequently, in most cases it is possible to continuously scan the entire abdomen and pelvis in one spiral run. Slice thicknesses between 3 and 5 mm at table speeds varying between 5 and 10 mm/s have been used to acquire a single spiral run. An examination separated into two scans entails the risk that the patient will move between the scans or that the second breathhold does not have the same depth as the first one, which means that a gap between the two spiral scans can occur. Hence, an accordingly large overlap zone of at least 3–4 cm should be included between the spiral scans.

Some authors suggest scanning the patient in prone and supine position (FENLON et al. 1998; HARA 1998). In a study of 48 patients with 51 colonoscopically proven polyps larger than 5 mm (HARA 1998), prone and supine image sets were compared to the supine image sets alone. A total of 12 additional polyps larger than 5 mm were detected on prone and supine exams compared to the supine exam only, a difference which was found to be statistically significant (p=0.004). Figure 6.8 demonstrates a non-distended sigmoid colon in which the lack of distension prevented detection of a 13-mm polyp in the first virtual endoscopic reconstruction of CT data obtained from a patient examined in the prone position. Only by repeating the spiral CT solely over the targeted area in the sigmoid colon without reinsufflation of carbon dioxide could the 13-mm polyp be unmistakably displayed.

However, it needs to be emphasised that by scanning the patient in supine and prone position, not only the radiation exposure is doubled (when CT is the imaging modality), but also the number of reconstructed images, the transmission time of the images to the workstation, the postprocessing and, of course, the interpretation time. After judicious consideration, one might, however, assume that with optimal patient preparation, optimal use of spasmolytic medication, careful and experienced rectal gas insufflation until immediately before scanning starts and optimal patient coaching during the breathhold, a second examination in the prone position is rarely needed. Most CT scanners today have almost instant image reconstruction so that the radiologist can decide, while the patient is still on the table, whether an additional scan, conceivably focused only on a limited part of the bowel, is required to assure ample evaluation of the entire bowel.

6.1.4.6.2 Magnetic Resonance Imaging

If MRI is intended to be used as the imaging modality, fast breathhold sequences, both T1- and T2-weighted, such as TSE, HASTE and FLASH-2D, have been proposed and evaluated. Additionally, examinations have been conducted to determine which contrast medium and in which dilution, if applied as a liquid enema in the large intestine, would result in optimal contrast between the bowel lumen and the bowel wall (LUBOLDT et al. 1998a).

6.1.4.6.3 Intravenous Contrast

The diagnostic value of intravenous contrast material in the history of computed tomography is well known, and its standard usage today belongs to state-of-the-art CT (ROGALLA et al. 1996). The benefits, especially in liver diagnostics and consequently for the detection of liver metastases, are indisputable. On the other hand, the issue of whether or not intravenous contrast material application is beneficial for virtual endoscopy has not been resolved.

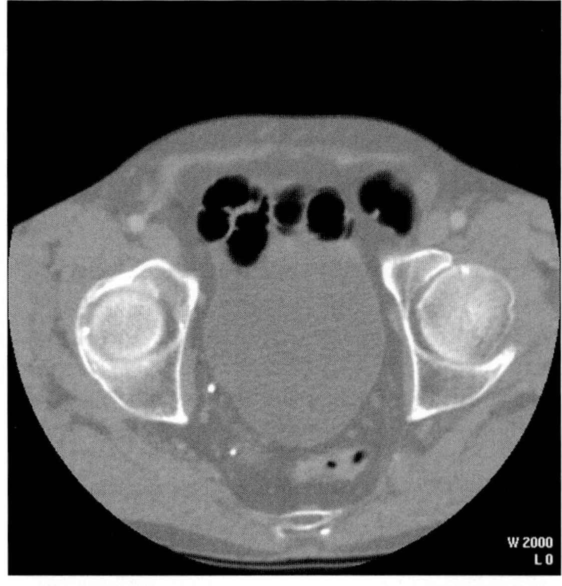

a

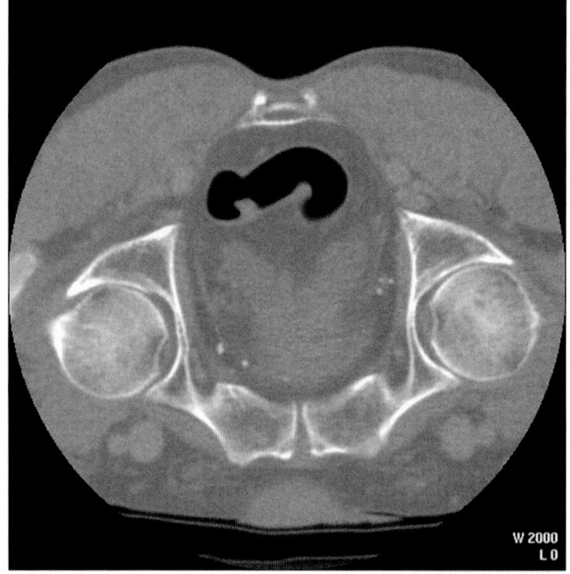

b

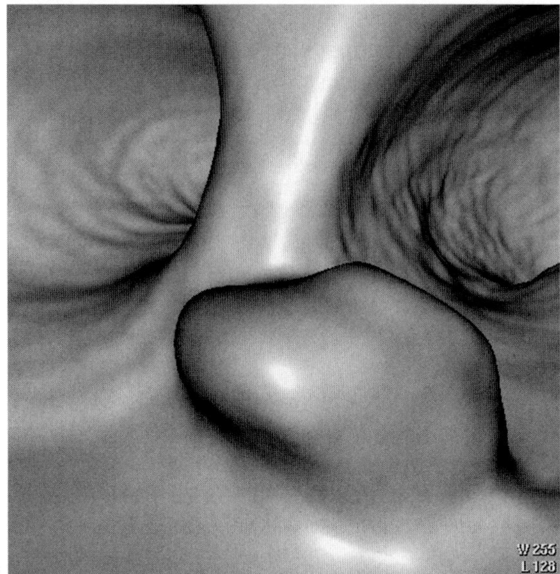

c

Fig. 6.8. During the first spiral examination in supine position (**a**), no polyp can be identified due to the partially collapsed sigmoid colon. After repositioning the patient in prone position (**b**), the 1-cm polyp in the sigmoid colon is clearly identifiable. **c** Virtual endoscopy of the polyp

Most investigators have refrained from giving i.v. contrast material since the already existing strong contrast in the CT (air against soft tissue) would not improve substantially by contrast material accumulation in a polyp. In one of our studies in which all patients received contrast material, the axial slices obtained were analogous to those of a standard diagnostic contrast-enhanced CT examination, and no limitations in the simultaneous evaluation of additional abdominal and pelvic organs were evident (Rogalla et al. 1998). The debate regarding the benefits of intravenous contrast has only begun, and an initial comparative study of 152 virtual coloscopies showed that by giving intravenous contrast material, the reader's confidence and, correspondingly, the diagnostic accuracy improved (Morrin et al. 1999a). The authors reported that – as expected – the advantage of intravenous contrast administration, especially with a suboptimally prepared colon, lies in the visible enhancement of the mucosa.

6.1.4.6.4
Faecal Tagging

In combination with respective postprocessing software, it could be sensible to use oral contrast medium in order to identify intestinal contents that, despite optimal bowel cleansing, are not always eliminated (Vining 1998). Two goals should be reached: firstly, all stools should be contrasted; secondly, remaining fluid in the bowels should be contrasted. Both can be achieved if the patient drinks 30 ml of water-soluble contrast material once the oral bowel preparation begins, in which case also newly formed stools become enhanced. An additional application of 30 ml oral contrast medium 1–2 h before the actual CT examination allows marking of the residual fluid in the intestines. With this procedure, also known as faecal tagging, remaining stool is easily recognised because of its high density, and polyps which would be covered by a contrasted fluid pool are then identifiable as contrast gaps. Through a software function (Fig. 6.9), the fluid can be subtracted so that, in addition to air, also contrast material appears to be transparent and an unobstructed view of the entire intestinal circumference is made possible (Wax et al. 1998).

6.1.4.7 Three-Dimensional Rendering Parameters

The actual innovation of the new imaging modality, apart from the modified image acquisition technique which has been adjusted to the requirements of virtual endoscopy, lies in this aspect of the techno-

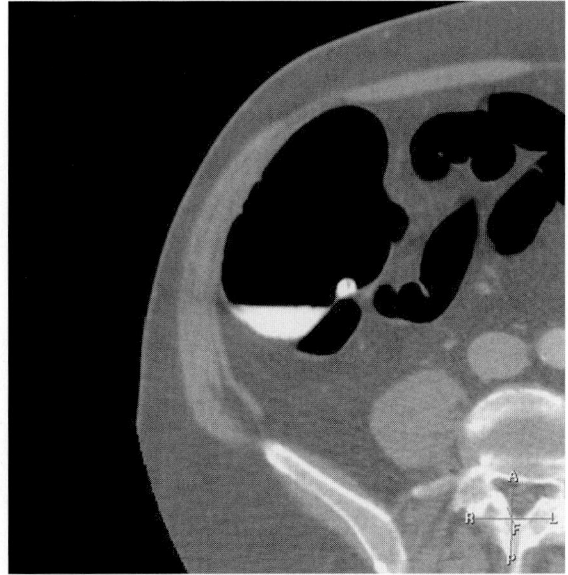

a

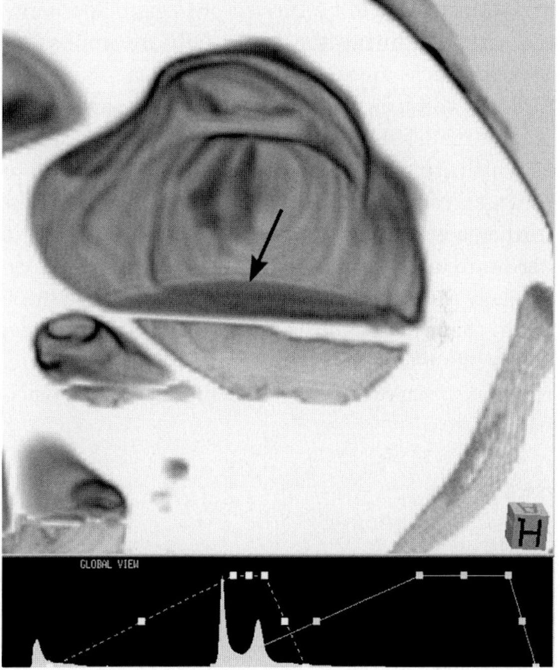

b

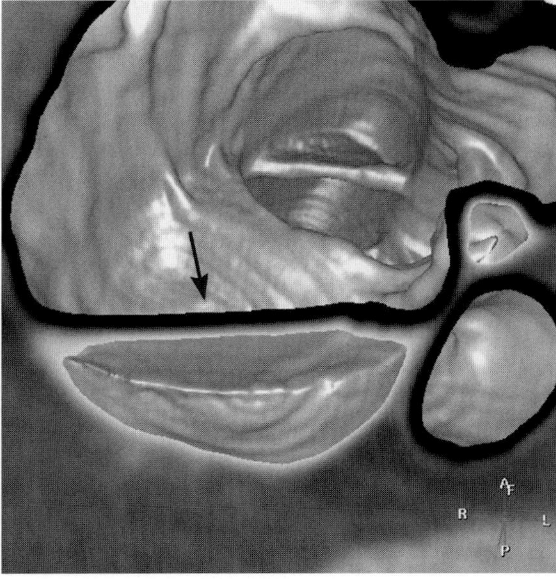

Fig. 6.9a–c. Faecal tagging technique: **a** The axial cross-sectional image shows the fluid level, which was labelled by giving contrast medium. Both virtual reconstructions (**b** Siemens workstation, Virtuoso; **c** Philips workstation, EasyVision) show a view both above and below the fluid level. Polyps can be virtually detected in this manner even when they are covered with contrast agent. For both workstations, avoiding the presentation of the transition zone between air and contrast material as a disturbing "membrane" remains a problem (*arrows*)

logical developments. As explained in the chapter on technical background, two notable postprocessing techniques are currently available: the surface rendering technique and the volume rendering technique. Due to the limited computing capabilities in the mid-1990s, most of the reconstructing occurred by means of surface rendering (Johnson et al. 1997; Royster et al. 1997; Satava 1996; Vining et al. 1994). With such a technique, it is also possible to attain a practically real-time navigation with inexpensive hardware. The boundaries of this reconstruction method lie in the limited spatial resolution and in the unconditional dependence on the initial segmentation procedure: if it fails to provide visualisation solely of the colonic lumen and, for instance, other sections are included in the segmentation, the segmentation needs to be carried out again. Spontaneous changes during the navigation are impossible with this technique.

For both reconstruction techniques – surface and volume rendering – a threshold value must be indicated which is either used as a basis for segmentation or as classification criterion, respectively. Although the further advances in data acquisition in CT and in hardware and software for the workstation were essentially prerequisites for the development and operation of virtual endoscopy, the many parameters which influence the type and quality of the volume-rendering images are far from being sufficiently elucidated.

6.1.4.7.1 Surface Rendering

The most important parameter for the surface rendering technique is the correct choice of thresholds for the segmentation process. The threshold determines a grey value (in CT density value), and all grey values above or below that predetermined value will either be included in the segmentation or not (binary display). If the threshold value is poorly chosen, the colon may appear to have artificial stenoses or holes in its walls.

6.1.4.7.2 Volume Rendering

The most important parameter for the volume rendering technique is the correct choice of an opacity map, which principally means that certain tissue types, expressed in CT as density values (HU), are assigned specific levels of opacity. All smooth transitions between 0% (completely transparent) and 100% (completely opaque) are possible, and it is simply a question of parameter adjustments by the radiologist, indicating which tissue types should appear to be transparent and which opaque. The deciding advantage of the volume rendering technique is that through assigning an opacity map to specific grey levels, the binary display can be circumvented and replaced by the depiction of depth information. If the opacity map were to be assigned a single grey value so that all values above and below appeared either transparent or opaque, this would represent the display by means of surface rendering, although the actual calculation technique differs. Selected software programs also use an approach in which the reconstruction method is based on the volume rendering technique; the surface, however, is represented as opaque in the same interactive display.

Figure 6.10 shows the effect of the choice of thresholds on the representation of diverticula and colonic folds. The corresponding image examples elucidate that poor settings of the threshold value may lead to decreased sensitivity with regard to detection of diverticula. Admittedly, potential holes ("pseudolucencies") in the intestinal wall or mucosal folds are depicted when the threshold values are set too high, but typical 'sharp' holes, as in the surface reconstruction, do not occur.

6.1.4.7.3 Threshold Fitting

Diverticula occur most commonly in the sigmoid colon, so that in this region of the colon a threshold of –550 Hounsfield units (HU) enables an optimal portrayal of the diverticula (Fig. 6.10d). Contrarily, the problem of "holes" in the mucosal folds occurs primarily in the ascending colon, since the orientation of the folds lies mostly in the axial plane, and in combination with an axial scanning direction in CT the partial volume effect becomes pronounced. Therefore, a threshold of –800 to –900 may be appropriate in the ascending colon. This situation can be resolved if the user adjusts the threshold to local conditions during the navigation through the intestines, in which case the cut-off values continuously change along the navigation route (threshold fitting).

6.1.4.7.4 Shading, Lights, Depth-Encoding, and Reflections

It is important to keep in mind that the surface in the virtual endoscopy does not reflect the true physiological surface. The natural colour impression, the aspects of single blood vessels in the mucosa, the characteristics of the mucus, etc. are unobservable in virtual endoscopy. The surfaces can be

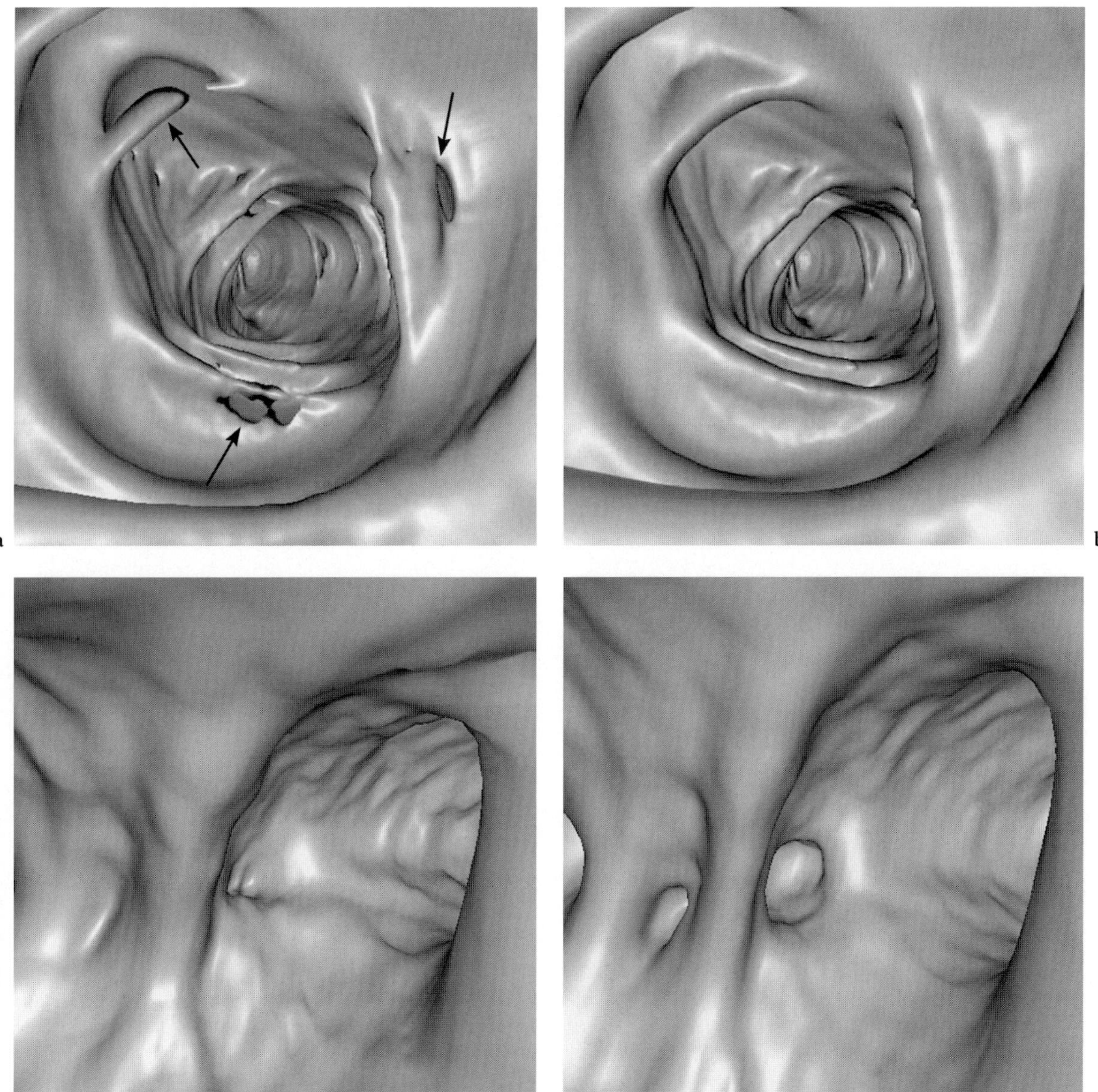

Fig. 6.10a–d. Threshold selection: for both surface and volume rendered reconstruction, proper selection of the threshold to define the colonic lumen is crucial. **a** If the threshold is set too high (above –600 HU), there is a danger that holes (pseudolucencies, *arrows*) will be perceived in the bowel wall or in bowel folds . **b** Same view, but with correct threshold setting at –750 HU. The pseudolucencies no longer appear. **c** If the threshold is too low, diverticula can escape detection. **d** After setting the threshold at –550 HU the diverticula in the sigmoid colon become clearly apparent

altered simply by changing the rendering parameters, demonstrating that the virtual surface has an artificial character. Nevertheless, all software producers strive to make the virtual pictures appear as realistic as possible, and a colour tone intended to approach the natural mucosal colour is offered by many software packages.

In order to simulate reality and to improve the three-dimensional effect, light sources are usually used that come either, like flexible endoscopy, directly from the viewing point or from a different angle (see Chap. 1). From the light source result shadow effects with which characteristics of the wall become strongly enhanced (Fig. 6.11a,b). Additionally, reflections can be imposed on surfaces that are exactly 90° to the viewing axis. As a result, the surface appears to shine. The degree to which the brightness diminishes with increasing distance from the viewer

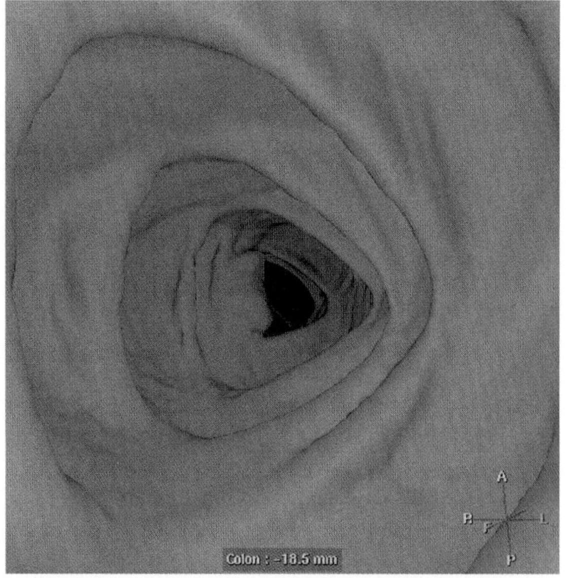

a

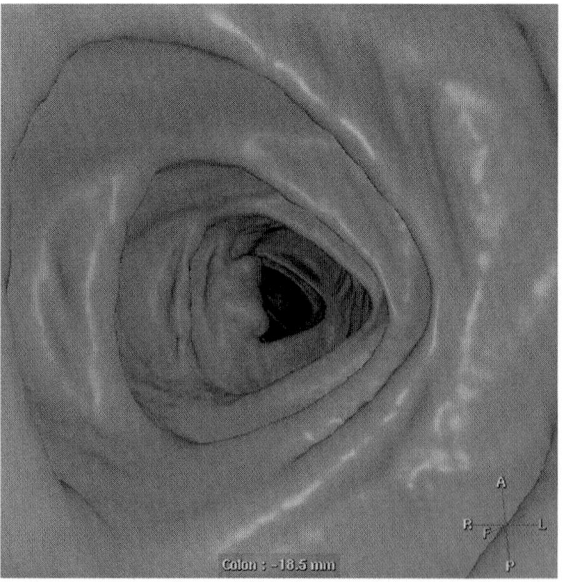

b

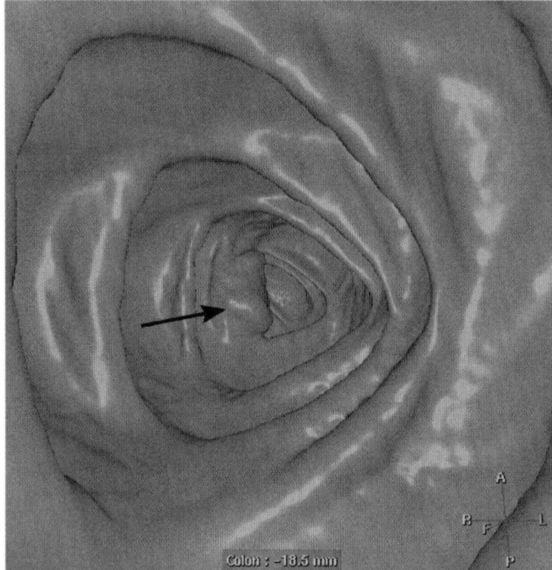

c

Fig. 6.11a–c. Three examples of the same virtual endoscopic view. Without light reflections (**a**), the mucosal surface appears relatively dull. By using calculated light reflections, the image appears much more natural (**b**). A variable darkening in the depths of the object can allow detection of deep-lying processes (**c**) from afar (colon carcinoma, *arrow*)

can also be varied (so-called depth encoding); in this way too, the endoscopic impression is embodied in the virtual reconstruction (Fig. 6.11c). It should once again be explicitly emphasised that conclusions regarding the attributes of the mucosa cannot currently be drawn from the computerised projection.

Presently the assignment of colour tones in the virtual endoscopic images is not diagnostically relevant, and a pure view of the images in grey tones is sufficient. This can change when multiple classifications should be detectable in one picture; for example, when radiodense fluid levels should be displayed in a colour other than that of the intestinal wall (Fig. 6.12). Adjusting the colour of the intestinal wall according to the type of tissue lying behind it is merely a question of coding. A thin wall can then be coded with a different colour than a thick wall. Although there is an appreciable potential in this technique, such colour coding is not yet commercially available.

6.1.4.8
Postprocessing and Navigation

Since the introduction of virtual endoscopy, the large intestine has proved especially favourable for real-time navigation (Parkins 1994); because of its long

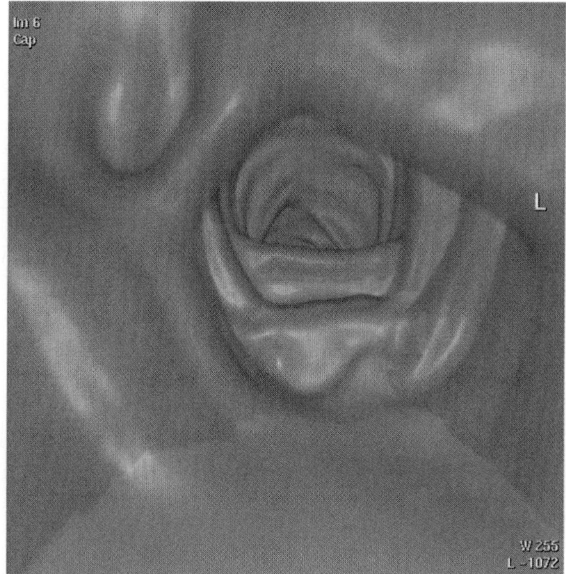

Fig. 6.12. Colour reconstruction: Remaining fluid in the intestine can be demonstrated in a colour other than that chosen for the intestinal lumen. In addition, the fluid is made to appear optically transparent. The advantage lies in the ability to clearly label remaining intestinal contents and, simultaneously, to recognise pathology through the liquid

and tubular structure and relatively simple anatomy (in contrast to the tracheo-bronchial tree), it is particularly suitable for a fly-through.

Numerous methods already exist to interpret virtual endoscopy. The ultimate goal must be, however, to obtain a complete overview of the pathology in the shortest possible time. This implies that for a screening method, all polyps in the colon must be detected. Not to be disregarded is the additional task of detecting further pathological changes in the abdomen which are not necessarily related to the primary goal of inspecting the colon. The illusion of a trip inside the patient's colon is currently made possible through two computer techniques:

- A perspective is superimposed onto the simple three-dimensional reconstruction of the colon including high-power magnification, so that objects closer to the radiologist's viewpoint appear larger than objects of similar size that are further from that viewpoint.
- Real-time rendering capabilities (generating three-dimensional images at a rate of 16–30 frames per second).

The currently available imaging tools which are discussed in the literature and run on various workstations generally encompass the following spectrum.

6.1.4.8.1 Panning Through Multiplanar Two-Dimensional Images

The simplest form is a run through the axial slices in the movie mode on the screen. Advantageous is that this technique does not require complex hardware and exists on every workstation in varying speeds. The greatest disadvantage, however, is that the viewer is presented with the complete axial image information at all times, and focusing on a single bowel loop is consequently difficult. Furthermore, all the bowel loops are more than unlikely to be met exactly orthogonally so that, despite the relatively simple anatomical structure of the large colon, it can be very problematic to systematically move from one region to the consecutive one. Initial success using this method has been reported for gastric diagnostics (Minami et al. 1999). A possible assistance is a hybrid projection from non-enlarged axial slices in combination with a perspective representation of the colon (Fig. 6.13). In this case, the insufflated regions of the colon, which also with optimal monitor settings appear black and therefore do not contain image information, would be filled in with the three-dimensional reconstruction of the intestinal surface. CT slices are ordinarily regarded from caudal so that consequently the view in the separate colon regions also follows from caudal. However, it is simply a question of the settings for the hybrid function and it is also possible, despite the "slice view" from caudal, to superimpose the intestinal view from cranial onto the CT image (Fig. 6.13b). By using this technique it is possible to view the colon from both directions without having to readapt from the customary view.

The benefit of this hybridisation is that no demands are made on the navigation system, and that after setting the respective parameters such as threshold, colour, shading options and reconstruction interval, all slices from the workstation, without additional interaction of the radiologist or the technologist, as in a batch mode, can be directly calculated without further human investment of valuable time.

6.1.4.8.2 Flying Through Surface Rendered or Volume Rendered Endoscopic Models

Either after segmentation of the large colon (usually through a threshold value) with the surface rendering method, or after classification (determining which tissue types should be transparent and which opaque) in the volume rendering method, the radiol-

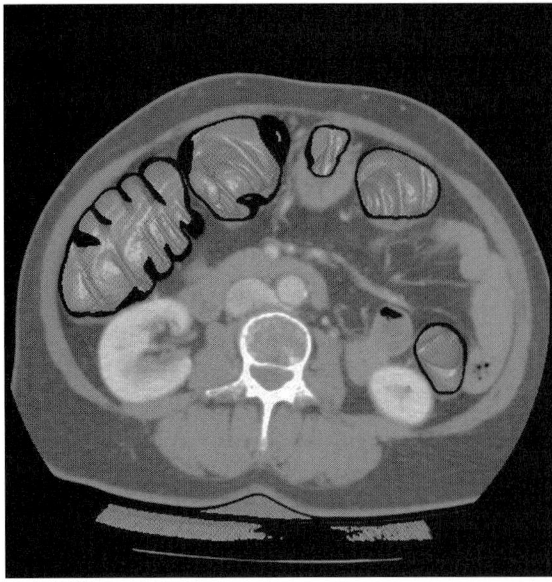

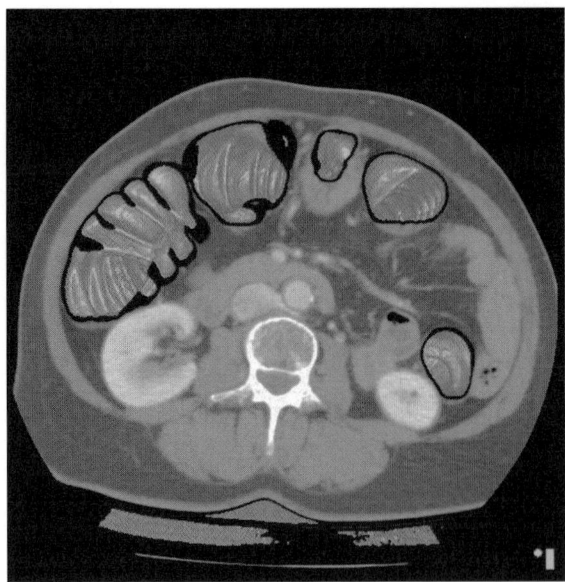

Fig. 6.13a, b. Same axial slice, but "filled" with different "virtual information": image **a** contains the three-dimensional colon when viewed from the bottom (as the axial slice); image **b** contains the view from top. The axial image remains unchanged. The *arrow* points towards a polyp

ogist can navigate through the colon, more or less in real time, by moving the mouse or with dedicated keys, according to the speed of the processor and the type of rendering method used. Most software systems allow viewing of the respective multiplanar reconstruction during the navigation, so that the external morphology is available at any time (Fig. 6.14).

If the software and hardware are fast enough to allow true real-time navigation with optimal diagnostic image resolution, this method may be regarded as ideal, since inspection and navigation combined with the possibility to interactively change views and focus on pathology if needed are combined in one step thus being time efficient. Although systems including such real-time navigation with possible diagnostic quality are currently not commercially available, it remains a question of time until the hardware will realise the necessary reconstruction speed. Initial reports on such attempts have already been published (Hoffmann et al. 1998).

6.1.4.8.3 Flying Through Colon Models with Semi-Automatic or Automatic Assistance of Navigational Aids (i.e., Automatic Path-Tracking Tools)

If real-time reconstruction with high image quality cannot be achieved, there are alternative methods to circumvent the existing waiting time on the workstation. Through semi-automatic or even almost fully automatic path-tracking tools the manual work of the radiologist on the workstation can be extensively reduced. (Paik et al. 1998b). Common to all approaches of the software is that the end-product will be a fly-through movie that runs through the entire colon (Horwich et al. 1999; Samara et al. 1999; Schmutz et al. 1999). The start and endpoint of the path can be set by a trained technologist, and the radiologist has the sole task of viewing the finished movie for diagnostic purposes (Okuda et al. 1998).

Trouble arises with automatic path-setting through stenoses and collapsed areas of the colon. The path-finding algorithm must place the path through the stenosis, either alone or interactively with guidance from the user. Of importance in this procedure is whether the shifting of tasks during the total postprocessing towards the technologist and the computer actually reduces the amount of time that the radiologist must dedicate to diagnosing the case.

In a comparison study, we opted to evaluate whether and how an automatic path-tracking tool for virtual colonoscopy could decrease the time the physician needed to reach a final diagnosis. The spiral CT data from 27 patients were used for virtual colonoscopy. A trained technologist performed automatic path tracking (prototype EasyVision workstation, Philips), limiting the task of the physician to interpretation of the images. The following terms were defined: human tasks (sum of technologist's

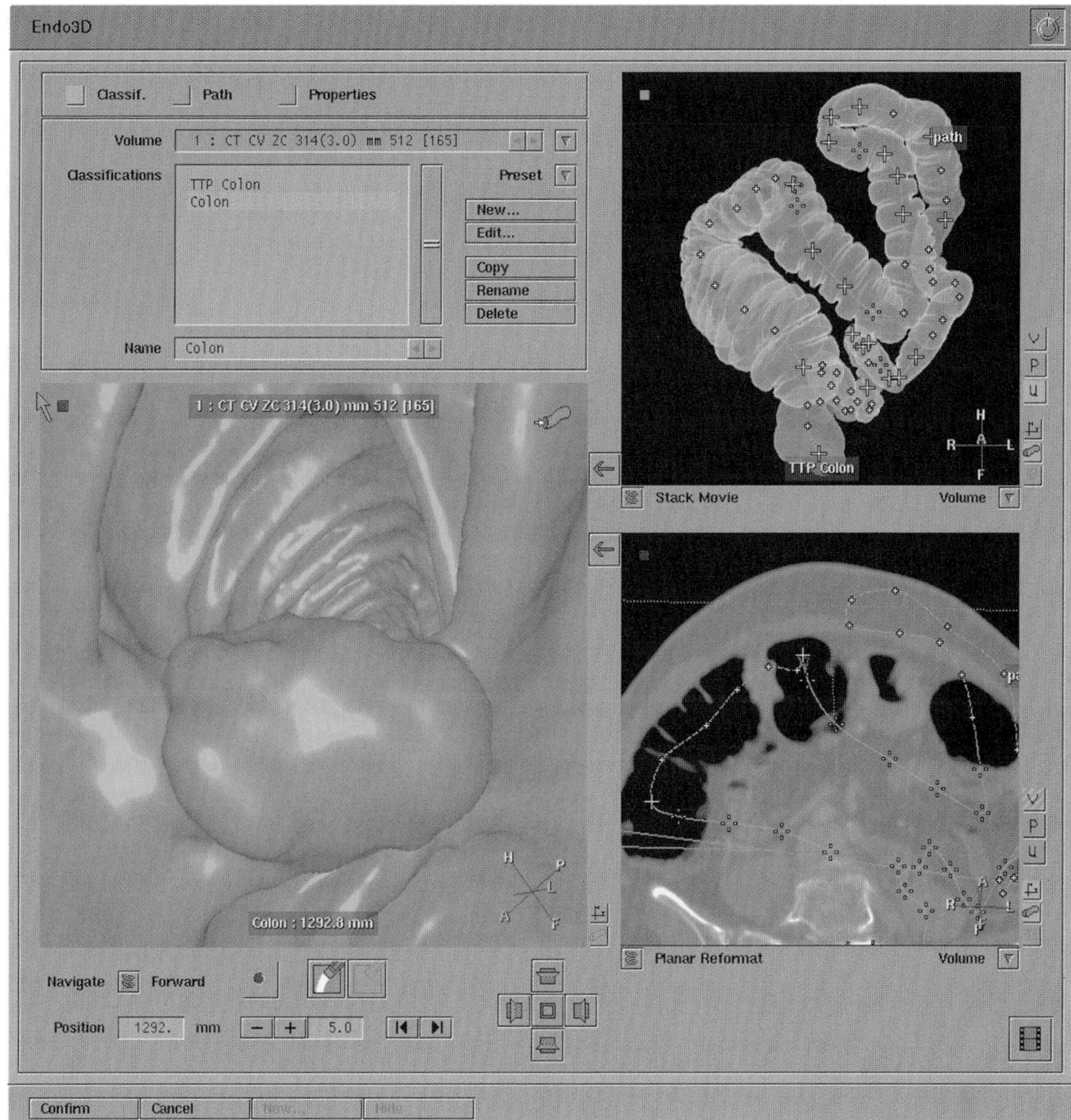

Fig. 6.14. Navigation panel. During manual navigation, the actual position of the viewpoint is referenced in a 3D image (TTP) and in a multiplanar reformatted image

and physician's tasks), and throughput (total time from arrival of the images on the workstation to final diagnosis). By setting the average manual navigation time of 32 min to 100%, the technologist's task required 14% (4.5 min), the physician's task 45% (14.5 min), the human task 59% (20 min), the off-line computation 122% (39 min), and the throughput time required 181% (58 min). In other words, the physician's tasks and the overall human tasks consumed significantly less time in the automated procedure ($p<0.05$) (Rogalla et al. 1999).

6.1.4.8.4 Unfolding, Unravelling or Splitting the Entire Colon

This technique departs from the expectation of imitating the flexible endoscopy. Figure 6.15 exemplifies the advantages of a fly-through video of the intestine, especially if the video is calculated or viewed in two directions (from the caecum to the anus and vice versa). Despite this possibility of viewing the colon from two opposing directions or of making use of a viewing angle greater than 90°, pol-

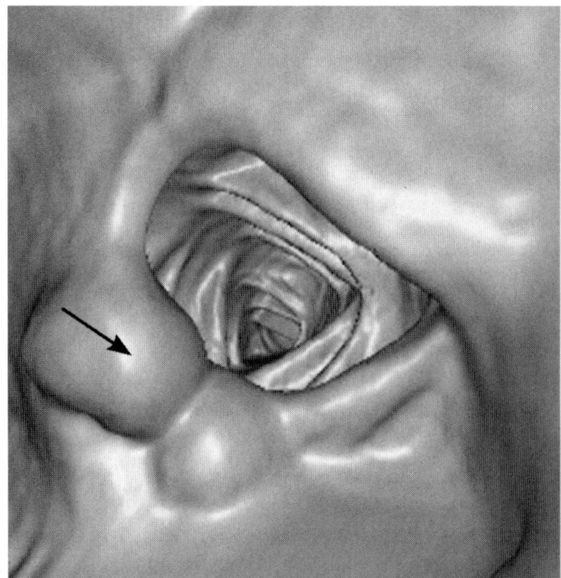

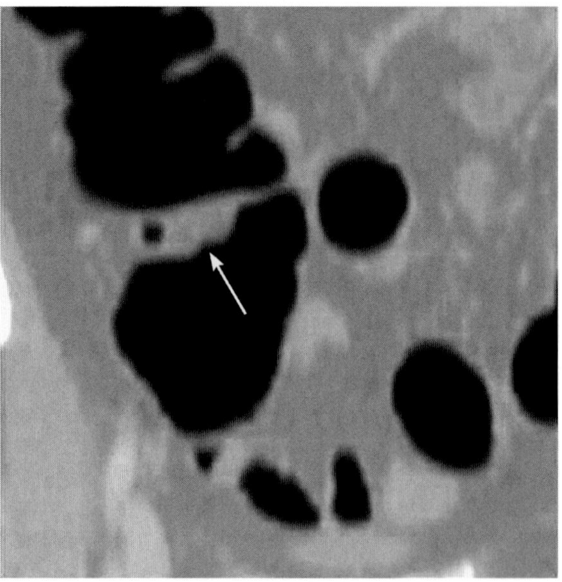

Fig. 6.15. a High-quality virtual reconstruction of a view from the caecum into the ascending colon. The image interpretation is highly facilitated due to the almost "natural" representation of the colon. The *arrow* points to the ileocaecal valve, which shows an ampullar thickening as a normal deviant. **b** The corresponding multiplanar reconstruction

yps which are hidden between two intestinal folds can nonetheless be overlooked (Fig. 6.16). Uncertainty remains, however, as to whether it is unquestionably necessary to imitate flexible endoscopy with its "tunnel view".

Several alternatives have already been recommended, including a digital unfolding or unravelling technique (McFarland et al. 1997; Wang et al. 1998). The authors proposed an electrical field-based method to unravel the convoluted colon, that is, to digitally straighten it with curved cross-sections and flatten it over a plane. After this procedure, the radiologist can browse through the colon (Beaulieu et al. 1999), with the advantage that the perspective distortion is negligible; also, direct measurements are possible. Another possibility is to simply slice the colon longitudinally and display it as if pressed flat onto the image plane (Fig. 6.17).

A further alternative, well known from the distorted display of geographical maps and world globes, is the Mercator projection (Paik et al. 1999). The authors of a study carried out to ascertain which of three visualisation techniques – one fly-through movie, two fly-through movies (forwards and backwards) and the new Mercator projection – best covers the entire surface of the colon, found that only 49.7% of the entire colonic surface was actually visualised with the single-direction movie, 74.2% with the double-direction movie, and 98.8% with the Mercator projection (Paik et al. 1998a). Although

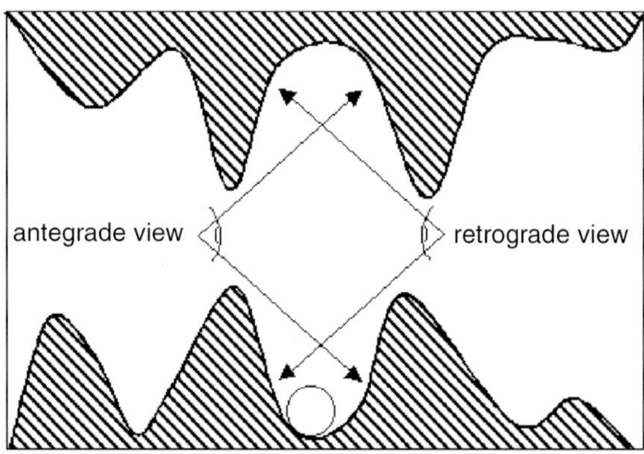

Fig. 6.16. Schematic drawing showing how "blind spots" arise: if the colon is observed forwards and backwards along a path, a polyp lying between two closely neighbouring folds can be easily overlooked. Several possible solutions exist for this problem: in addition to the forwards and backwards view, four additional side views along the path can be reconstructed. The reader must then view six movies simultaneously. Next to other projection techniques such as the Mercator projection (see Sect. 6.1.4.8.4), an automatic recognition of the "blind spots" seems feasible. The areas not inspected on the forwards and backwards view could be colour coded in a 3D model. The reader would then know which intestinal segments require further investigation

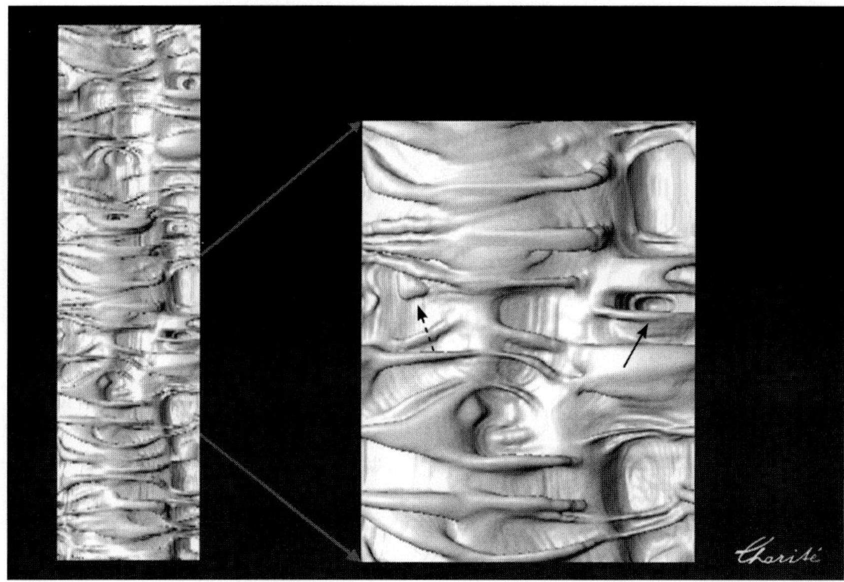

Fig. 6.17. Panoramic view of the colon. The bowel wall is split along its longitudinal axis and laid out in a flat plane. Since bends in the bowel are no longer displayed, notable image distortion results, preventing reliable, direct distance measurements. The *dashed arrow* indicates a small polyp, which becomes very obvious in the panoramic view. The *second arrow* indicates a small diverticulum

these results are highly promising, whether such unusual projections actually facilitate the detection of pathology for the radiologist still needs to be investigated. In any case, all the mentioned new visualisation techniques would require some time for the radiologist to get acquainted with them before they could be implemented safely, accurately and reliably.

6.1.4.8.5 Competing Visualisation Techniques

In a similar manner to that inwhich fly-through movies attempt to imitate flexible endoscopy, cross-sectional imaging data can be reconstructed by means of volume rendering to create the impression of a DCBE, a procedure named "tissue transition projection" (Fig. 6.18). Unlike reconstructions that are based on the CT attenuation value of single volume elements (voxels), such as surface shaded displays or maximum-intensity projections, tissue transition projection (TTP) is calculated solely from gradients in the volume of interest (Höhne et al. 1990), i.e. from the differences in attenuation values of neighbouring voxels. The gradients in the volume are calculated directly from the volume data at arbitrary positions (Terwisscha van Scheltinga et al. 1997), and at sample locations along a ray in the direction of the selected view, grey values and gradients are calculated (see also Chap. 1). A translucency value is then modulated by the gradient strength at that position (Levoy 1988). The voxels at the front of the ray are projected first, and partially obscure voxels at the back of the ray.

The resulting three-dimensional object can finally be viewed from all sides and directions, enlarged, and varied in brightness and contrast. In an initial assessment (Rogalla et al. 1998) of 34 patients with a total of 28 colorectal cancers, the tissue transition projections depicted, corresponding with the virtual colonoscopy, all tumours. However, 17% more diverticula were visible in virtual colonoscopy than on TTP, suggesting that due to the gradient calculation in the volume, the images are interpolated to a greater extent and the detail resolution is comparatively reduced. The extent to which TTP is suitable for polyp detection in a screening setting has not yet been satisfactorily investigated.

6.1.4.8.6 Computer-Assisted Polyp Detection

Automatic detection of polyps is, at the current stage of development, not feasible. The technique of virtual endoscopy is, compared with other current procedures for colon imaging, still very young. Its strong potential is far from fully recognised and explored. Thus, it is quite conceivable that, with continual technical development, especially in the field of pattern recognition, neuronal networks and artificial intelligence, computer-assisted polyp detection will become practicable within the next decade.

Despite the rapid expansion of new visualisation techniques, viewing the intestine in a fly-through video will nonetheless continue to gain acceptance. This is most likely because the similar images from flexible endoscopy have become well accepted, and both sur-

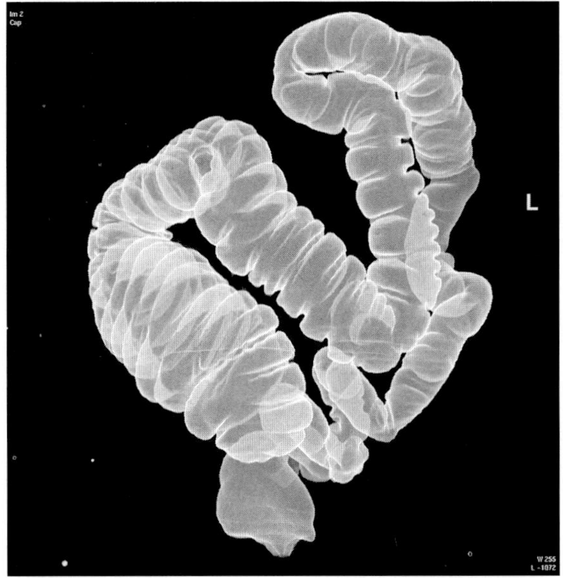

a

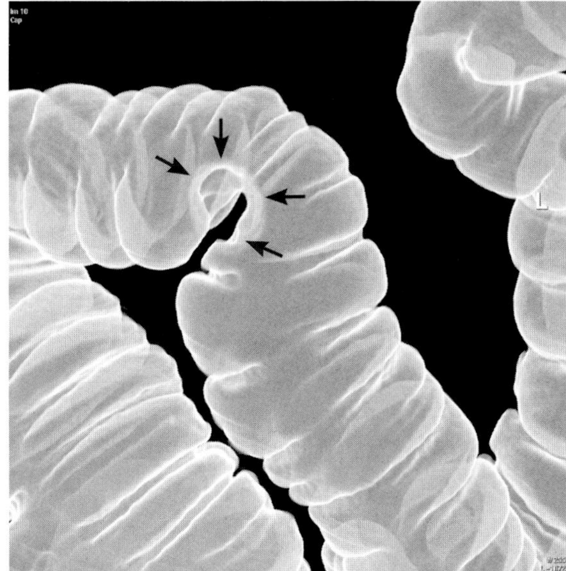
b

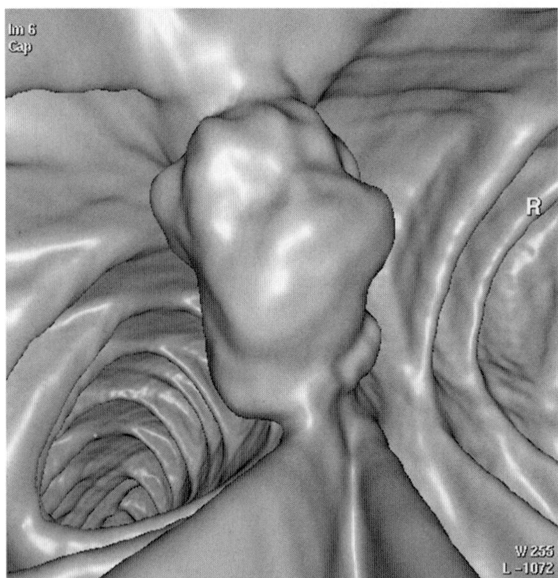

c

Fig. 6.18. a TTP image of the colon. A large, polypous tumour reaching almost 2 cm in size is detectable in the transverse colon (*arrows*). **b** Appreciation of the form and size of the polyp is substantially better in the enlargement. **c** Display of the same polyp in the virtual endoscopy. With a viewing angle of 100°, it is possible to look in both directions along the transverse colon

geons and gastroenterologists are more apt to accept a new technique when the presented images do not appear to be too abstract or ambiguous. Although the primary goal is assisting the radiologist in reaching a diagnosis, the findings must eventually be presented to the clinicians and such a demonstration should be simple and convincing. Undoubtedly a flight through the colon, similar to the flexible endoscopy video, is more impressive and convincing than a flat, two-dimensional presentation.

6.1.4.9 Image Interpretation and Pitfalls

Regardless of which new technique is used to visualise the colon, the goal for the radiologist remains the identification of all polyps in the minimal amount of time. Additionally, one of the greatest problems in judging whether or not a procedure is suitable for screening (including satisfactory sensitivity and specificity) is deciding what should be used as a gold standard for comparison.

6.1.4.9.1
Gold Standards

Theoretically, the ideal method to verify the findings in virtual endoscopy would be intraoperative confirmation (Fig. 6.4). In practice, however, this is plausible only in selected cases and only in circumstances where surgical intervention will follow. The majority of researchers in this field have used flexible colonoscopy for comparative purposes; comments regarding its accuracy have already been made in this chapter. An interesting alternative was examined in a study in which artificial polyps were "implanted" in a spiral CT (Karadi et al. 1998). In a blinded reading, three radiologists confirmed that the artificial, digital polyps did not differ from the true polyps in the scans. In the end, the prepared spiral CT scans could be used as usual for virtual reconstructions.

6.1.4.9.2
Solitary Polyp/Adenoma

A large series of polyps resected at colonoscopy shows that about 4% (range 2–6%) of adenomatous polyps consist of invasive carcinoma (Fenoglio and Pascal 1982). As already mentioned, the likelihood of cancer in a polyp increases with the polyp's size and with the fraction of the polyp that is comprised of villous tissue. Adenomatous polyps (adenomas) are classified histologically as tubular, tubulovillous, or villous, depending on the proportion of villous tissue. All adenomas have some degree of histological dysplasia that is now usually classified as being either low- or high-grade. The risk of cancer spreading to the lymph nodes in colorectal adenomas has been evaluated in a careful histological study of surgically and colonoscopically resected specimens. Studies indicate that because lymphatic channels do not penetrate the muscularis mucosa layer, "focal" or "intraepithelial" mucosal cancers that do not invade this layer have virtually no chance of metastasising lymphatically (Fenoglio et al. 1973). Several prospective series of patients with resected polyps containing these intramucosal cancers confirm that simple polypectomy is most certainly a decisive therapy for such lesions (Haggitt et al. 1985).

Figure 6.19 shows a 1.6-cm, partially pedunculated polyp which was resected in an endoscopic session following virtual endoscopy. The histology of the polyp did not show any high-grade dysplasia, which meant that immediate follow-up was deemed unnecessary. Noteworthy is that due to the lack of ability to manipulate the intestine in virtual endoscopy, precise presentation of the polyp stalk is not attainable. Only once the polyp is hanging freely in the intestinal lumen is it also possible to present the peduncle on virtual endoscopy. Figure 6.20 shows a polyp 10 cm in length which could not be removed in

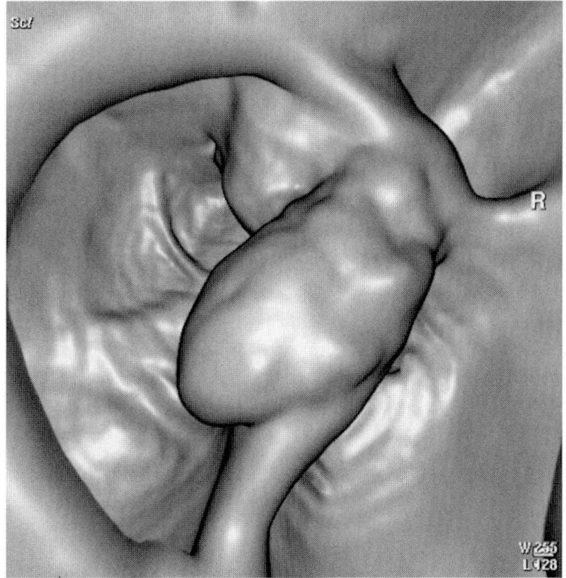

a

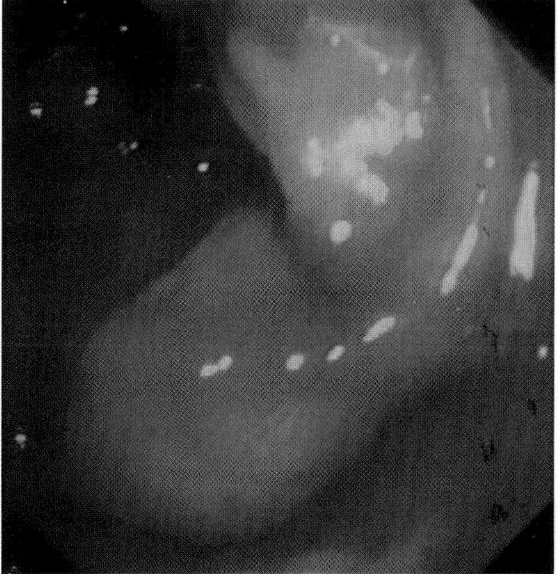

b

Fig. 6.19. a Virtual endoscopic view onto the 1.6-cm pedunculated polyp in the transverse colon. The polyp is lying directly on the bowel wall, so that the peduncle cannot be freely demonstrated. **b** The same view of the 1.6-cm adenomatous polyp on flexible endoscopy. The polyp was removed during the same session with an electric loop

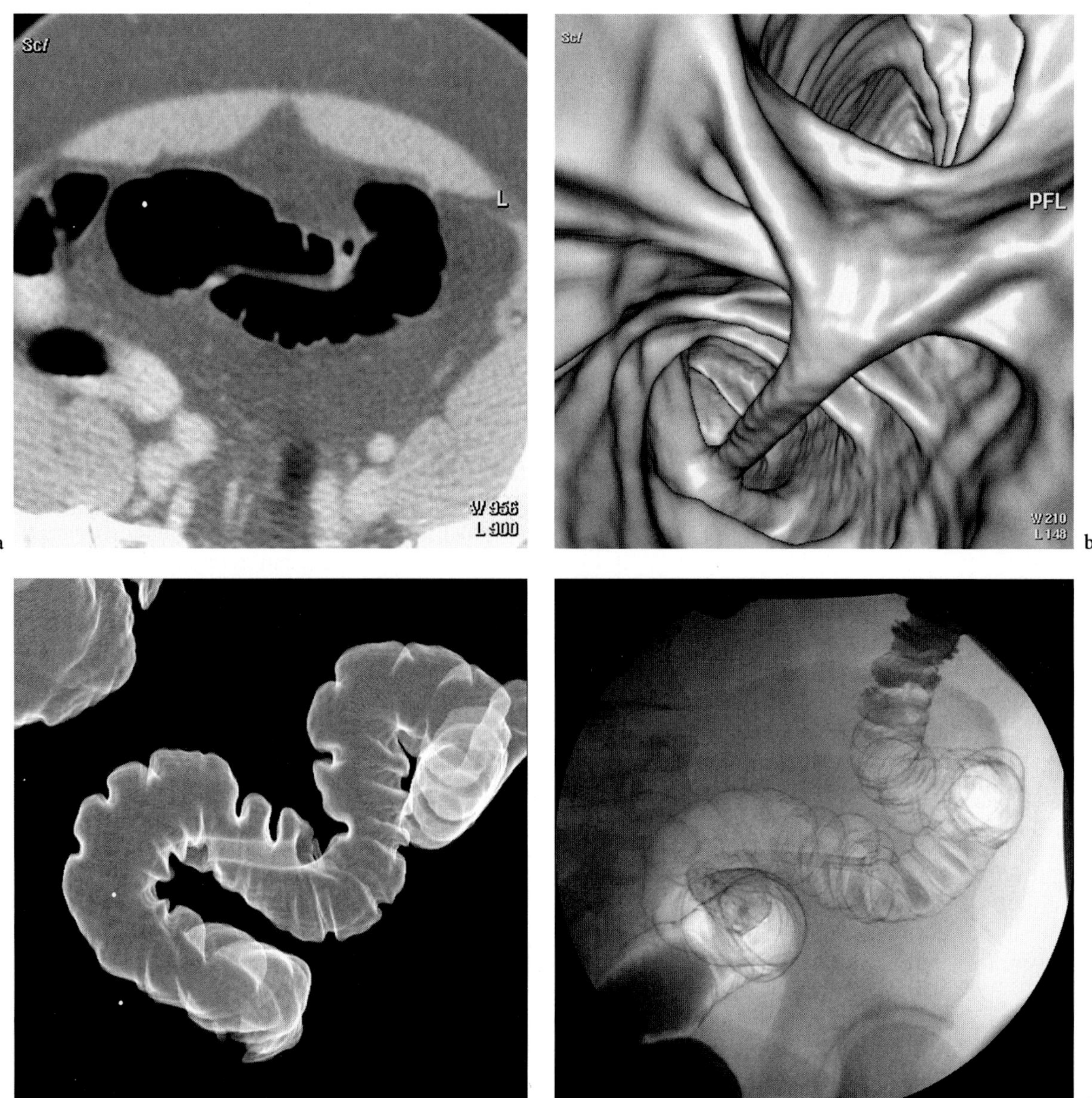

Fig. 6.20. a Axial CT slice through the sigmoid colon in a patient referred for surgical removal of a giant colon polyp. The preoperative CT image demonstrated the pedunculated tumour; however, the shape is very difficult to identify without a 3D reconstruction. Imaging parameters: 3 mm slice thickness, 2 mm reconstruction interval. **b** Virtual endoscopy with view out of a sigma loop onto the polyp: the peduncle pulls a mucosal fold distally. Viewing parameters: 90° viewing angle, 2% depth encoding, volume rendering technique. **c** Corresponding TTP reconstruction. **d** Corresponding double-contrast barium enema of the same polyp equally demonstrating the 10-cm pedunculated tumour. DCBE, being a dynamic examination, showed that the suspended polyp was freely movable in the lumen. The final histology after endoscopic polyp removal revealed a haemangioma

the course of ambulatory endoscopy because of its size. The patient was therefore sent for operative removal of the polyp. Only after the long stalk was seen on virtual endoscopy and, at the insistence of the surgeons, also in a DCBE study, was the polyp removed in a repeat flexible endoscopy by means of an electric loop. The histology showed haemangioma.

Of primary interest, however, are small polyps, especially those approximately 1 cm in size, since the probability of a malignant transformation increases with the magnitude of the polyp. Figure 6.21 shows a 3-mm polyp located shortly before the splenic flexure in the transverse colon. The small polyp sits exactly on a fold and is therefore easy to recognise. A

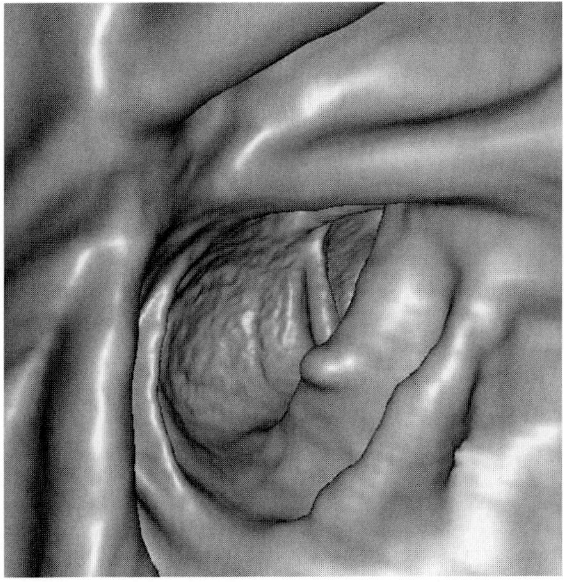

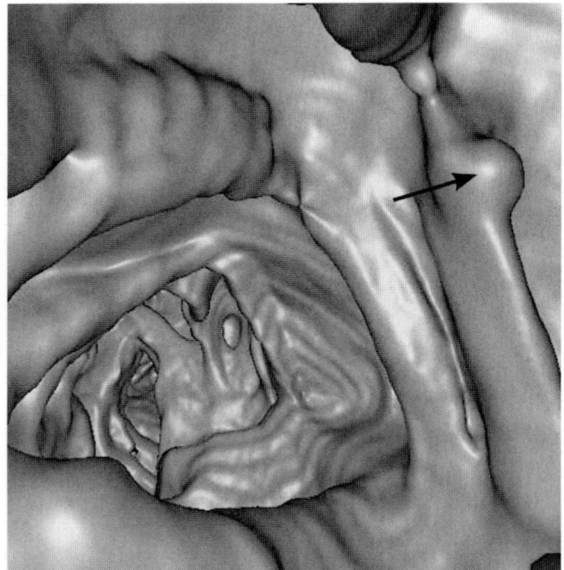

a

Fig. 6.21. Image of a 3-mm polyp immediately proximal to the left flexure. Due to its location upon a fold, the polyp is easily recognised

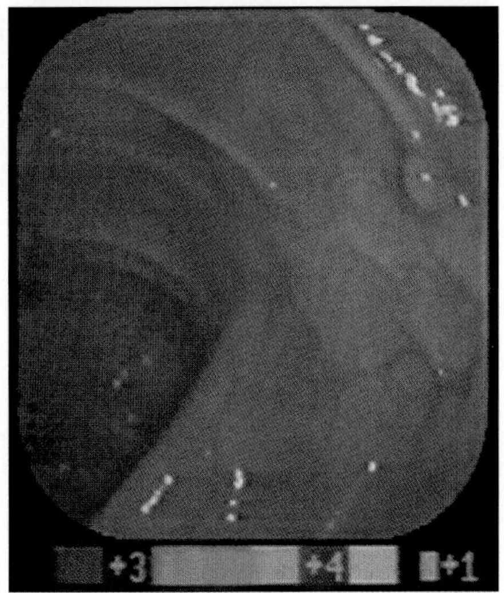

b

Fig. 6.22a, b. Presentation of a 3-mm adenomatous polyp in the ascending colon in a patient who was not very well prepared (stool remnants and much mucus remained in the bowel). Such small polyps can be easily overlooked when the intestine is inadequately emptied. Corresponding view on flexible endoscopy, also displaying the 3-mm polyp. One of the strategic advantages of true endoscopy is that small amounts of stool and fluid can be immediately removed

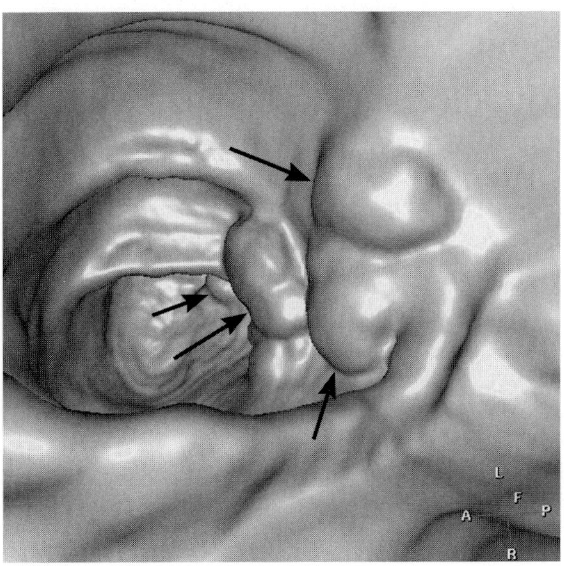

Fig. 6.23. Multiple small polyps (*arrows*) in a patient with familial adenomatous polyposis. Primary scan parameters: 3 mm slice thickness, 5 mm/s table speed, 2 mm reconstruction interval

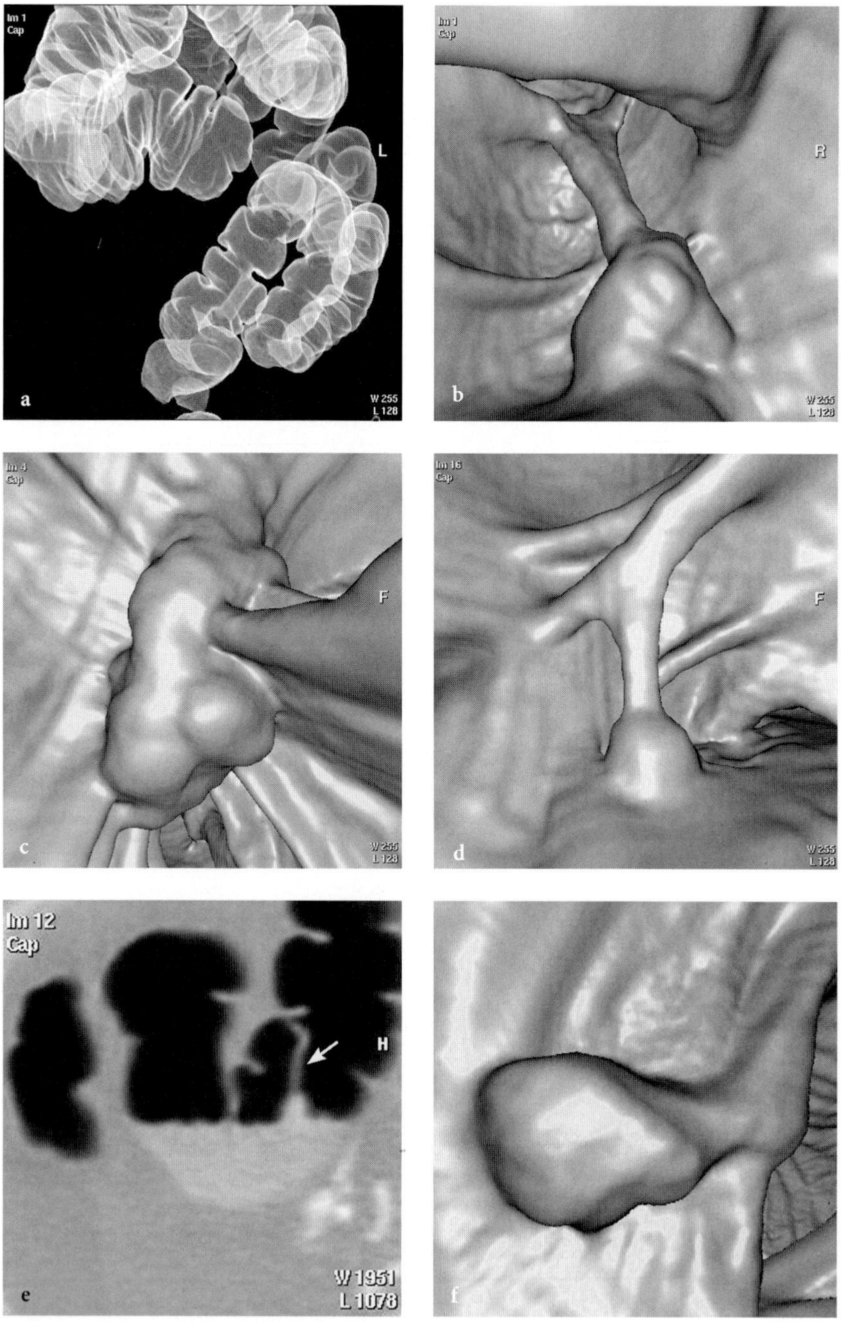

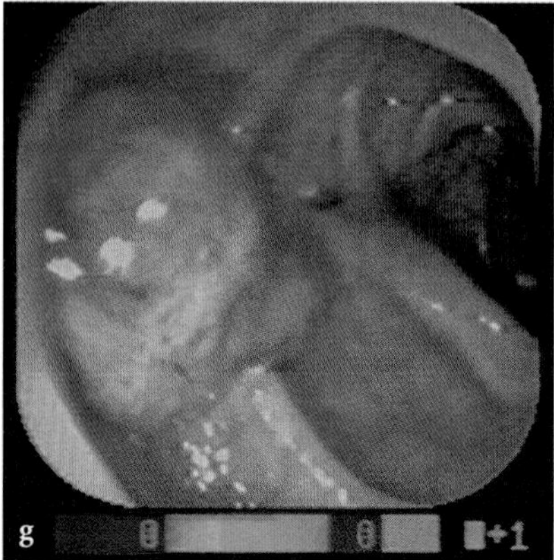

Fig. 6.24a–g. A 59-year-old man with multiple pedunculated polyps. The TTP reconstruction (**a**) nicely visualises the stalk of the polyp, and on the corresponding virtual reconstruction, the entire polyp can be presented three-dimensionally (**b**). Images **c** and **d** represent further pedunculated polyps in the same patient. Image **e** shows the suspended polyp (*arrow*) from **d** in an axial plane. The tip of the polyp is submerged in the remaining fluid. Images (**f**) and (**g**) demonstrate the morphological correlation between virtual and flexible endoscopy, although the flexible endoscopy is especially advantageous for examining pedunculated polyps since the possibility of manipulating and characterising the polyps exists. The virtual endoscopy is only a momentary image, yielding limited information as to the length of the peduncle. All polyps from this patient were endoscopically removed and not a single malignant transformation was detected

more difficult constellation is when the quality of the virtual endoscopy is limited due to artefacts, be it continuous breathing motions of the patient or non-optimal colonic cleansing (see Sect. 6.1.4.9.13). Figure 6.22 shows the correlation between flexible and virtual endoscopy of a 3-mm polyp which, although detected on virtual endoscopy, was not classified with certainty as a polyp. However, due to its small size the polyp was of no significance.

6.1.4.9.3 Multiple Adenomas

The occurrence of multiple polyps is also possible (Fig. 6.23). Patients with multiple adenomas that are larger than 1 cm (Fig. 6.24), and show tubulovillous or villous histology, or even high-grade dysplasia, have a 3–6 times greater risk of developing colorectal carcinoma (Winawer et al. 1993). On virtual endoscopy it is possible to put forward the diagnosis of "multiple adenomas" only if the anamnesis and clinical data have ruled out the presence of other pathological conditions (see below) and multiple polyps are displayed. Figure 6.25 shows a patient with multiple adenomas. Due to the described increased risk for colorectal carcinoma it should be recommended that, after successful polypectomy of all suspicious adenomas, leading to the so-called "clean colon", the patient returns for a follow-up examination in 3 years.

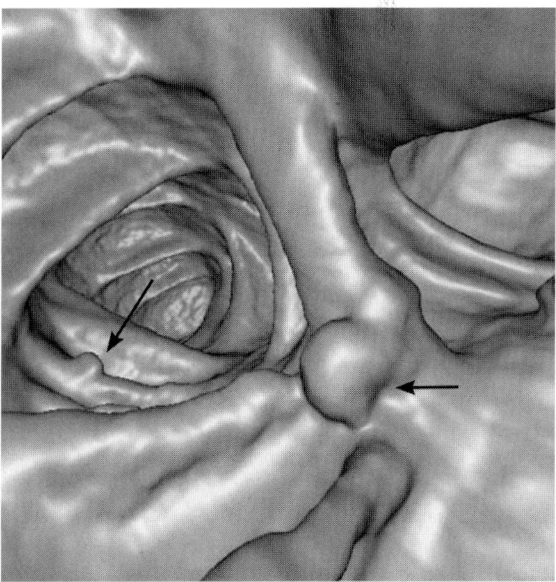

Fig. 6.25. A 43-year-old man with evidence of 17 polyps. The image shows a 3-mm and an 11-mm polyp (*arrow*)

6.1.4.9.4 Lynch Syndrome

If, in a family of at least two generations, a colorectal carcinoma is diagnosed in at least three members, of whom one is younger than 50 years upon diagnosis and at least one is a first-degree relative of both others, the so-called Amsterdam criteria have been met and the presence of Lynch syndrome is probable (Lynch et al. 1993). Mutations on chromosomes 2, 3, and 7 are responsible for the inheritance with high penetrance of this hereditary non-polyposis colorectal cancer (HNPCC), which accounts for approximately 5% of all colorectal carcinomas.

The goal of virtual endoscopy must be restricted to the confirmation or ruling out of colorectal carcinoma. The diagnosis of HNPCC can be completed only with the assistance of the anamnestic data. If this information is known and the Amsterdam criteria are filled, then the presence of a carcinoma must also be investigated in young patients. To date, it has been recommended that the members of afflicted families be examined every 1–2 years starting from 20 years of age and undergo annual coloscopy from the age of 40, in which case virtual colonoscopy is a possible alternative. In a Scandinavian study, the development of six carcinomas was observed in a study population of 251 individuals who underwent endoscopic examinations triennially over a 10-year period (Järvinen et al. 1995).

6.1.4.9.5 Familial Adenomatous Polyposis

This condition is inherited in an autosomal dominant manner with a high degree of penetrance, but can also occur as a result of a spontaneous mutation. Starting from the second or third decade of life, hundreds or thousands of adenomas can be detected throughout the large intestine. An inevitable consequence, if the disease is left untreated, is malignant maturation into colorectal carcinoma, frequently before the age of 40 years. Circa 1% of all colorectal cancers have their origin in familial adenomatous polyposis (FAP). Screening children of parents who have been identified as having FAP poses an additional challenge, since neither colonoscopy nor virtual endoscopy is an optimal procedure; in this case, however, molecular genetic analysis might preclude any unnecessary long-term monitoring for 50% of the children.

Virtual endoscopy is well designed to display the multiple adenomas of familial polyposis (Fig. 6.23). However, the same problem exists for virtual as for flexible endoscopy: the isolated inspection permits no conclusion regarding the benign or malignant

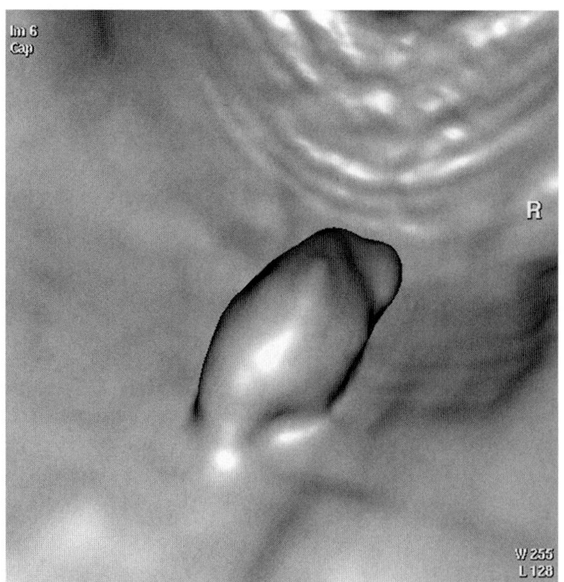

a

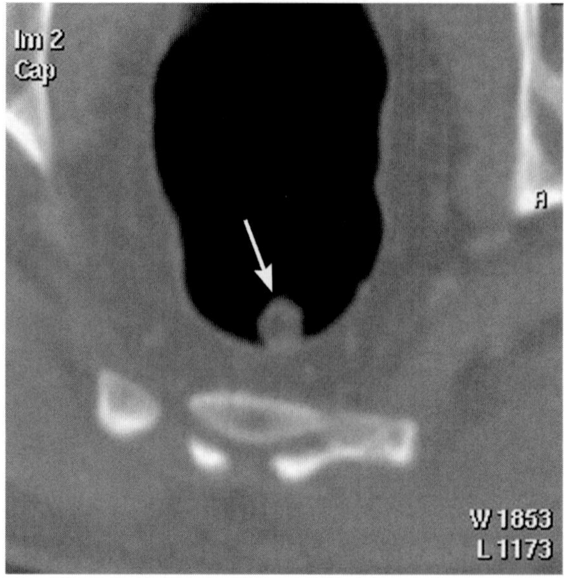

b

Fig. 6.26 a, b. An example of a hamartoma in the recto-sigmoid colon. The small polyp consists predominantly of fatty tissue (CT density: –67 Hounsfield units). The following flexible endoscopy with polyp removal confirmed the suspected hamartoma

nature of the polyps, so a biopsy remains obligatory. Yet, since only a limited number of polyps can be histologically examined, it is quite possible that a neighbouring unexamined polyp is dysplastic. In this respect, even a negative biopsy allows no peace of mind, leaving the indication for preventive colectomy considerable.

6.1.4.9.6 Peutz-Jeghers Syndrome, Hamartoma Polyposis, Juvenile Polyposis

Peutz-Jeghers syndrome is characterised by multiple hamartomas dispersed primarily in the small intestine, rarely in other portions of the gastrointestinal tract, and by altered pigmentation of the skin and mucosa (perioral skin, lips, oral mucosa). Female patients are commonly afflicted with tumours of the breast and urogenital area. Even if the hamartomas are pathologically not considered, in up to 10% of cases a carcinoma will appear in the gastrointestinal tract, principally in the stomach or small intestine, rarely in the colon (Giardiello et al. 1987).

Hamartoma polyposis is a rare condition that is inherited in an autosomal dominant fashion. The manifestation is usually in childhood, but is possible until 20 years of age, and is characterised by symptoms caused by the voluminous polyps, including intestinal obstruction and gastrointestinal bleeding.

Also rare is hereditary juvenile polyposis, where carcinomas are detected in approximately 10% of the patients. A malignant transformation seems to occur via an intermediate dysplasia of isolated hamartomas (Jass et al. 1988).

For all three diseases, the differential diagnostic contribution of virtual endoscopy is limited; its value is confined to identifying and depicting the hamartomas (Fig. 6.26) and polyps. For further histological validation a biopsy is mandatory. Currently, there is little experience regarding whether hamartomas can be adequately differentiated from dysplastic polyps. The present situation does not foresee the possibility, except when being implemented for initial diagnostics of an affected patient, that virtual colonoscopy could be recommendable for these patients, although precisely such individuals with a long history of repeated colonoscopies are mostly willing and interested in an alternative method.

6.1.4.9.7 Ulcerative Colitis

The indication for endoscopic monitoring of ulcerative colitis patients is critically discussed (Von Herbay et al. 1994). It was postulated in older publications that up to 50% of the patients present with colorectal carcinoma 30 years after disease manifestation (Jass et al. 1988). According to more recent investigations, the risk of developing a colorectal malignancy, even after 20 years, appears to be twice as high as in the general population (Langholz et al. 1992; Pinczowski et al. 1994). The observation that histologically detected dysplasias are often associated with carcinomas led to a further expansion of the coloscopic monitoring programmes. It is presently accepted that a patient with the histological diagnosis of high-grade dysplasia should be treated with a colectomy (Choi et al. 1993; Woolrich et al. 1992).

The virtual endoscopy can exclude the presence of a colorectal carcinoma, but also that of polyps. Consequently, if the indication for an examination is the exclusion of carcinoma or polyps, virtual endoscopy could be considered a component of such a tracking programme. Yet, the assistance of virtual endoscopy goes further: the ability to judge the thickness of the intestinal wall in all sections of the colon by viewing the axial or multiplanar slices allows assessment of any existing inflammatory processes (Fig. 6.27). Moreover, pseudopolypous changes, often found in the course of inflammatory

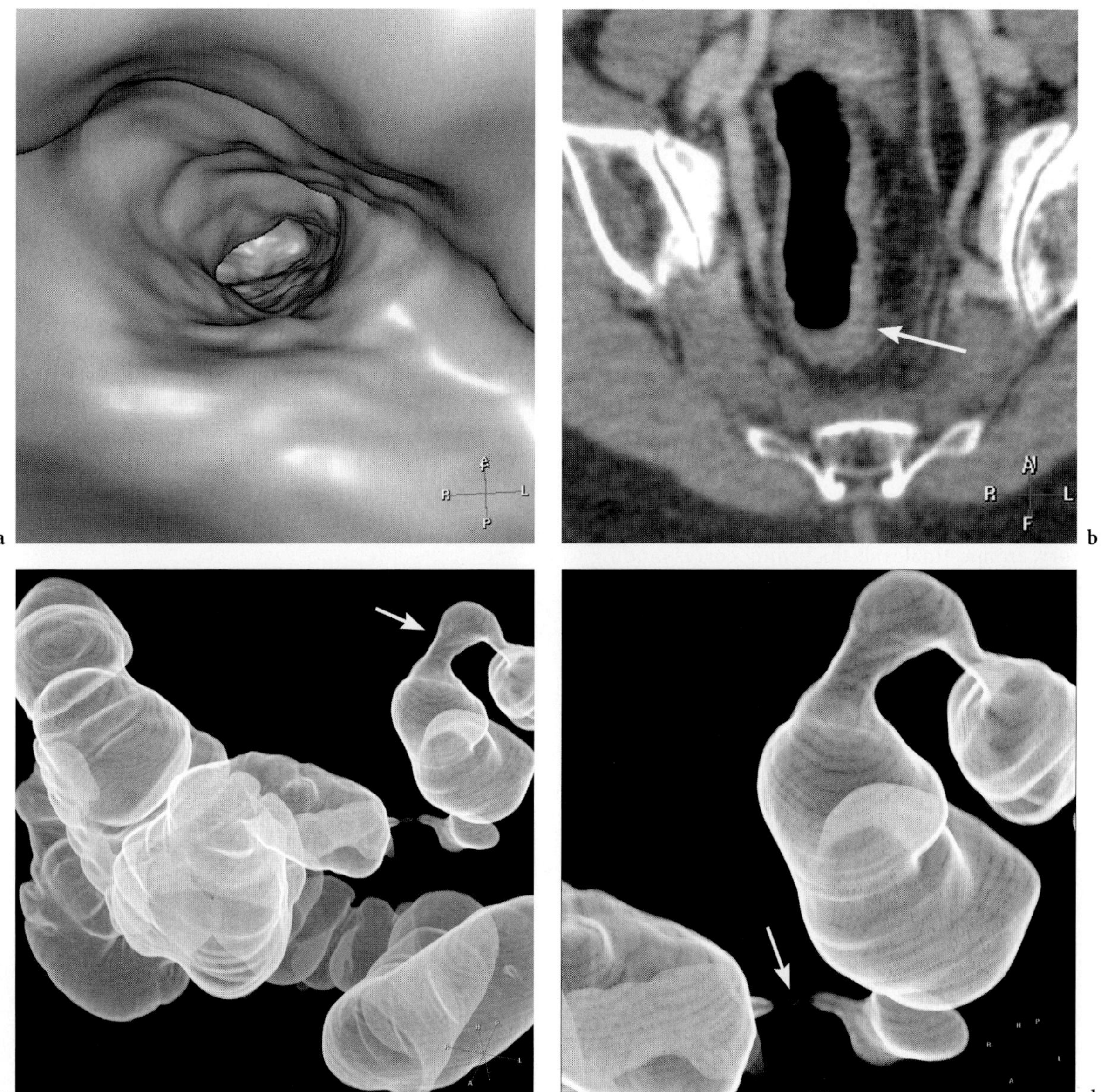

Fig. 6.27a–d. A 65-year-old woman with a long history of ulcerative colitis. The patient refused further flexible endoscopies due to the extreme pain experienced during passage of the endoscope through the multiple stenoses. The virtual endoscopy (**a**) shows a coarse mucosal surface, supporting the suspicion of a stenosis. The axial image (**b**) at the level of the rectosigmoid colon clearly shows the inflammatory wall thickening (*arrow*). In the TTP reconstructions (**c**, **d**), the segmental pattern of the longstanding colitis (for more than 30 years) with the impressive stenotic changes are best appreciated as an overview (*arrows*)

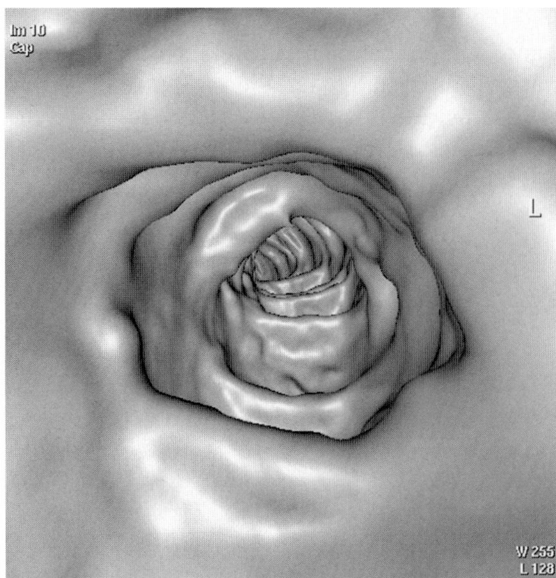

a

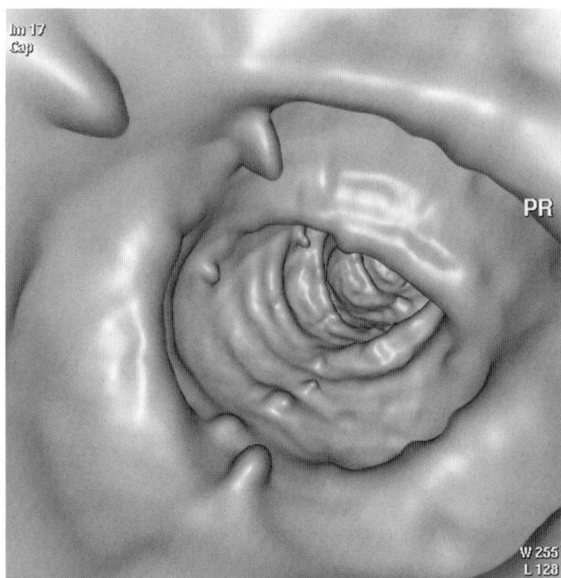

b

Fig. 6.28a, b. Multiple so-called pseudopolyps in the descending colon in a patient with histologically proven colitis. Note the coarse surface of the intestinal wall

affections described in terms of "postinflammatory polyposis" or "cobblestone appearance", can also be revealed on virtual endoscopy (Fig. 6.28). In such instances histological classification based solely upon virtual endoscopy is, of course, not possible; however, in combination with the often known clinical history, an intestinal wall thickening corresponding to the duration of illness, in combination with proliferative fatty tissue (creeping fat), an inflammatory pericolic infiltration and the demonstration of multiple small polyp-like structures, the diagnosis can be stated with confidence.

The status after colitides has a typical presentation on virtual endoscopy as well: the scarcity of haustra, otherwise known as "featureless" colon, can be impressively documented (Fig. 6.29). This has been shown to be favourable for virtual endoscopic imaging. Due to the reduced mucosal folds in the "burned-out" colonic areas, less fluid is retained in the intestine and as a result it is possible to obtain an essentially free, unobstructed view over a large segment of the colon. One notable advantage of virtual endoscopy in patients with inflammatory intestinal diseases, especially in the affected areas, is that the mechanical and often painful irritation caused by flexible endoscopy can be circumvented. The patients with ulcerative colitis examined in our hospital were especially euphoric about the painless examination; most patients with these chronic diseases are traumatised by the repetitive endoscopies. If the virtual endoscopy reveals that the colon is free of polyps, all sections of the large bowel are well viewable, no secondary signs exist indicating a previous inflammation and the patient is asymptomatic, then flexible endoscopy need not be performed.

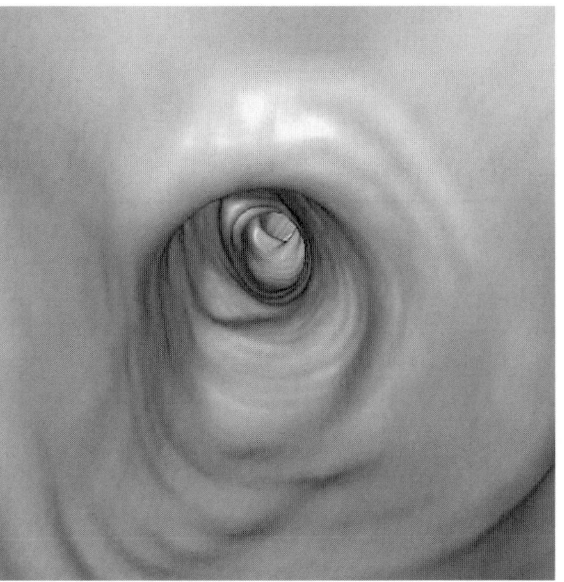

Fig. 6.29. Example of a "featureless colon" in a patient with longstanding colitis. Note the almost complete loss of haustra in the descending colon

6.1.4.9.8
Crohn's Disease

Patients with Crohn's disease also have an increased risk of suffering from colorectal cancer. No studies investigating which stage of illness and which timc interval are best for endoscopic surveillance are not yet available. The risk of developing a malignancy is further increased by extensive or total colitis and by early onset of the disease with the first manifestation occurring before the 30th birthday (Gillen et al. 1994). In these cases, a monitoring programme similar to that of patients with ulcerative colitis should be considered.

Since patients with Crohn's disease tend to be rather young, the use of ionising radiation should be considered with reservation. In an acute case, for example a clinically acute abdomen, the indication for CT is indisputable, albeit with a different clinical purpose than in virtual endoscopy: of acute interest is the exclusion of complications such as abscess or fistulas, with exclusion of a tumour a secondary goal. Furthermore, intestinal cleansing is hardly achievable in acute instances. In such circumstances, MRI can play a valuable role, particularly because of the absence of radiation exposure. As yet there is no experience to show whether an MRI examination protocol that allows for adequate image quality to diagnose complications can simultaneously provide data employable for virtual endoscopic postprocessing.

In essence, virtual endoscopy can also provide valuable information for patients with Crohn's disease. It is possible by an endoscopically impassable stenosis of the proximal intestine to image the colon beyond the stenotic area and rule out a tumour or any other manifestations occurring as a result of the underlying disease (Fig. 6.30). Furthermore, virtual endoscopy offers the possibility to distinguish pseudoulcerations, which on flexible endoscopy, due to the absence of optical depth information, cannot be differentiated from fistulas. This ability to appreciate depth penetration is not a strength of virtual endoscopy per se, but rather of the cross-sectional imaging; through multiplanar reconstructions, one level can be positioned exactly in the area of interest in order to portray the path of an ulcer or a fistula. Importantly, although the diagnosis of this disease is greatly facilitated by imaging modalities, the proof lies invariably in the histological analysis, which requires a true endoscopic examination (Fig. 6.31). Because isolated mucosal changes are often the main pathology in Crohn's disease and these changes are not visible in virtual endoscopy, the diagnostic value of virtual endoscopy for this disease must be critically evaluated.

6.1.4.9.9
Colorectal Cancer

Since the presence of colorectal cancer is largely associated with lesions larger than 1 cm in diameter (Muto et al. 1975; Winawer et al. 1997), detection of colorectal cancer can be considered to be the second goal (following polyp detection) of virtual endoscopy and is, due to the expected larger size of the lesions, comparatively simple to realise. In a prospective study, 63 patients with clinical or endoscopic suspicion of colorectal cancer were examined with spiral CT after bowel cleansing, premedication with 40 mg *N*-butylscopolamine and rectal insufflation of CO_2 gas. Virtual endoscopy was calculated using the volume-rendering technique. The images were interpreted without knowing the true endoscopy findings, and all carcinomas diagnosed were surgically resected.

In 51 patients, a total of 53 carcinomas were found in all stages (pT1: n=4; pT2: n=22; pT3: n=21; pT4: n=6), resulting in a calculated sensitivity of 100%; however, the smallest tumour had a size of 0.8 cm. Furthermore, due consideration must be paid to the highly selected patient collective in this examination; the results can hardly be extrapolated to a randomised, unselected population in a screening setting. The specificity is another question that deserves further evaluation: in this series, the results from virtual and true endoscopy (including biopsy) aroused suspicion of a stage T4 sigmoid tumour in one patient, but massive chronic diverticulitis was found upon histopathology after surgical resection.

Reconstruction of the data with the TTP technique can very impressively show the surgeon where the carcinoma is localised (Fig. 6.32). With assistance of a path that extends through the distended bowel, exact information as to the distance from the anus is possible. Another aspect has become apparent through the use of virtual endoscopy: due to the necessary modifications of the examination protocol, i.e. the use of particularly thin slices compared to standard CT of the abdomen and pelvis, more precise classification of the tumor stage is made possible: the reduced partial volume effect in thinner slices leads to improved presentation of tissue boundaries, and an infiltration of the tumour into the surroundings can be diagnosed with greater confidence (Fig. 6.33). Preliminary evaluation of the staging in the above-mentioned series showed that preoperative differentiation between stages T2 and T3 and between stages T3 and T4 was in better accordance with the histopathological staging results than the intraoperative palpation and inspection by the surgeons.

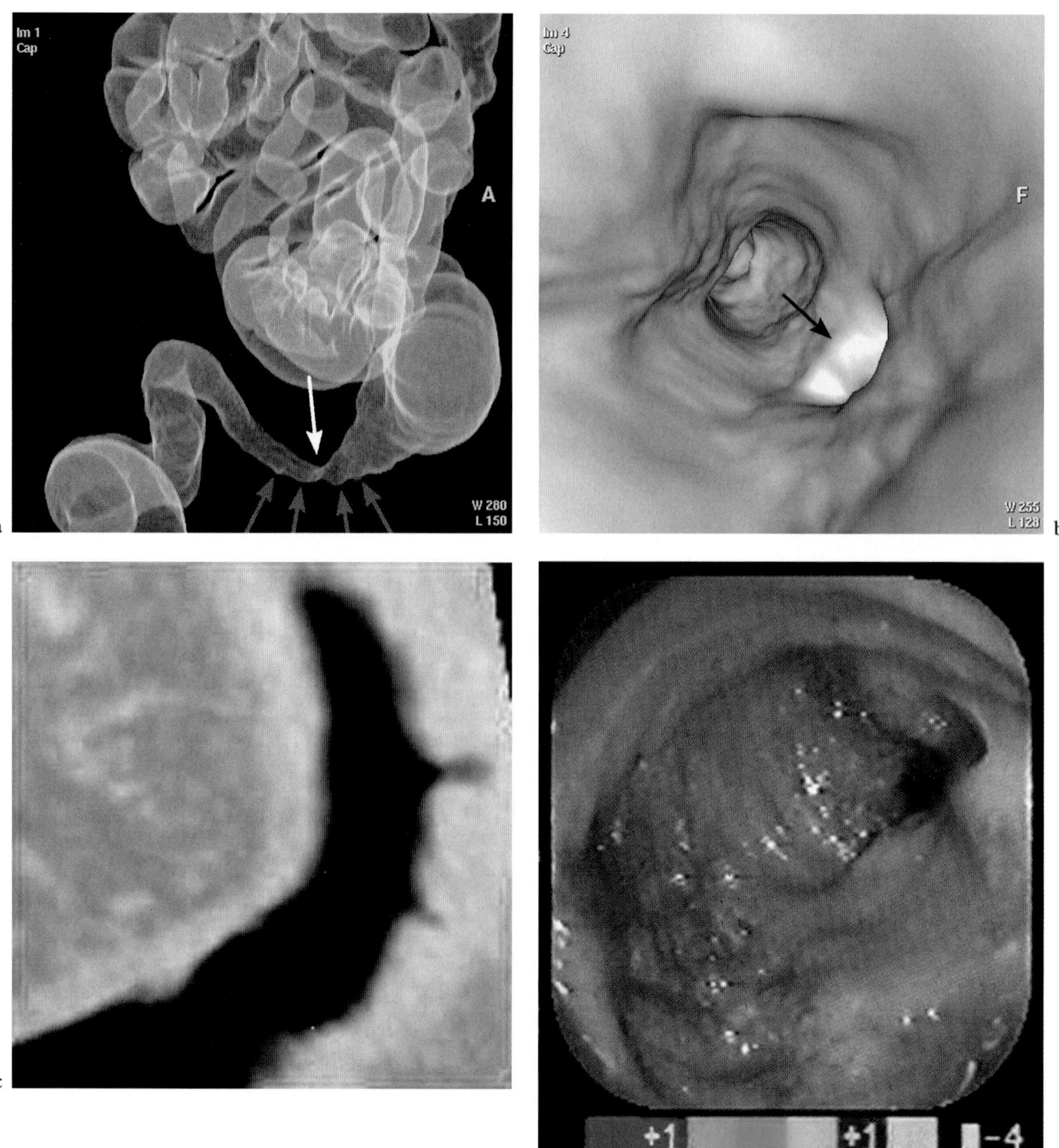

Fig. 6.30a–d. Young female patient with Crohn's disease. The TTP image (**a**) demonstrates the high-grade stenosis (*arrow*) in the sigmoid colon that could not be passed with a flexible endoscope. The *red arrows* show multiple "pseudoulcerations", which typically arise in Crohn's disease. Note also the prestenotic dilatation, which is nicely visible in this type of display. **b** In the virtual endoscopy, the ulcerations (*arrow*) are also easily identified. The view is directed from distal to proximal towards the stenosis. **c** In an enlargement of the multiplanar reconstruction of the sigmoid colon distally to the stenosis the distinctive wall thickening and deep pseudoulcerations are clearly recognisable. Fistulas are not present. **d** Display of the stenosis in the flexible endoscopy. The detected lumen remainder in the upper right corner was too narrow for the passage of the flexible endoscope

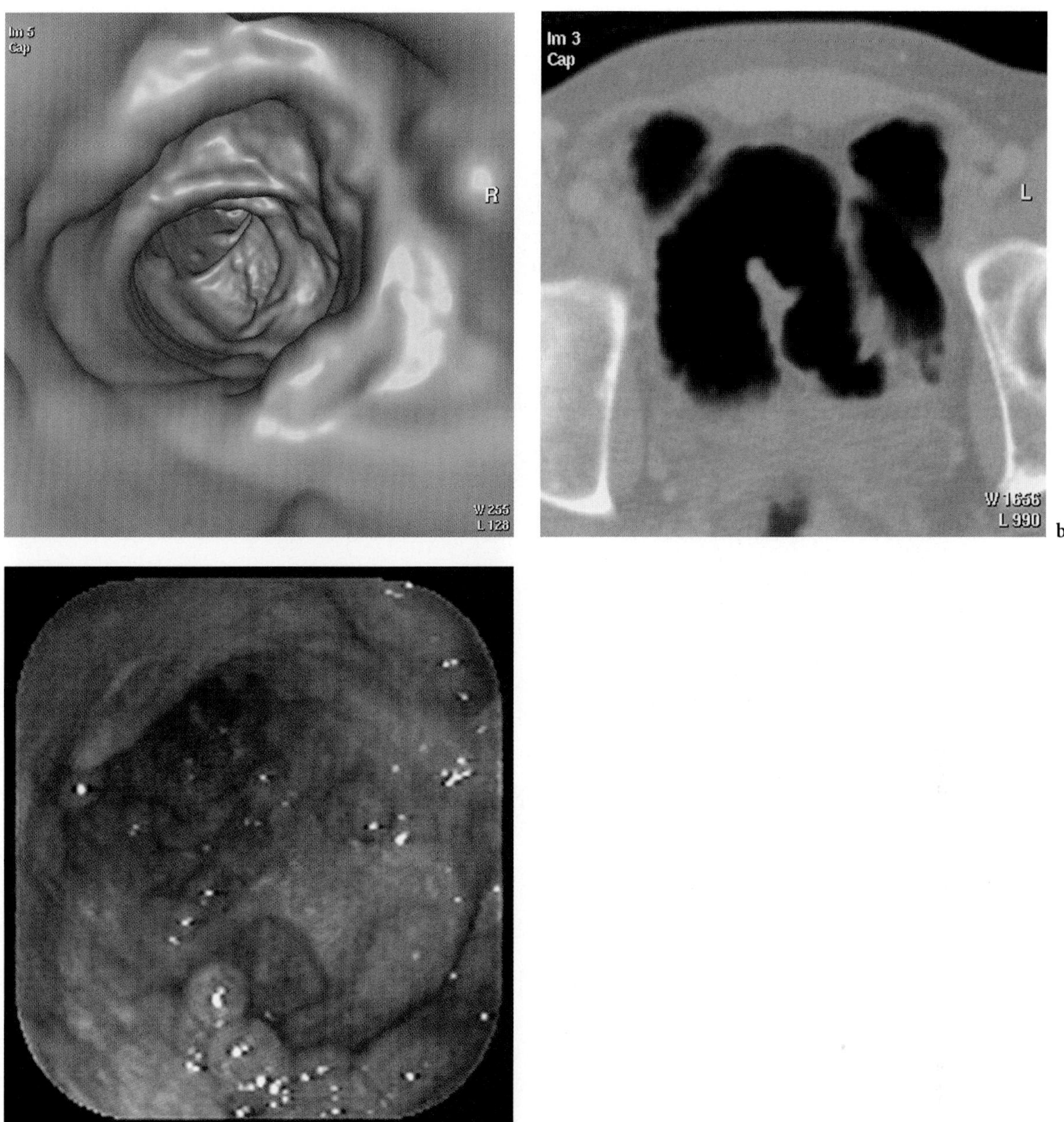

Fig. 6.31a–c. A 36-year-old man with Crohn's disease. The multiple unspecific pseudopolypous inconsistencies in the virtual endoscopy (**a**) are clearly identifiable, and in combination with the multiplanar reconstructions (axial image, **b**) it is possible to express the suspicion of Crohn's disease from the morphology. The ultimate diagnosis can, however, first be established after flexible endoscopy (**c**) and subsequent biopsy. Note, however, the strong morphological correlation between virtual and flexible endoscopy

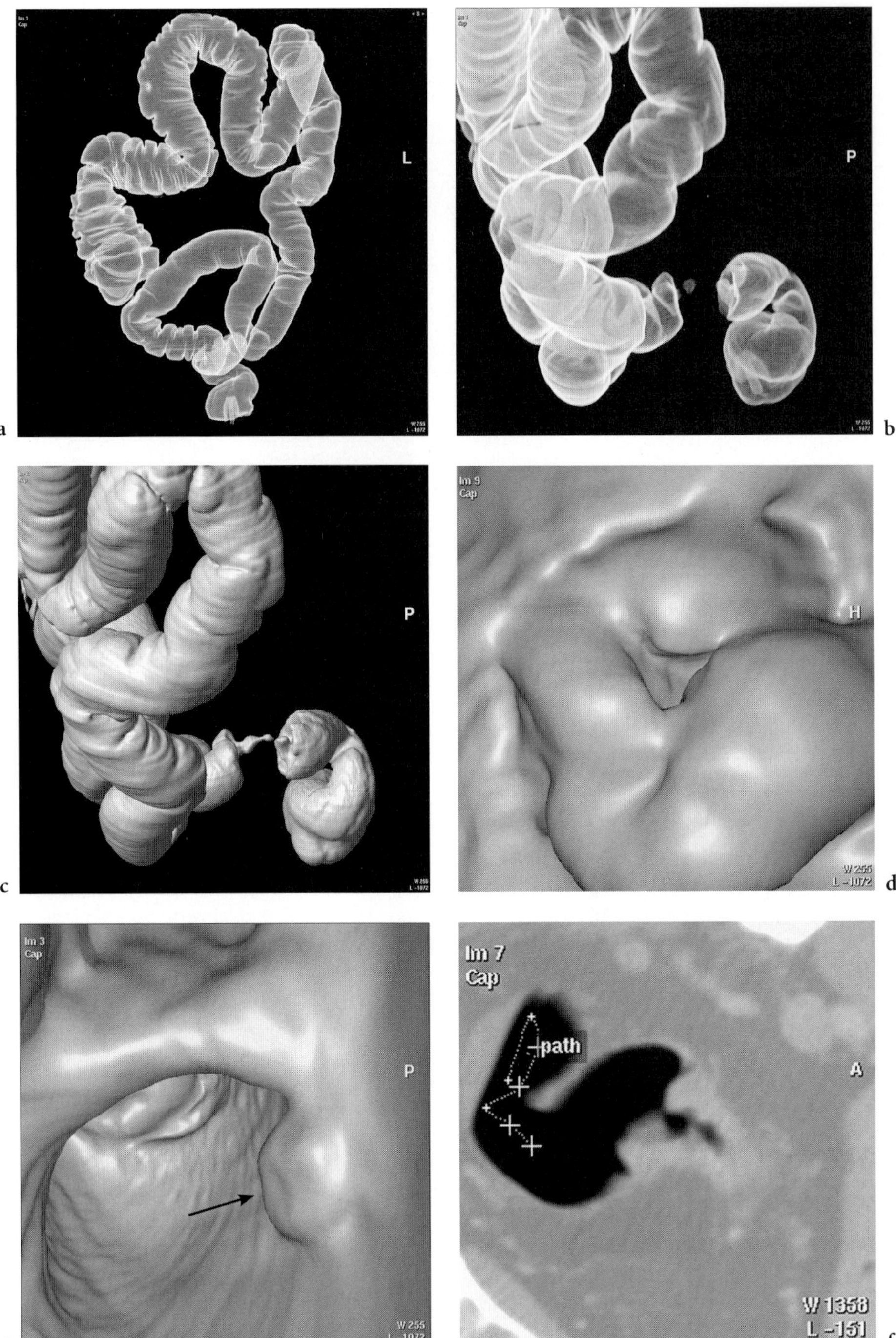

Fig. 6.32a–f. A 69-year-old man with endoscopically ascertained but impassable carcinoma in the sigmoid colon. The overview image (**a**) in TTP technique initially does not show the tumour; however, once the bowels have been rotated the tumour stenosis can be impressively displayed (**b**). In this case, a 3D surface-rendered display (**c**) is also implementable because in this display too the tumour is well visible. The virtual endoscopy (**d**) shows the stenosing tumour that can be virtually bypassed. Proximal to the tumour (**e**) a smaller 6-mm polyp was detected (*arrow*). The multiplanar reconstruction (**f**) is diagnostically indispensable since only in this presentation can the depth of infiltration be judged. Through the path placed along the intestine, it is possible to reliably estimate the location of the tumour in centimetres ab ano

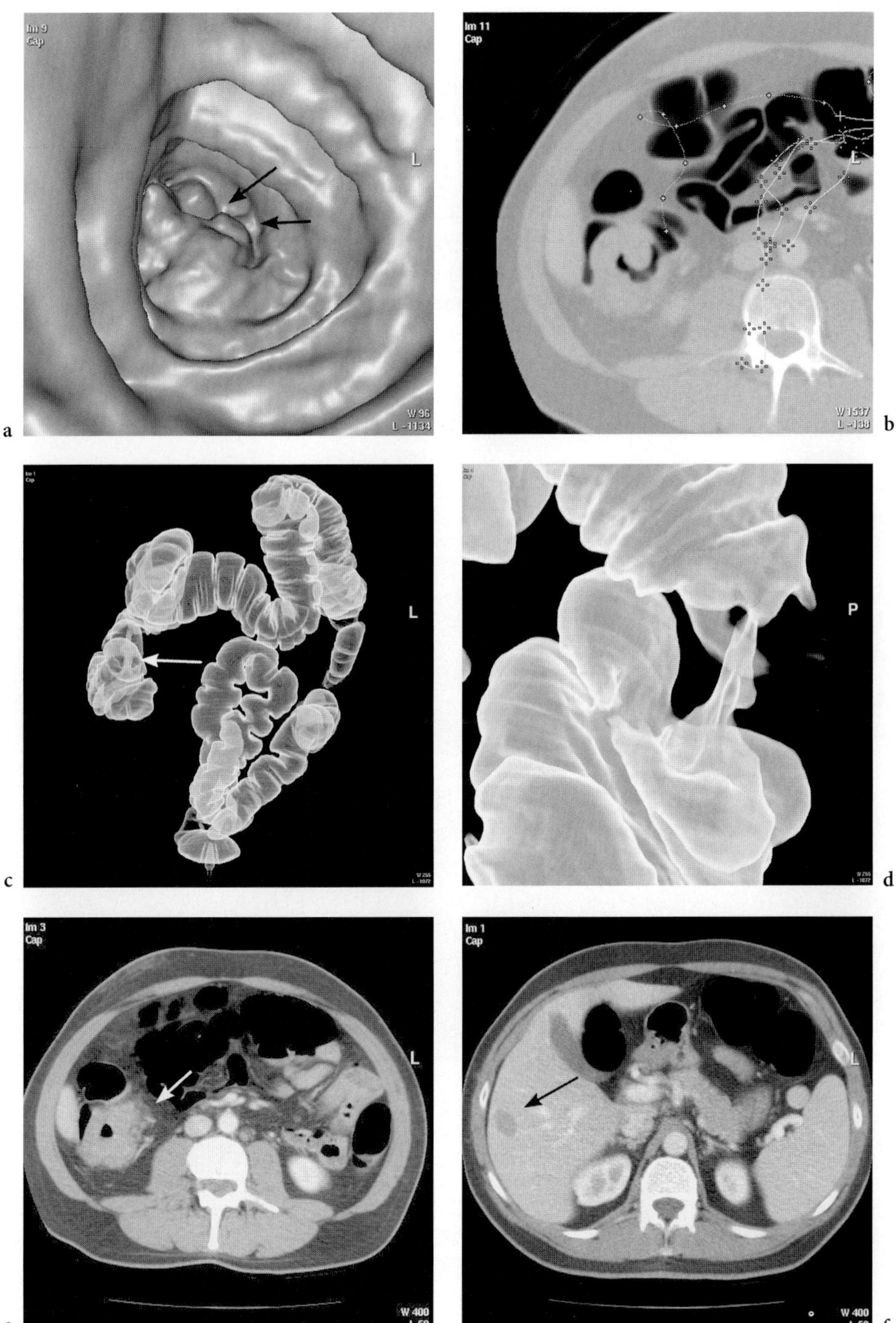

Fig. 6.33a–f. A 47-year-old man with a carcinoma in the ascending colon. The virtual endoscopy (**a**) is a view from distal onto the nodular-stenotic growing tumour (*arrows*). The path in the axial cross-section (**b**) traces the path taken by the virtual endoscope approaching from a distal point in the colon. The overview in TTP technique (**c**) permits visualisation of the stenosis (*arrow*) in the ascending colon through the transparent bowel wall; a TTP image from the left dorsolateral side shows effectively the full extent of the tumour (**d**). Because intravenous contrast material was given for this examination, the tumour growth beyond the colonic wall (*arrow*) can also be portrayed in the axial image (**e**) using a soft tissue window/level setting (400/50). In addition, the locally affected lymph nodes are depicted (stage N1). In the liver (**f**) a single hepatic metastasis is shown (*arrow*). The tumour was staged as T3N1M1

Virtual endoscopy appears to have multiple properties that are advantageous for the investigation of suspected colorectal carcinoma and for preoperative assessment. With a great degree of certainty, the tumour can be detected, precisely localised, well demonstrated and simultaneously staged. In addition, by administering intravenous contrast medium preoperatively, staging of distant metastases can be achieved. Independent of which modality, CT or MRI, is used for virtual endoscopy, the exclusion of liver metastases can be accomplished concurrently with the customary diagnostic certainty.

A further current demand on imaging modalities is the indication to carry out DCBE in order to determine whether a carcinoma causing an intestinal stenosis, a second tumour, or a synchronous carcinoma in the large bowel exists. If the tumour stenosis is too restrictive and the flexible endoscope is not able to pass this obstacle, it is necessary to rule out a synchronous carcinoma preoperatively (Fig. 6.34). The occurrence of a synchronous carcinoma is reported to be 1.6–9.3% in the literature (Isabel-Martinez et al. 1988). In a study on 29 patients with colorectal cancers that were endoscopically not traversable, not only all 29 cancers were detected, but also two synchronous cancers and a total of 24 polyps proximal from the occlusive carcinoma, all of which were later, if not surgically removed, confirmed either by fol-

a

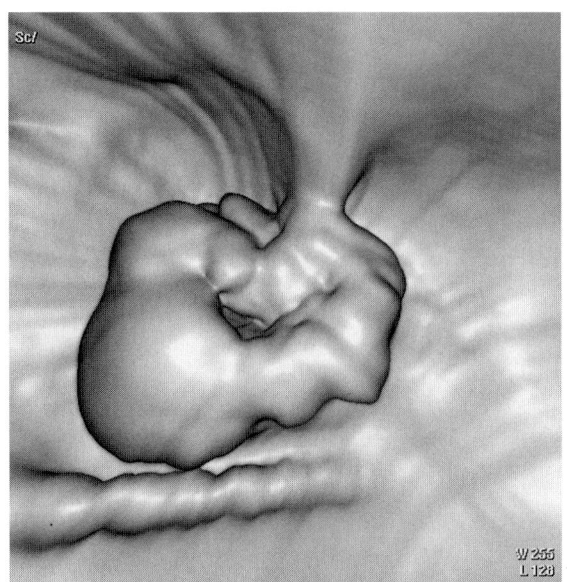

b

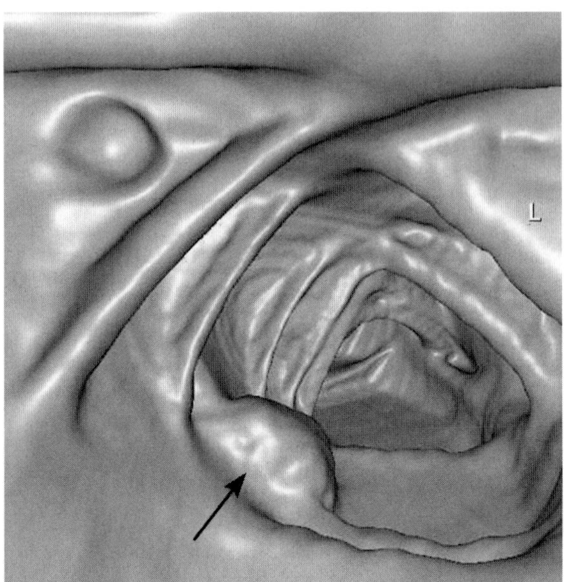

c

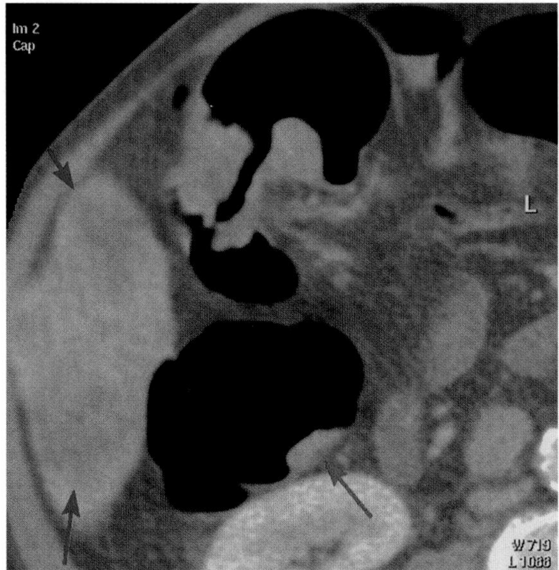

Fig. 6.34a–c. Stenotic colon carcinoma in the right flexure. The presence of a synchronous carcinoma was to be ruled out preoperatively. **a** The virtual endoscopic view from distal onto the carcinoma, which could not be passed endoscopically. **b** Proximal to the tumour two further findings can be observed: a 5-mm polyp and a small second carcinoma (*arrow*). **c** The axial slice demonstrates the tumour growth beyond the bowel wall; the *red arrow* indicates the small proximal concurrent tumor. Both tumour manifestations enhance with intravenous contrast material. Note also the simultaneous depiction of disseminated hepatic metastases (*blue arrows*)

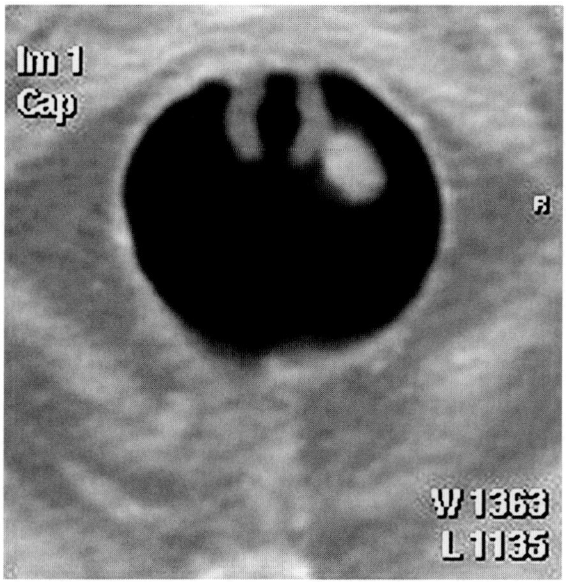

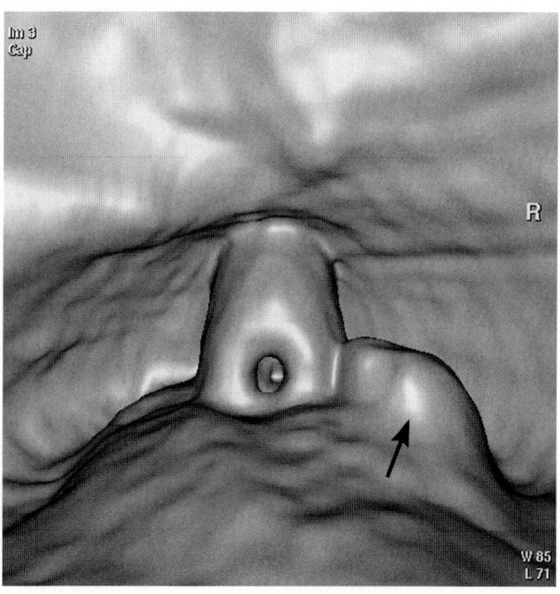

Fig. 6.35a, b. Example of an 8-mm rectal polyp. **a** The tip of the rectally inserted tube has already come into contact with the polyp. **b** Viewing back upon the rectal ampulla the polyp (*arrow*) located in close proximity to the rectal tube can be easily overlooked

low-up endoscopy or barium enema examination (Fenlon et al. 1999a). Preoperatively conducted barium enemas did not allow the complete evaluation of the proximal colon; in other words, neither colonoscopy nor barium enema examination were successful in detecting the two synchronous cancers in that series.

Deep-lying polyps and rectal carcinomas represent a special scenario since they are easily overlooked on virtual endoscopy (Fig. 6.35). Firstly, the placed intestinal tube can disguise the tumours so that only a "retrospective" view prompts suspicion of a tumour. In addition, especially with intravenous contrast agent administration, both tumour tissue and haemorrhoids are enhanced, in which case differentiation is possible neither morphologically nor with contrast agent dynamics. In this respect, it is necessary to perform rectal palpation before positioning the rectal tube. This should serve the purpose not only of ruling out a deeply seated carcinoma (Fig. 6.36), but also, in the event of such a carcinoma, of avoiding perforation during placement of the intestinal tube.

6.1.4.9.10
Follow-Up After Polypectomy and Surgery

The diagnosis of a solitary adenomatous polyp or flat adenoma with a size of less than 1 cm followed by an endoscopic polypectomy in healthy individuals does not increase the probability of being afflicted with a colorectal cancer. For this reason, a single tubular adenoma need not, especially in elderly individuals, imply special after-care. Even for individuals who undergo occasional sigmoidoscopies, the presence of a tubular adenoma less than 1 cm in size is associated with a probability of less than 1% of presenting with a colorectal cancer. Also, the likelihood of development of a carcinoma at a future date does not differ from that in individuals with an average risk (Atkins et al. 1992).

If a polyp has been removed and does not show any histological evidence of high-grade dysplasia, there appears to be no special indication for follow-up or repeated virtual or flexible endoscopy. These circumstances change, however, upon detection and therapy of a colorectal carcinoma, because metachronous carcinomas (i.e. carcinomas that develop 6 months or more following discovery of the first tumour) occur with a frequency of 2%. Here the role of virtual endoscopy is especially appreciable, since a local recurrence (Farouk et al. 1998; Thoeni 1997) and distal metastases can be ruled out simultaneously in the framework of a postoperative follow-up visit (Freeny 1986; Harned et al. 1994; Ott et al. 1998). In this regard, follow-up programmes can be critically revised (Romano et al. 1995), not to mention the fact that there is controversy in the literature concerning the value of an intensive after-care programme following operative removal of colorectal carcinoma (Giess et al. 1998). In a current study on

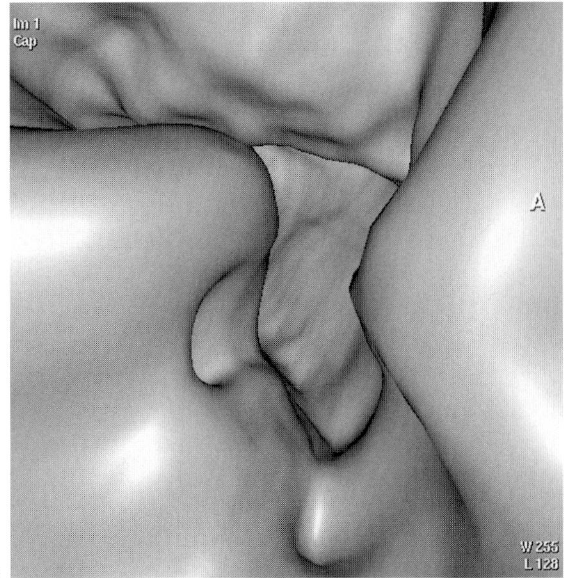

a

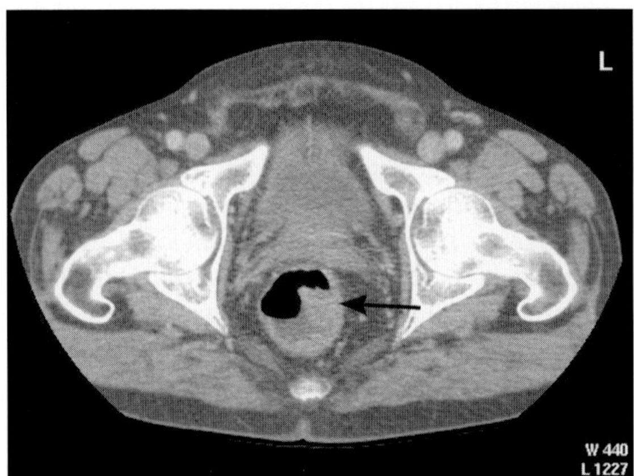

b

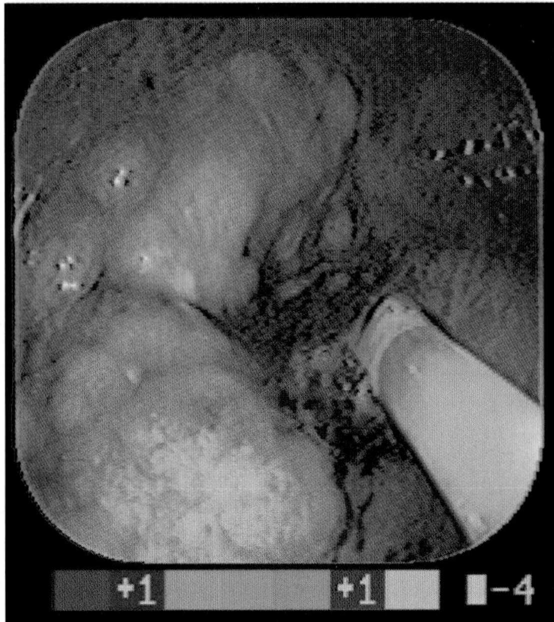

c

325 patients, an improvement in the 5-year survival rate could not be shown with intensive after-care consisting of annual colonoscopy, liver CT and chest radiography (Schoemaker et al. 1998). Intensive follow-up programmes are also disputable from the viewpoint of cost-effectiveness (Biggs and Ballantyne 1994).

An upcoming interesting field of research will be when metabolic information from positron emission tomography (PET) can be fused with morphological information obtained through CT or MRI (Ogunbiyi et al. 1997; Tempero et al. 1995). It is conceivable that PET information will also be able to be superimposed upon virtual endoscopic images, thus adding functional information to endoscopic views.

6.1.4.9.11 Diverticula, Normal Variants

Colon diverticula are very common among older generations in Western, industrialised countries. An estimated 33–48% of the population older than 50 years are afflicted (Hughes 1969; Manousos et al. 1967). At the age of 70 years, up to 60% suffer from diverticula (Painter and Burkitt 1975). Although right-sided colonic diverticula occur and are common in the Orient, in Western societies the problem is predominantly that of left-sided and particularly sigmoid diverticula. Approximately 10–30% of the patients are symptomatic (Almy and Howell 1980; Parks 1975; Pohlmann 1988), about 1 in 70 of this group require hospitalisation, and 1 in 200 undergo surgical intervention (Hughes 1975). Diverticula are also not uncommon in younger individuals; for example, ca. 10% of the patients between the ages of 30 and 50 years who receive barium enemas also have diverticula. Morbidity and death due to diverticulitis relate to the degree of sepsis at presentation, compounded by coincidental degenerative diseases in aged patients, which may be reduced by optimal operative and supportive treatment but cannot be

Fig. 6.36a–c. A 56-year-old patient with a deep-seated rectal carcinoma. The tumour was palpated digitally and the rectal tube was removed after insufflation of carbon dioxide and prior to the CT acquisition. Otherwise, the tumour would have been traversed by the tube, preventing its detection. **a** The virtual endoscopy view, which corresponds with the true endoscopic view taken during biopsy (**c**). The axial scan (**b**) demonstrates the rectal carcinoma, which can be differentiated from the remaining rectal fluid due to the enhancement caused by the contrast material (*arrow*)

eliminated. In a condition in which the great majority of patients do not require surgery, the challenge in management is timely identification of patients who will benefit from operation whilst minimising the frequency of unnecessary and inappropriate interventions.

The concept that acquired sigmoid diverticular disease represents a consequence of dietary deficit in vegetable fibre is widely accepted (Painter and Burkitt 1975). Moreover, factors such as the morphological changes in the colonic wall associated with hyperelastosis (Whiteway and Morson 1985) and altered collagen structure (Wess et al. 1995) related to ageing contribute to its progression. An active lifestyle with physical exercise supplements the protective effect of the reduced intraluminal pressure associated with a high fibre diet in terms of a reduced incidence of diverticular disease (Aldoori et al. 1995).

All in all, diverticula are easily identified by virtual endoscopy (Fig. 6.37). They show the characteristic appearance that is exactly parallel to the flexible endoscopy presentation. TTP also allows simple and unproblematic recognition of diverticula. Most often, however, the corresponding axial CT slice is even more useful for diagnostic purposes and shows the full extension of the herniation. Axial slices are required in order to identify an accompanying inflammation based on a swelling of the intestinal wall, the colonic folds, or in order to diagnose infiltration of the surrounding adipose tissue. In relation to the remaining colon, swollen folds are also well discernible in virtual endoscopy, but often the sigmoid colon remains incompletely distended. In such cases adequate sigmoid distension can be achieved either through additional gas insufflation or alternatively by re-examining the patient in prone position. The consequent additional examining time, the postprocessing workload and, if CT is used, the increased radiation exposure have already been mentioned.

The administration of intravenous contrast material produces sufficient diagnostic information for the exclusion or detection of an abscess formation in the pericolic region of symptomatic patients. Last but not least, the foundation is supplied for discussing with the surgeons the indication for placement of a drain under CT guidance, and, if so decided, CT-guided drainage in the same session. Extremely extensive, inflammatory pericolic infiltrates remain difficult to differentiate from a tumour. In one case of massive obstruction with corresponding clinical symptoms, flexible endoscopy with simultaneous biopsy initiated the suspicion of an advanced colorectal carcinoma; virtual endoscopy even postulated the suspicion of infiltration from a carcinoma in the neighbouring organs (tumor stage T4). At operation, conglomerate tumours were resected under oncological recommendation. It was only the subsequent histological examination that produced the correct diagnosis of chronic diverticulitis with no evidence of malignancy.

The symptoms of diverticulitis can, as already discussed, be very similar to those of colorectal carcinoma. The value of virtual endoscopy in patients with abdominal pain and occult blood in the stools is firstly to rule out a malignant tumour and then to provide a basis for recommendations of possible therapeutic alternatives. Since the exclusion of malignancy within an immensely inflamed intestinal wall is difficult almost to the point of impossibility, the possibility of repeating the examination after clinical control of the symptoms and initiation of the appropriate therapy should be considered.

6.1.4.9.12
Side Findings

"Side findings", defined as relevant findings that are entirely unsuspected and have nothing to do with the existing intestinal symptoms, or abdominal findings of purely incidental nature, are not infrequent. Among 296 patients, 39 had side findings (13.2%), varying greatly in aetiology. Next to aneurysmal widening of the aorta, vertebral columnar changes, haemangiomas in the liver and pancreatic pseudocysts, leiomyomas of the uterus, mature teratomas (Fig. 6.38) in female patients and, in one case, a urothelial cell carcinoma (Fig. 6.39) were detected. Common to these patients is that the use of intravenous contrast material proved indispensable; the resulting diagnoses otherwise may have remained undescribed. Whether this alone justifies the general application of i.v. contrast material is questionable, especially if the virtual endoscopy is being implemented as a screening modality. In such a setting, the prevalence of side findings is even more limited than that of intestinal pathology. Therefore, one could argue that only in the case of questionable findings should re-examination with contrast material be considered. As already mentioned in Sect. 6.1.2, "Screening for Colorectal Polyps", a prerequisite for any screening technique is cost-effectiveness, and with this in mind the general use of contrast medium should be restrictively considered.

6.1.4.9.13
Artefacts

Anatomic Distortion. Any data acquisition from the human body represents a data sampling technique,

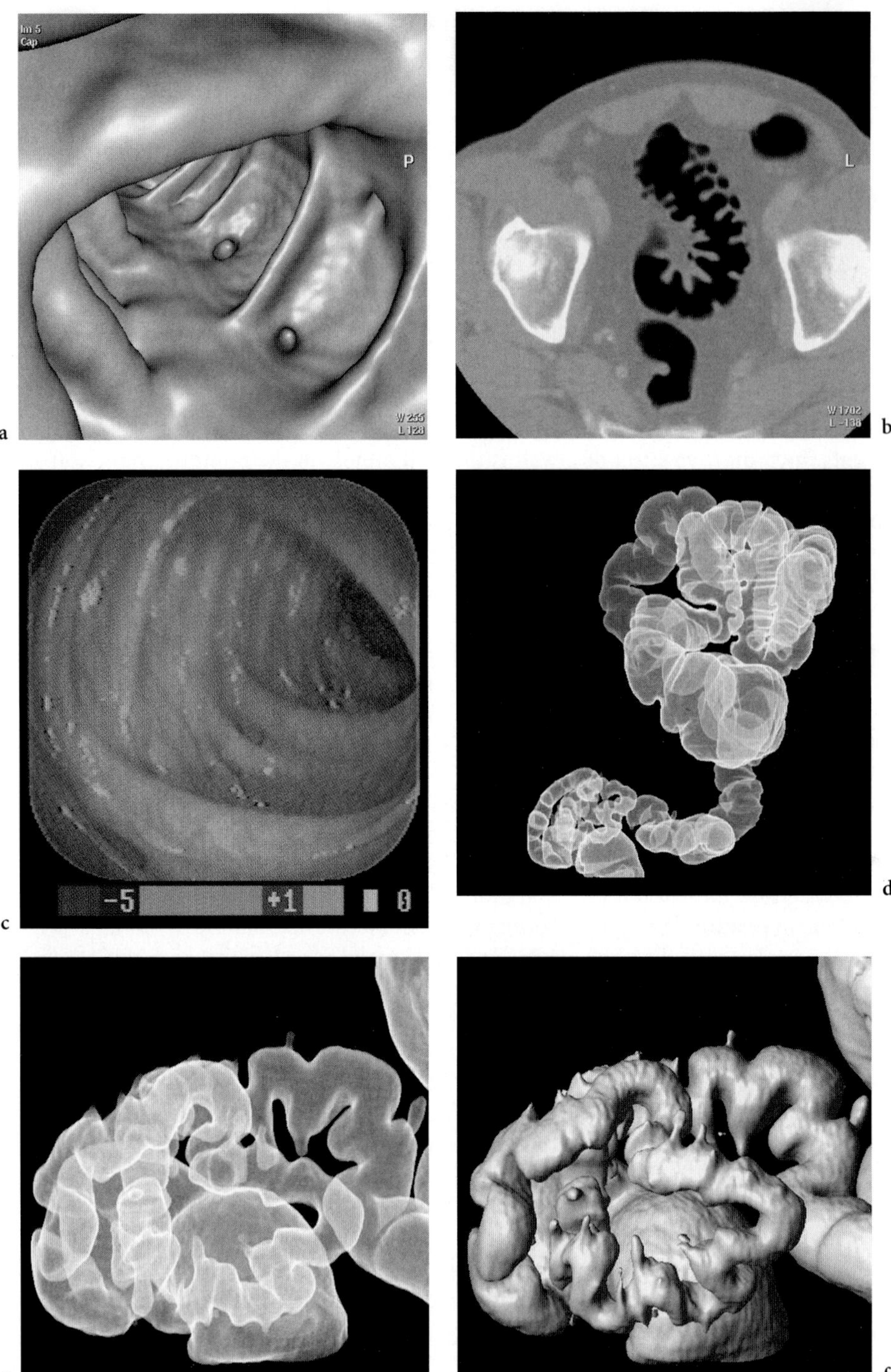

Fig. 6.37a–f. A massive diverticulosis can be well demonstrated in virtual endoscopy (**a**) as well as in the axial slices (**b**). Furthermore, a strong correlation exists between virtual and fibreoptic endoscopy (**c**). The TTP images (**d, e**) impressively show the entire sigmoid colon with its numerous diverticula in one image. The diagnosis of diverticulosis is also irrefutable in the surface-shaded display (**f**)

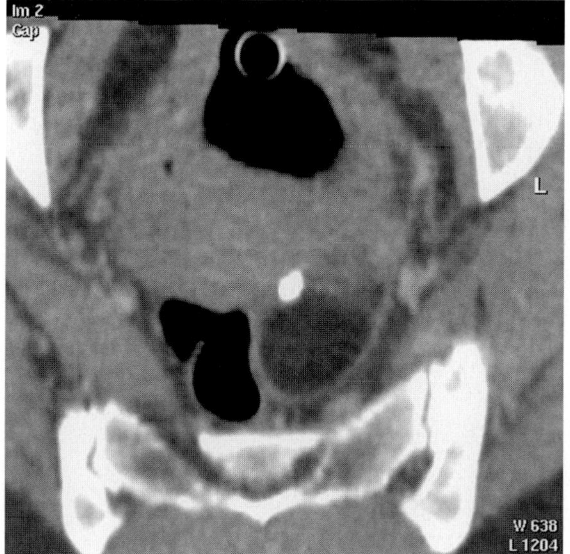

a

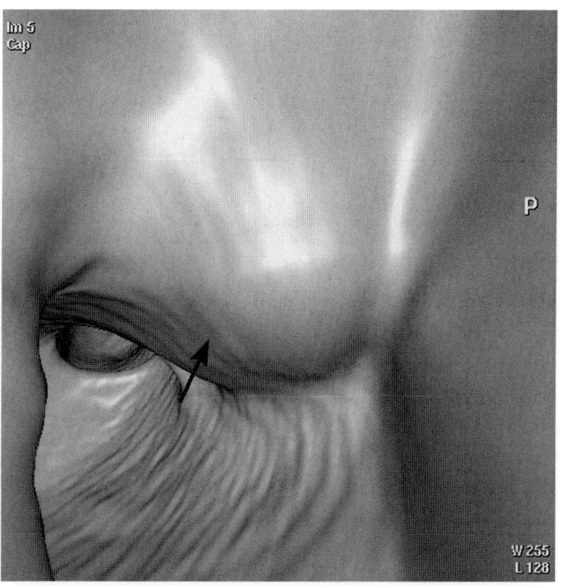

b

Fig. 6.38a, b. A 43-year-old woman who refused a flexible endoscopic examination. The multiplanar slice (**a**) clearly depicts a 4-cm tumour containing regions with fatty tissue and a small tooth. In the virtual endoscopy (**b**), a flat indentation of the colonic lumen can be seen, caused by the space-occupying effect of the teratoma (*arrow*)

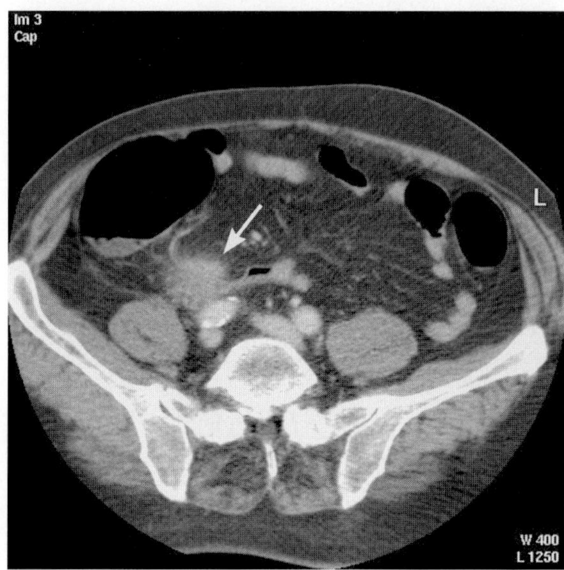

Fig. 6.39. A 60-year-old asymptomatic patient in whom virtual colonoscopy was indicated to rule out a colorectal cancer. The bowel was unremarkable; however, a 2.5-cm urothelial carcinoma was found incidentally (*arrow*). Some faecal residue is seen in the caecum

and the higher the sampling frequency – in other words, the more the information from the images per volume available – the better the anatomical display and the better the details that are visible in the virtual endoscopy. In accordance with the Nyquist theorem, the visual representation of a structure, for example a polyp, requires at least two independent slices in order to actually display it in a reconstruction.

In spiral CT, the slice thickness in essence determines the spatial resolution, and the pitch factor describes the table speed in relation to the revolving speed of the gantry. With higher pitches, the sampling rate over the volume decreases and anatomical distortions increase (Fig. 6.40). This effect is well known for spiral CT and extensively described in general relation to this modality (Kalender et al. 1994; Polacin et al. 1994) and also for virtual endoscopy (Beaulieu et al. 1998).

Motion Artefacts, Breathing Artefacts. General consensus has been reached that a spasmolytic agent, i.e. *N*-butylscopolamine, should be administered in order to achieve optimal distension of the large bowel. For CT, intestinal motility during the scanning does not play a notable role, since due to the short acquisition time for a single slice – of 1 s or even less – slow intestinal peristaltic waves are of no consequence. For MRI, the bowel peristalsis is an important issue despite breathhold sequences: in contrast to CT, which obtains the image data sequentially, the complete volume is obtained during one breathhold in MRI, and intestinal motility compromises the quality of the entire image.

An identical problem exists for breathing motions. Because of the still prolonged total scanning

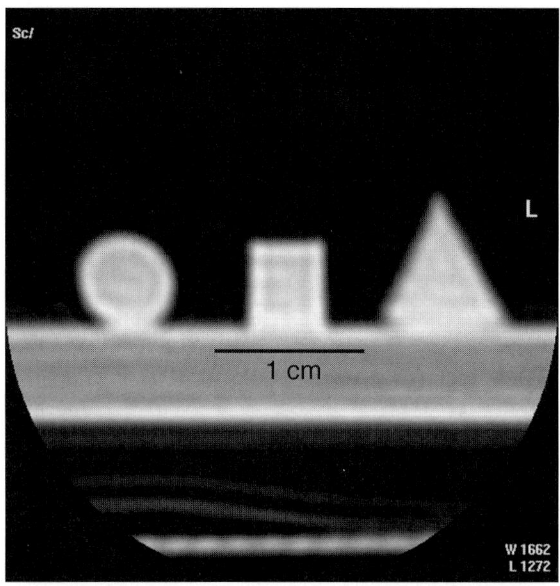

a

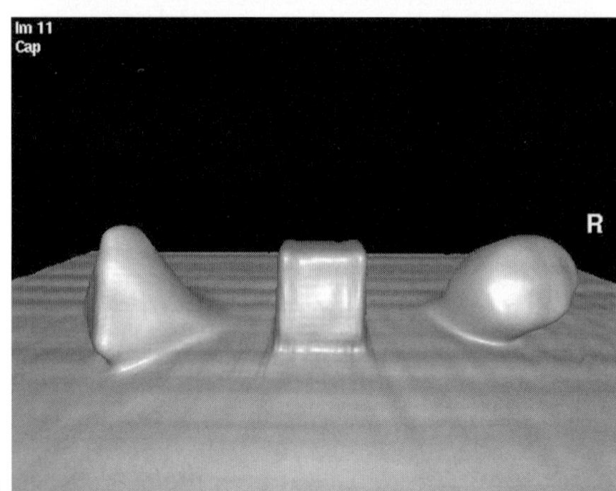

b

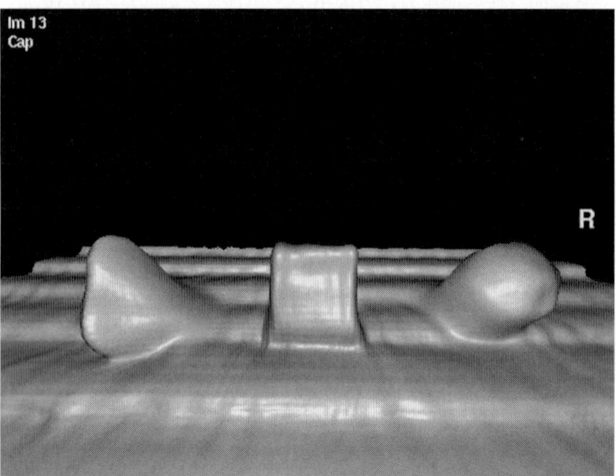

c

Fig. 6.40a–c. Phantom consisting of three different elementary forms. **a** A typical axial slice through the phantom. Imaging parameters: 5 mm slice thickness, 2 mm reconstruction interval. **b** Virtual reconstruction based on a pitch of 1:1 (table feed: 5 mm/s). **c** Virtual reconstruction based on a pitch of 2:1 (table feed: 10 mm/s). Remaining parameters were identical. Note the tremendous extent of pitch artefacts in **c**

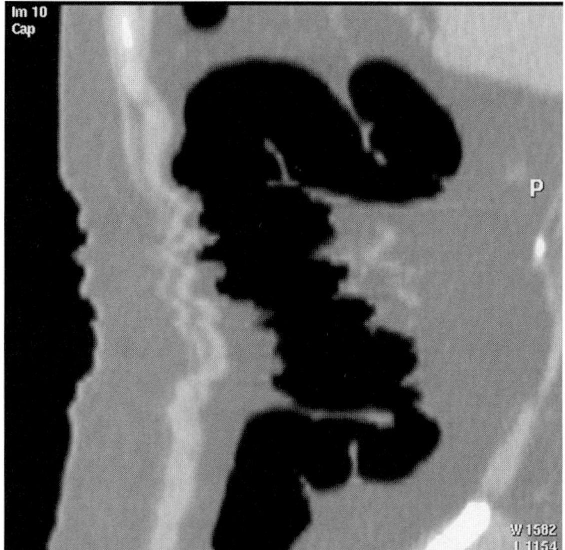

a

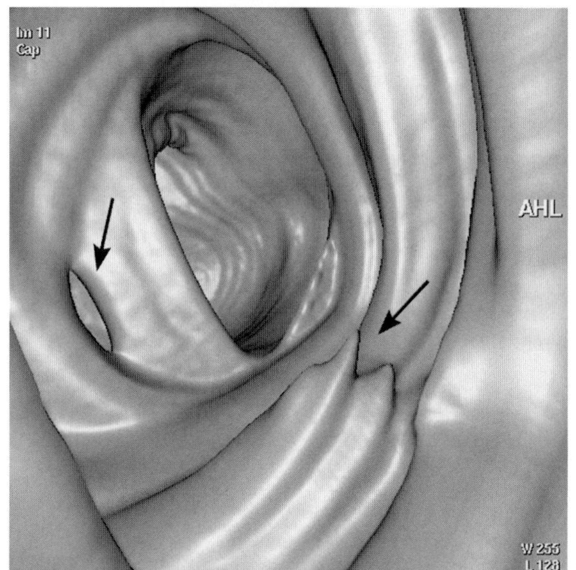

b

Fig. 6.41a, b. Example of a patient who could not maintain a breathhold for longer than 15 s. Since scanning direction was from top to bottom, the upper part of the sagittal reconstruction (**a**) shows no artefacts, whereas the middle part is heavily distorted due to breathing excursions. As scanning progresses to the pelvic region, the breathing has less effect. **b** The virtual reconstruction demonstrates two artefacts: arteficial holes in folds and cogwheel-like figures (*arrows*). However, there is little risk of confusing breathing artefacts with true findings because of their characteristic appearance

time in spiral CT (up to 50 s) it occasionally occurs that patients cannot hold their breath for the whole period. Examining the patient in a direction from cranial to caudal avoids a quality compromise due to breathing motions towards the end of the spiral acquisition. Nevertheless, there are still patients that cannot even hold their breath for 10 s (Fig. 6.41) or are absolutely unable to control their breathing. Reduction in image quality is inevitable under these circumstances; however, the artefacts customarily have a characteristic form and are as such generally identifiable.

Image Noise. One characteristic of all imaging techniques is image noise. When attempting to minimise the radiation exposure for the patient by reducing the radiation dose, the image noise becomes a dominant problem in CT. There are differences across the world in societies' sensitivity towards radiation exposure; in Europe, particularly in Germany, especially high sensitivity prevails. Generally, a reduction in radiation exposure is recommended as long as the image quality is not compromised to such an extent that loss of diagnostic information results or artefacts become so dominant that findings become disguised or artificially created. If CT is being used, a virtual colonoscopy will require an examination of the pelvic region, i.e. the vicinity of the reproductive organs in female patients. Although this represents an ideal occasion to apply a low-dose technique, in this region, due to the skeletal structure and its oval form, the image noise is increased even in standard CT. The effect of image noise is illustrated in Fig. 6.42. Along with the technical improvements in gantry designs, the development of new solid-state detector materials with their increased sensitivity to X-rays (detector efficacy), the improved section sensitivity profiles and many more developments such as modulation of the tube current according to the patient's body geometry, an ultimate goal for CT might be radiation exposure for virtual colonoscopy of approx. 1 mSv. For comparison, the annual, natural radiation exposure in Austria ranges between 3 and 6 mSv.

Bowel Collapse. Undistended or partially collapsed parts of the bowel might represent the most prominent problem in virtual endoscopy, because where no contrast exists, virtual endoscopy is impossible. As already explained, some authors suggest scanning the patient in supine and prone position for that reason, accepting all the disadvantages of doubling the workload etc. Careful insufflation of rectal gas and immediate scanning after the insufflation certainly helps to prevent a bowel collapse, which mainly occurs in the sigmoid colon. Also, in our experi-

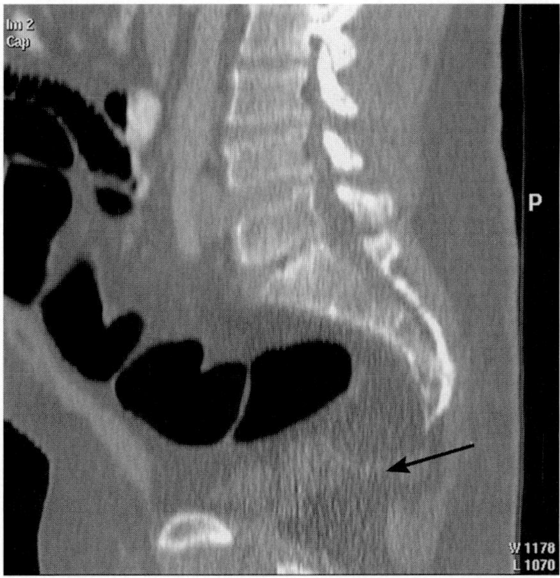

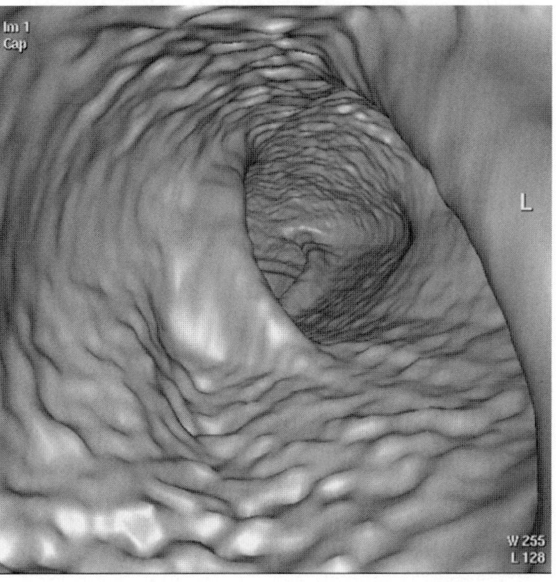

Fig. 6.42a, b. Example of a virtual colonoscopy using 120 kV and 25 mAs, 3 mm slice thickness, pitch 1.7:1, 2 mm reconstruction interval. In the sagittal reconstruction (**a**), pronounced image noise is visible, particularly in the pelvic region (*arrow*). In the virtual endoscopic display (**b**), the bowel wall has an irregular surface and appears to have multiple flat polyps. It may become difficult to differentiate a true polyp from the artificially "rough" surface

ence, uncontrolled or forced insufflation leads to a higher likelihood of spastic reaction, and intensive training of the nurses and technologists seems crucial for optimal patient preparation, timing and scanning.

Partially filling the bowel with contrast material, either through oral or rectal administration, might be another solution; however, it requires the double thresholding feature that makes transparency of both air and contrast material possible (Fig. 6.9). Currently, there is no software available that allows the elimination of the "transition bar" that originates from grey values partially representing air and partially contrast material. Since these bars are mostly horizontal and could be automatically detected and removed, it can be expected that this problem is in principle soluble (Wax et al. 1998). Caution is always advisable when features of an image are automatically removed by a computer, since small polyps or relevant anatomical details and pathology may disappear and remain unrecognised by the radiologist. It should be emphasised that collapsed bowel parts represent the main cause of overlooked polyps. Even i.v. contrast material is not always the answer, since not only the polypous tissue but also the intestinal wall absorbs the contrast agent, preventing differentiation.

Fluid Levels and Residual Faeces. It would be inaccurate to describe fluid levels and faecal residue as imaging artefacts; both are real, existing matter and can only lead to misinterpretation of the images. Fluid levels are a source of error that is unavoidable despite optimal patient preparation. Fluid levels occur in practically every patient, but with varying intensity. They are most commonly found in the caecum, between a few folds in the transverse colon, in the first sigmoid flexure and in the rectum (Fig. 6.12; Fig. 6.43). For the most part, the fluid levels in the rectum can be avoided if the patients are asked to go to the toilet immediately before placement of the rectal tube and this is immediately followed by the examination.

Conducting the CT without i.v. contrast material and without oral labelling (see Sect. 6.1.4.6.4, Faecal Tagging) bears the consequence that polyps beneath the fluid level are concealed. The application of i.v. contrast material allows for differentiation and demarcation of not only the mucosa but also the polypous structures from the water (Fig. 6.44). If oral contrast material is given, the software on the workstation should have the above-mentioned double threshold function, in order to facilitate an undisturbed glance under the fluid level. Oral administration of contrast medium also allows good differentiation between true polyps and residual faecal matter.

Rendering Artefacts. This category accounts for a large variety of artefacts, for example the rippling artefact, which emerge through the rendering algo-

a

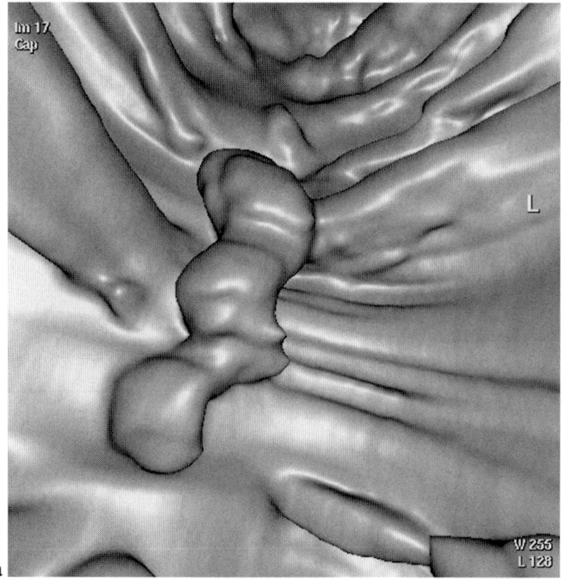

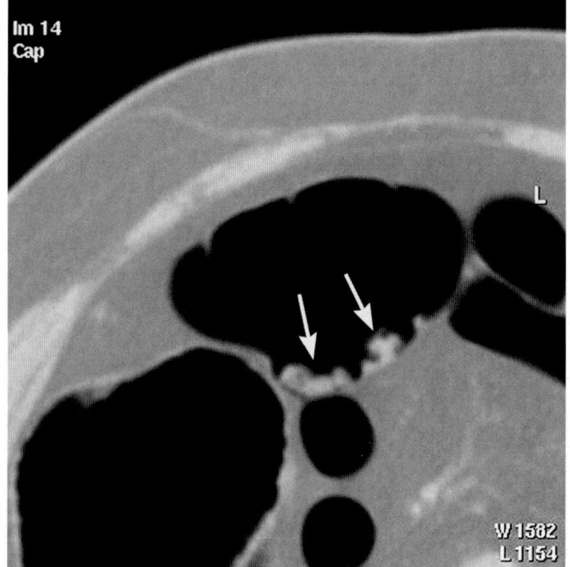

Fig. 6.43. The virtual endoscopic view (**a**) permits recognition of a long "formation", which is never typical of a polyp or carcinoma. In the axial slice (**b**), the "fluffy" consistency is evident (*arrow*), leaving no doubt that the object represents faecal residue

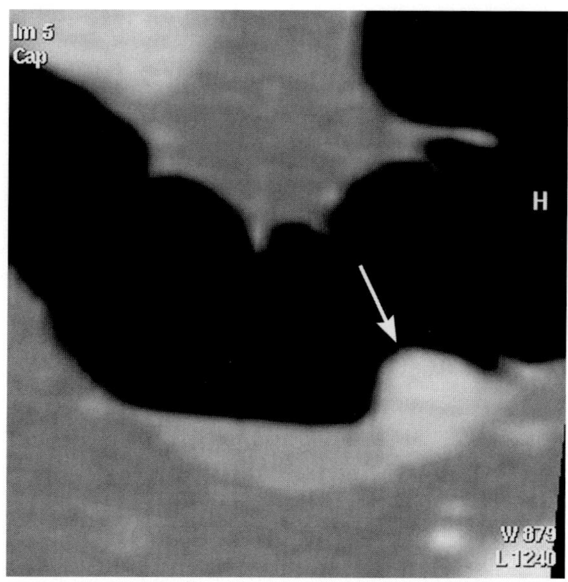

Fig. 6.44. Remaining fluid in the bowel partly covers a polyp. After administration of intravenous contrast material the polyp (*arrow*) can be distinguished from water

rithm and are not included in the original slices as image information. Further details of these artefacts and how they originate can be found in Chap. 1.

6.1.4.10 Clinical Results

Virtual colonoscopy has not yet gained widespread acceptance among radiologists or gastroenterologists. In addition, the clinical results available to date, although often including a correlation with flexible endoscopy or surgery, have all been conducted with selected patient populations; none have been carried out on a true "screening population" having a lower prevalence of colorectal cancer or adenomatous polyps. Despite the possibility of calculating sensitivities and specificities also in small populations, a low specificity for virtual endoscopy in a screening setting would have the consequence that many false-positive patients would have to be re-examined with flexible endoscopy. The costs incurred by false-positive test results are substantial and must be included when assessing the cost-effectiveness of virtual endoscopy.

Initially, sensitivity for polyps represented the focus of most research. In an original study measuring sensitivity, the authors found 83% sensitivity for polyps with a size of 8 mm that were artificially implanted in an intestine. The slice thickness used in this study was 5 mm. Another group, in an initial assessment of sensitivity and specificity, found: for polyps larger than 10 mm, 75% sensitivity and 90% specificity; for polyps between 5 and 10 mm, 66% sensitivity and 63% specificity; and for polyps smaller than 5 mm, 45% sensitivity and 80% specificity (Hara et al. 1997). These data are based on examinations of 70 patients with a total of 115 adenomatous polyps, who additionally underwent CT with 5 mm slice thickness; flexible endoscopy served as the gold standard. The relatively large slice thickness allows one to comprehend why polyps 5 mm in diameter or less could not be reliably detected.

In another examination of 44 patients, overall sensitivity of 93% and specificity of 86% were calculated; the slice thickness was again 5 mm (Dachman et al. 1998). Using oral contrast material for labelling the fluid residues in the colon, the sensitivity for all lesions was 67% and the specificity 50% in a population consisting of 35 patients with 11 patients having space-occupying lesions. However, the sensitivity and specificity were better for patients with polyps larger than 5 mm (100% and 63% respectively), and patients with polyps larger than 1 cm (100% and 84%). The positive and negative predictive values of virtual endoscopy were also computed in this study, with the following results: for any given polyp size, 48% and 93%; for polyps larger than 5 mm, 44% and 95%; and for polyps larger than 1 cm, 57% and 100%. The authors concluded that subtle patient preparation with the adjunct of oral contrast material to label the residual fluid and faecal matter results in improved polyp detection.

In our own series, we prospectively imaged 67 patients for whom either colonoscopic or surgical correlation existed. The primary slice thickness was 3 mm with a pitch factor of 1.7. For all patients who participated in the study, there was either strong clinical suspicion of a colorectal carcinoma or evidence of tumour from a flexible endoscopy carried out elsewhere. The results of the histopathology indicated that a total of 57 patients indeed had a colorectal carcinoma; all were detected in the virtual endoscopy. A total of 17 polyps were found; the smallest malignant tumour had an 8-mm diameter. From these data, the sensitivity of virtual endoscopy can be calculated as 100% for colorectal carcinoma, independent of tumour stage at the time of detection, and specificity as 98%, since one case of exacerbated, extensive diverticulitis in the sigmoid colon was misinterpreted as colon carcinoma. The overall sensitivity for polyps amounted to 92%, with specificity of 83%.

It may be concluded that currently virtual endoscopy on the basis of spiral CT data can achieve sensitivity of 80–95% for polyps of sufficient size, starting from 5 mm. With improved data acquisition (i.e., thinner slices) stable values ranging between 90% and 95% are attainable (FENLON et al. 1999b). Initial results using MRI as the imaging source have led to the recognition that similar values with respect to polyp detection can be obtained when the bowel is thoroughly filled with contrast material. In contrast, the specificity is very much dependent on how well faecal residues and imaging artefacts can be differentiated from true polyps. This is undoubtedly an area where improvement is called for, especially if virtual endoscopy is to be implemented as a screening method in a population with a low prevalence of polyps.

6.1.5 The Whole Picture: Is There a Role for Virtual Colonoscopy?

Research and development in the field of virtual colonoscopy have shown that this technique has the potential to detect polyps with acceptable precision and certainty and thus meets important prerequisites for a screening technique. The question which remains to be answered is how large a polyp must be in order to be detected with certainty; the declared, strict opponents of this method argue that occasionally even a small polyp can already have undergone malignant transformation, and this cannot be registered by virtual endoscopy.

These critics object that virtual endoscopy:

- Cannot detect small polyps with enough certainty. However, even the gold standard, i.e. flexible endoscopy, has a 27% margin of error for polyps smaller than 5 mm (REX et al. 1997).
- Methodologically cannot detect small flat adenomas. However, these tumours are also difficult to recognise in flexible endoscopy, and special techniques are necessary to achieve an improvement (JARAMILLO et al. 1995).
- Is incapable of obtaining information about the aetiology even when a small polyp is detected, and as a result, such patients must undergo flexible endoscopy with biopsy anyway.
- Does not depict early inflammatory changes or allow recognition of small ulcerations, since the surface is artificial and includes no information as to the composition of the mucosa.
- Represents only a snapshot, failing to provide information on movement or motility. Also, for example, mucus and stool residues cannot be removed during the examination.
- Goes hand in hand with ionising radiation. This is true if CT is used, but is inapplicable if MRI is the examination technique.

On the other hand, the supporters of virtual endoscopy reason that it:

- Can be implemented simply and reliably.
- Boasts high patient acceptance, since the complete examination lasts only a few minutes, the scanning procedure alone lasting one single breathhold.
- Is much less painful, since the mechanical manipulation is relatively limited.
- Requires no sedation, eliminating the associated risks.
- Bears no noteworthy risk of perforation (flexible diagnostic endoscopy: 1:1000 to 1:5000).
- Is cheaper than flexible endoscopy in various Western countries.
- Not only offers the possibility to see the bowels from within, but also represents an opportunity to concurrently conduct a complete abdominal assessment with the possibility of detecting side findings; if a colorectal carcinoma is present, the staging can be accomplished simultaneously.
- Is handicapped by limitations with respect to sensitivity and specificity which are merely a question of the technology and can be expected to be ameliorated by concrete improvements in the near future (multislice CT, tissue-specific contrast agents for MRI etc.).

Fibreoptic flexible endoscopy remains the most important and currently the only possibility to histologically identify a colorectal carcinoma preoperatively. Furthermore, for many other non-malignant conditions, such as inflammatory bowel diseases, Crohn's disease and ulcerative colitis, the final diagnosis cannot be made without flexible endoscopy. The value of flexible endoscopy is undiminished, and currently there is absolutely no indication that its position as a tool for medical diagnostic purposes can be questioned.

Nevertheless, one should not disregard the fact that flexible endoscopy has failed to reach one very important goal: acceptance among the general population as a screening method. Even such fine, elaborated diagnostic methods as chromoscopy or microscopic endoscopy (JARAMILLO et al. 1995) cannot significantly improve acceptance. Lastly, this method is invasive and requires sedation, with the attendant risks.

Two questions remain to be answered:

1. What is the value of an excellent diagnostic

method such as flexible endoscopy if an individual is clearly at risk but does not attend screening examinations?
2. Is it foreseeable that virtual endoscopy, its advantages and disadvantages considered, could improve the accessibility and attractiveness of a screening programme?

A predominant reason for the sceptical and negative attitude of the population towards flexible endoscopy is the associated discomfort, and exactly this point attracts patients to virtual endoscopy. The unsatisfactory sensitivity and specificity should be an incentive for all researchers to strive for technological and methodological improvements (REX 1998). One important difference, however, remains: a biopsy cannot be taken during virtual endoscopy, and the surrounding tissue remains invisible for the flexible endoscope. This leads to a further indication for virtual endoscopy: preoperative evaluation, be it for cancer staging or for assessment of the colon proximal to a stenotic area. In these specific settings, little resistance can be expected from medical professionals as no satisfactory alternative exists.

Today, the time investment for a radiologist engaged in viewing and diagnosing the virtual endoscopy images is far too long, and certainly is not adequately reimbursed by the health care providers (SONNENBERG et al. 1999). It has been shown for flexible endoscopy that a trained nurse might perform as well as a gastroenterologist in conducting the enteral examination (MAULE 1994), thus reducing the cost of the procedure. It might also be anticipated that virtual endoscopy, including patient preparation, scanning, networking the data and reconstruction of a virtual flight movie or any similar type of presentation could be performed by a trained technician, and the radiologist could focus on image interpretation rather than having to concern him- or herself with various technical aspects of software solutions.

Virtual endoscopy and flexible endoscopy can only narrow-mindedly be viewed as competing methods (REX et al. 1999). In light of the immense threat posed by colorectal cancer and the problems associated with its prevention and preoperative patient evaluation, it is important to recognise how well the two procedures can complement one another (MCFARLAND and BRINK 1999). Focusing on the patient in the centre, the strengths of the individual methods should not be viewed separately, but together. The outcome is less room for question and doubt and an otherwise unattainable improvement in patient care.

6.1.6
Summary – How to Perform a Virtual CT Colonoscopy

The complete procedure of virtual endoscopy can be separated into three parts: (1) data acquisition; (2) data processing; (3) data viewing. Although each part is functionally independent of the others, it is possible, for example, that a certain software function can change the requirements for data acquisition. If the software contains a tool to remove various contrast gradients, the patient can then be additionally prepared with oral contrast material in order to mark the residual fluids (see subsection Fluid Levels and Residual Faeces, in Sect. 6.1.4.9.13, Artefacts).

Data Acquisition
The data acquisition step can be divided into preparation of the patient and choice of the correct scanning parameters. For patient preparation, there are two main goals:
- Get a clean colon: This necessitates preparation starting at least 12 h, ideally 24 h, before the examination. For this purpose there are numerous preparations on the market (see Sect. 6.1.4.3, Patient Preparation) of which two deserve mention: GoLytely is an agent widely used in the US, and Fleet is reported to give the best cleansing results, coinciding with our own experience. The patient should be advised to explicitly follow the directions in the instruction leaflet. If your workstation supports a faecal tagging function, you may give the patient 30 ml oral contrast material at the beginning of the cleansing procedure and another 30 ml 1–2 h before the initiation of scanning.
- Get the colon distended: After rectal intubation, the possibility exists to use room air (which is cheap and readily available) or carbon dioxide (which requires certain safety equipment) for insufflation. A second choice should be made between the two spasmolytic agents mentioned previously, Buscopan and glucagon, with consideration given to contraindications. The insufflation should be as gentle as possible and should be terminated only shortly before initiating the spiral scan.

The optimal scanning parameters must be used. Depending on the scanner capabilities, the primary selection should be the thinnest beam collimation that does not require a pitch factor higher than 2:1 and still allows coverage of the entire abdomen within one single breathhold. For most spiral CT units with a limitation of 60 revolutions of the gantry in one period, a slice thickness of 5 mm with a table speed of up to 8 mm/s cannot be avoided.

Whenever possible, the beam collimation should be reduced to 3 mm or less; with multislice CT, 2.5 mm or less presents no problem for the implementation. The reconstruction interval should be selected according to the workstation. A goal of 30%–40% of the effective slice thickness would in most cases indicate a 2-mm reconstruction interval. Using a 1-mm reconstruction interval has little effect on the image quality but burdens the workstation considerably.

The following decisions pertain to the usage of i.v. contrast material and scanning in the supine or prone position, or even both. Since these issues are currently under research, there are currently no general recommendations or guidelines.

Data Processing

All major hardware producers in this field currently offer a workstation with an endoluminal viewing function. Although there are quite visible differences in quality, a general judgement as to which equipment is the best is not made in this book. The two main hardware platforms are Silicon Graphics or Sun Sparcstation based. Each system has advantages and disadvantages, and the systems differ considerably in price. When evaluating various workstations, the workload for the computer should not be underestimated and the computation time should be carefully checked, since much of one's own valuable time can be taken up waiting for the computer to finish its job.

The only currently acceptable transfer protocol is naturally DICOM. The possibility of exporting data not only in DICOM but also in a PC- or Macintosh-compatible format deserves additional consideration. Finally, a colour documentation option is also desirable.

Data Viewing

Broad consensus (or the smallest common denominator) exists that viewing the axials serves as a reference to which one can always return should the findings in any other viewing technique be vague or dubious. Otherwise, the viewing technique is the current research field for virtual endoscopy, and any general recommendation would be meaningless since new software developments tomorrow can make today's recommendations obsolete.

Acknowledgements. Our thanks are expressed towards Mrs. S. Wedel, MD, Mr. H. Ernst, MD, PhD and Mrs. M. Ortner, MD (Department of Gastroenterology, Charité) for their fabulous support during the clinical studies and for contributing the flexible endoscopic images.

References

Ahlquist DA, Hara AK, Johnson CD (1997) Computed tomographic colography and virtual colonoscopy. Gastrointest Endosc Clin N Am 7:439–452.

Aldoori WH, Giovannucci EL, Rimm EB, et al. (1995) Prospective study of physical activity and the risk of symptomatic diverticular disease in men. Gut 36:276–282.

Almy TP, Howell DS (1980) Diverticular disease of the colon. N Engl J Med 320:325–331.

Anderson N, Cook HB, Coates R (1991) Colonoscopically detected colorectal cancer missed on barium enema. Gastrointest Radiol 16:123–127.

Atkins WS, Morson BC, Cuzick J (1992) Long-term risk of colorectal cancer after excision of rectosigmoid adenomas. N Engl J Med 326:658–660.

Baron JA, Gerhardsson de Verdier M, Ekbom A (1994) Coffee, tea, tobacco, and cancer of the large bowel. Cancer Epidemiol Biomarkers Prev 3:565–570.

Beaulieu CF, Jeffrey RB, Jr., Karadi C, Paik DS, Napel S (1999) Display modes for CT colonography. Part II. Blinded comparison of axial CT and virtual endoscopic and panoramic endoscopic volume-rendered studies. Radiology 212:203–212.

Beaulieu CF, Napel S, Daniel BL, et al. (1998) Detection of colonic polyps in a phantom model: implications for virtual colonoscopy data acquisition. J Comput Assist Tomogr 22:656–663.

Biggs CG, Ballantyne GH (1994) Sensitivity versus cost effectiveness in postoperative follow-up for colorectal cancer. Curr Opin Gen Surg :94–102.

Blakeborough A, Sheridan MB, Chapman AH (1997) Complications of barium enema examination: a survey of UK consultant radiologists 1992–4. Clin Radiol 52:142–148.

Bolin S, Franzen L, Nilsson S, Sjodahl R (1988) Carcinoma of the colon and rectum: tumors missed by radiologic examination in 61 patients. Cancer 61:1999–2008.

Bond JH (1995) Small flat adenomas appear to have little clinical importance in Western countries. Gastrointest Endosc 42:184–186.

Boring CC, Squires TS, Tong T (1993) Cancer statistics. CA Cancer J Clin 43:7–26.

Bowdy M (1998) Lag in colorectal screening rates prompts innovation. JNCI 90:886–887.

Brady AP, Stevenson GW, Stevenson I (1994) Colorectal cancer overlooked at barium enema examination and colonoscopy: a continuing perceptual problem. Radiology 192:373–378.

Burkitt DP (1971) Epidemiology of cancer of the colon and rectum. Cancer 28:3–13.

Burt RW (1997) Screening of patients with a positive family history of colorectal cancer. Gastrointest Endosc Clin N Am 7:65–79.

Byers T, Levin B, Rothenberger D, et al. (1997) American Cancer Society guidelines for screening and surveillance for early detection of colorectal polyps and cancer: update 1997. CA, Cancer J Clin 47:154–160.

Cancer Facts and Figures ACS (1999) 2. American Cancer Society, Inc., Atlanta, USA.

Choi PM, Nugent FW, Schoetz DJ (1993) Colonoscopic surveillance reduces mortality from colorectal cancer in ulcerative colitis. Gastroenterology 105:418–424.

Chu DZ, Glacco G, Martin RG, Guinee VF (1986) The significance of synchronous carcinoma and polyps in the colon and rectum. Cancer 57:445–450.

Chu KC, Tarone RE, Chow WH (1994) Temporal patterns in colorectal cancer incidence, survival, and mortality from 1950 through 1990. J Natl Cancer Inst 86:997–1006.

Chui DW, Gooding GA, McQuaid KR, Griswold V, Grendell JH (1994) Hydrocolonic ultrasonography in the detection of colonic polyps and tumors. N Engl J Med 331:1685–1688.

Cittadini G, Sardanelli F, De Cicco E, Casiglia M, De Cata T, Parodi RC (1998) Compared effect of a genetically engineered glucagon and hyoscine *N*- butylbromide on double-contrast barium meal study. Eur Radiol 8:449–453.

Crucitti F, Sofo L, Ratto C, et al. (1995) Colorectal cancer. Epidemiology, etiology, pathogenesis and prevention. Rays 20:121–131.

Dachman AH, Kuniyoshi JK, Boyle CM, et al. (1998) CT colonography with three-dimensional problem solving for detection of colonic polyps. AJR Am J Roentgenol 171:989–995.

Debinski HS, Love S, Spigelman AD, Phillips RKS (1996) Colorectal polyp counts and cancer risk in familial adenomatous polyposis. Gastroenterology 110:1028–1030.

Devesa SS, Chow WH (1993) Variation in colorectal cancer incidence in the United States by subsite of origin. Cancer 71:3819–3826.

Drew PJ, Hughes M, Hodson R, et al. (1997) The optimum bowel preparation for flexible sigmoidoscopy. Eur J Surg Oncol 23:315–316.

Eddy DM (1990) Sceening for colorectal cancer. Ann Int Med 113:373–384.

Eide TJ (1986) Prevalence abd morphological features of adenomas of the large intestine with and without colorectal carcinoma. J Histopathol 10:111–118.

Elliot MS, Levenstein JJ, Wright JP (1984) Faecal occult blood testing in the detection of colorectal cancer. Br J Surg 71:785–786.

Farouk R, Nelson H, Radice E, Mercill S, Gunderson L (1998) Accuracy of computed tomography in determining resectability for locally advanced primary or recurrent colorectal cancers. Am J Surg 175:283–287.

Fenlon HM, Clarke PD, Ferrucci JT (1998) Virtual colonoscopy: imaging features with colonoscopic correlation. AJR Am J Roentgenol 170:1303–1309.

Fenlon HM, McAneny DB, Nunes DP, Clarke PD, Ferrucci JT (1999a) Occlusive colon carcinoma: virtual colonoscopy in the preoperative evaluation of the proximal colon. Radiology 210:423–428.

Fenlon HM, Nunes DP, Schroy PC, 3rd, Barish MA, Clarke PD, Ferrucci JT (1999b) A comparison of virtual and conventional colonoscopy for the detection of colorectal polyps. N Engl J Med 341:1496–1503.

Fenoglio CM, Kaye GI, Lane N (1973) Distribution of human colonic lymphatics in normal, hyperplastic and adenomatous tissue: its relationship to metastasis from small carcinomas in pedunculated adenoma. Gastroenterology 64:51–58.

Fenoglio CM, Pascal PR (1982) Colorectal adenomas and cancer: pathologic relationships. Cancer 50:2601–2608.

Fink AM, Aylward GW (1995) Buscopan and glaucoma: a survey of current practice [published erratum appears in Clin Radiol 1995 Oct;50(10):740]. Clin Radiol 50:160–164.

Fork FT (1981) Double contrast enema and colonoscopy in polyp detection. Gut 22:971–977.

Fork FT (1983) Reliability of routine double contrast examination of the large bowel: a prospective study of 2590 patients. Gut 24:672–677.

Fork FT (1988) Radiographic findings in overlooked colon carcinomas: a retrospective analysis. Acta radiol 29:331–336.

Frager DH, Frager JD, Wolf EL, Beneventano TC (1987) Problems in the colonoscopic localization of tumors: continued value of the barium enema. Gastrointest Radiol 12:343–346.

Freeny PC (1986) Colorectal carcinoma evaluation with CT: preoperative staging and detection of postoperative recurrence. Radiology 158.

Frommer DJ, Kapparis A, Brown MK (1988) Improved screening for colorectal cancer by immunological detection of occult blood. Br Med J 296:1092–1094.

Frühmorgen P, Pfähler A (1990) [Complications in 39397 endoscopic examinations - a 7 year prospective decumentation about type and incidence]. Leber Magen Darm 3:20–32.

Fuchs CS, Giovannucci EL, Colditz GA, et al. (1999) Dietary fiber and the risk of colorectal cancer and adenoma in women. N Engl J Med 340:169–176.

Fujiya M, Maruyama M (1997) Small depressed neoplasm of the large bowel; its radiographic visualization and clinical significance. Abdominal Imaging 22:325–331.

Gaglia P, Atkin WS, Whitelaw S, et al. (1995) Variables associated with the risk of colorectal adenomas in asymptomatic patients with a family history of colorectal cancer. Gut 36:385–390.

Giardiello FM, Welsh SB, Hamilton SR, et al. (1987) Increased risk of cancer in the Peutz-Jeghers-Syndrome. N Engl J Med 316:1511–1514.

Giess CS, Schwartz LH, Bach AM, Gollub MJ, Panicek DM (1998) Patterns of neoplastic spread in colorectal cancer: implications for surveillance CT studies. AJR Am J Roentgenol 170:987–991.

Gilbertsen VA (1974) Proctosigmoidoscopy and polypectomy ind reducing the incidence of rectal cancer. Cancer 34:936–940.

Gillen CD, Andrews HA, Prior P, et al. (1994) Crohn's disease and colorectal cancer. Gut 35:651–655.

Giovannucci E (1998) Meta-analysis of coffee consumption and risk of colorectal cancer. Am J Epidemiol 147:1043–1052.

Giovannucci E, Ascherio A, Rimm EB, Colditz GA, Stampfer MJ, Willett WC (1995a) Physical activity, obesity, and risk for colon cancer and adenoma in men. Ann Intern Med 122:327–334.

Giovannucci E, Egan KM, Hunter DJ, et al. (1995b) Aspirin and the risk of colorectal cancer in women. New Engl J Med 333:609–614.

Glick SN, Teplick SK, Balfe DM, et al. (1989) Large colonic neoplasms missed by endoscopy. Am J Roentgenol 152.

Goei R, Nix M, Kessels AH, Ten Tusscher MP (1995) Use of antispasmodic drugs in double contrast barium enema examination: glucagon or buscopan? Clin Radiol 50:553–557.

Granqvist S (1981) Distribution of polyps in the large bowel in relation to age. A colonoscopic study. Scand J Gastroenterol 16:1025–1031.

Haggitt RC, Glotzbach RE, Soffer EE (1985) Prognostic factors in colorectal carcinomas arising in adenomas: implications for lesions removed by endoscopic polypectomy. Gastroenterology 89:328–336.

Hara AK (1998) Mayo clinic experience: polyp detection. Proceedings of the first international symposium on virtual colonoscopy, Boston, Oct. 1998 :35–37.

Hara AK, Johnson CD, Reed JE, et al. (1997) Colorectal polyp detection using CT colography: initial assessment of sensitivity and specificity. Radiology 205:59–65.

Hara AK, Johnson CD, Reed JE, Ehmann RL, Ilstrup DM (1996) Colorectal polyp detection using computed tomographic colography: two- versus three-dimensional techniques. Radiology 200:49–54.

Hardcastle JD, Roginson MHE, Moss SM, et al. (1996) Randomised controlled trial of faecal occult blood screening for colorectal cancer. Lancet 348:1472–1477.

Harned RK, 2nd, Chezmar JL, Nelson RC (1994) Recurrent tumor after resection of hepatic metastases from colorectal carcinoma: location and time of discovery as determined by CT. AJR Am J Roentgenol 163:93–97.

Haseman JH, Lemmel GT, Rahmani EY, Rex DK (1997) Failure of colonoscopy to detect colorectal cancer: evaluation of 47 cases in 20 hospitals. Gastrointest Endosc 45:451–455.

Hobbs FDR, Cherry RC, Fielding JWL, et al. (1992) Acceptability of opportunistic screening for occult gastrointestinal blood loss. BMJ 304:483–486.

Hoffmann KR, Samara Y, Fiebich M, Lan L, Doi K, Dachmann A (1998) Workstation for rapid interpretation of CT colon studies. Proceedings of the first international symposium on virtual colonoscopy, Boston, Oct. 1998 :97.

Höhne KH, Bomans M, Pommert A, et al. (1990) 3D visualization of tomographic volume data using the generalized voxel model. The Visual Computer 6:28–36.

Horwich PJ, Chen D, Li B, Wax MR, Gindi GR, Liang JZ (1999) The centerline of the colon: automating a key step in virtual colonoscopy. Radiology 213(P):258.

Hughes LE (1969) Postmortem survey of diverticular disease of the colon. Gut 10:336.

Hughes LE (1975) Complications of diverticular disease: Inflammation, obstruction and bleeding. Clin Gastroenterol 4:147.

Hundt W, Braunschweig R, Reiser M (1999) Evaluation of spiral CT in staging of colon and rectum carcinoma. Eur Radiol 9:78–84.

Husband JE, Hodson NJ, Parson CA (1980) The use of computed tomography in recurrent rectal tumors. Radiology 134:667–682.

Imray CHE, Radley S, Davis A, et al. (1992) Biliary bile acid profiles in patients with colorectal cancer or polyps. Gut 33:1239–1245.

Isabel-Martinez L, Chapman AH, Hall RI (1988) The value of a barium enema in the investigation of patients with rectal carcinoma. Clin Radiol 39:531–533.

Jaramillo E, Watanabe M, Slezak P, et al. (1995) Flat neoplastic lesions of the colon and rectum detected by high-resolution video colonoscopy and chromoscopy. Gastrointest Endosc 42:114–122.

Järvinen HJ, Mecklin JP, Sistonen P (1995) Screening reduces colorectal cancer rate in families with hereditary nonpolyposis colorectal cancer. Gastroenterology 108:1405–1411.

Jass JR, Williams CB, Bussey HJR, et al. (1988) Juvenile polyposis - a precancerous condition. Histopathology 13:619–621.

Johnson CD, Hara AK, Reed JE (1997) Computed tomographic colonography (Virtual colonoscopy): a new method for detecting colorectal neoplasms. Endoscopy 29:454–461.

Johnson CD, Ilstrup DM, Fish NM, et al. (1996) Barium enema: detection of colonic lesions in a community population. Am J Roentgenol 167:39–43.

Kalender WA, Polacin A, Suss C (1994) A comparison of conventional and spiral CT: an experimental study on the detection of spherical lesions [published erratum appears in J Comput Assist Tomogr 1994 Jul-Aug;18(4):671]. J Comput Assist Tomogr 18:167–176.

Karadi C, Beaulieu CF, Jeffrey RB, Paik D, Napel S (1998) Synthesis and insertion of polyps into helical CT data of the colon: technique and evaluation. Proceedings of the first international symposium on virtual colonoscopy, Boston, Oct. 1998 :96.

Kewenter J, Breringe H, Engaras B, Haglind E (1995) The value of flexible sigmoidoscopy and double contrast barium enema in the diagnosis of neoplasms in the rectum and colon in subjects with positive hemoccult: results of 1831 rectosigmoidoscopies and double contrast barium enemas. Endoscopy 27:159–163.

Kronborg O, Fenger C, Olsen J, et al. (1996) Randomised study of screening for colorectal cancer with fecal occult blood test. Lancet 348:1467–1471.

Kronborg O, Fenger C, Sondergaard O, et al. (1987) Initial mass screening for colorectal cancer with fecal occult blood. Scand J Gastroenterol 22:877–686.

Kudo S (1993) Endoscopic mucosal resection of flat and depressed types of early colorectal cancer. Endoscopy 25:455–461.

Kudo S, Tamura S, Nakajima T, et al. (1995) Depressed type of colorectal cancer. Endoscopy 27:54–57.

Landis HS, Murray T, Bolden S, Wingo PA (1998) Cancer statistics, 1998. Ca J Clin 48:6–30.

Langholz E, Munkholm P, Davidsen M (1992) Colorectal cancer risk and mortality in patients with ulcerative colitis. Gastroenterology 103:1444–1451.

Lanspa SH, Rouse J, Smyrk T, et al. (1992) Epidemiologic characteristics of the flat adenoma of Muto: A prospective study. Dis Colon Rectum 35:543–547.

Laufer I, Smith NCW, Mullens JE (1976) The radiologic demonstration of colorectal polyps undetected by endoscopy. Gastroenterology 70:167.

Leitzmann C (1998) [Colorectal cancer: the value of diet for prevention]. Onkologe 4:5–7.

Levoy M (1988) Display of surfaces from volume data. IEEE Computer Graphics and Applications 8:29–37.

Lieberman D (1991) Cost-effectiveness of colon cancer screening. Am J Gastroenterol 86:1789–1794.

Limberg B (1990) Diagnosis of large bowel tumors by colonic sonography. Lancet 335:144–146.

Luboldt W, Bauerfeind P, Wildermuth S, Marincek B, Debatin JF (1998a) Contrast optimization for assessment of the colonic wall and lumen in MR-colonography (MRC). Eur Radiol 9:145.

Luboldt W, Debatin JF (1998) Virtual endoscopic colonography based on 3D MRI. Abdom Imaging 23:568–572.

Luboldt W, Fröhlich J, Schneider N, Wildermuth S, Marincek B, Debatin JF (1998b) Enema optimization in MR-colonography (MRC). Eur Radiol 9:145.

Luboldt W, Steiner P, Bauerfeind P, Pelkonen P, Debatin JF (1998c) Detection of mass lesions with MR colonography: preliminary report. Radiology 207:59–65.

Lynch HT, Smyrk TS, Watson P, et al. (1993) Genetics, natural history, tumor spectrum, and pathology og hereditary nonpolyposis colorectal cancer: an updated review. Gastroenterology 104:1535–1549.

Mandel JS, Bond JH, Church TR, et al. (1993) Reducing mortality from colorectal cancer by screening for fecal occult blood. New Engl J Med 328:1365–1371.

Manousos ON, Truelove SC, Lumsden K (1967) Prevalence of colonic diverticulosis in the general population of Oxford area. Br Med J 3:762.

Maule WF (1994) Screening for colorectal cancer by nurse endoscopists. N Engl J Med 330:183–187.

McFarland EG, Brink JA (1999) Helical CT colonography (virtual colonoscopy): the challenge that exists between advancing technology and generalizability. AJR Am J Roentgenol 173:549–559.

McFarland EG, Wang G, Brink JA, Balfe DM, Heiken JP, Vannier MW (1997) Spiral computed tomographic colonography: determination of the central axis and digital unravelling of the colon. Acad Radiol 4:367–373.

Miller RE, Lehmann G (1978) Polypoid colonic lesions undetected by endoscopy. Radiology 129:295.

Minami H, Yoshioka N, Akahane M, Miyazawa M, Sato N, Ohtomo K (1999) New virtual CT endoscopy synchronized with multi-planar reconstruction: efficacy in detection, characterization and staging of gastric cancer. Eur Radiol 9:395.

Modan B, Barell V, Lubin F, et al. (1975) Low fibre intake as an aetiological factor in cancer of the colon. J Natl Cancer Inst 55:15–18.

Morrin MM, Kruskal JB, Farrell RJ, Reynolds BS, Raptopoulos VD (1999a) Intravenous contrast material enhances the diagnostic accuracy of CT colonography. Radiology 213(P):257.

Morrin MM, Kruskal JB, Farrell RJ, Reynolds KF, Raptopoulos VD (1999b) Does Glucagon improve colonic distention and polyp detection during CT colonography. Radiology 213(P):341.

Morson BC (1966) Factors influencing the prognosis of eraly cancer of the rectum. Proc R Soc Med 59:607–608.

Murakami R, Tsukuma H, Kanamori S, et al. (1995) Natural history of colorectal polyps and the effect of polypectomy on occurrence of subsquent cancer. Int J Cancer 46:159–164.

Muto T, Bussey HJR, Morson BC (1975) The evolution of cancer of the colon and rectum. Cancer 36:2251–2270.

Nakamura K (1994) [Carcinoma de novo and diagnostic criteria of colorectal carcinoma]. I-to-Cho 29:151–159.

Norfleet RG, Ryan ME, Wyman JB, et al. (1991) Barium enema versus colonoscopy for patients with polyps found during flexible sigmoidoscopy. Gastrointest Endosc 37:531–534.

Obrecht WF, Wu WC, Gelfand DW, et al. (1984) The extent of successful colonoscopy: a second assessment using modern equipment. Gastrointest Radiol 9:161.

O'Donovan AN, Somers S, Farrow R, Mernagh J, Rawlinson J, Stevenson GW (1997) A prospective blinded randomized trial comparing oral sodium phosphate and polyethylene glycol solutions for bowel preparation prior to barium enema. Clin Radiol 52:791–793.

Ogunbiyi OA, Flanagan FL, Dehdashti F, et al. (1997) Detection of recurrent and metastatic colorectal cancer: comparison of positron emission tomography and computed tomography. Ann Surg Oncol 4:613–620.

Okuda S, Kettenbach J, Schreyer A, et al. (1998) Virtual colonoscopy application with automated fly-through trajectory. Proceedings of the first international symposium on virtual colonoscopy, Boston, Oct. 1998 :92.

Ott DJ, Wolfman NT, Scharling ES, Zagoria RJ (1998) Overview of imaging in colorectal cancer. Dig Dis 16:175–182.

Paik DS, Beaulieu CF, Jeffrey RB, Karadi C, Napel S (1999) Evaluation of radiologist performance in polyp detection using map projection virtual colonoscopy. Radiology 213(P):241.

Paik DS, Beaulieu CF, Jeffrey RB, Karadi CA, Napel S (1998a) Panoramic virtual colonoscopy using the mercator projection. Proceedings of the first international symposium on virtual colonoscopy, Boston, Oct. 1998 :93.

Paik DS, Beaulieu CF, Jeffrey RB, Rubin GD, Napel S (1998b) Automated flight path planning for virtual endoscopy. Med Phys 25:629–637.

Painter NS, Burkitt DP (1975) Diverticular disease of the colon, a 20th century problem. Clin Gastroenterol 4:3–22.

Parkins T (1994) Computer lets doctor fly through the virtual colon. JNCI 86:1046–1047.

Parks TG (1975) Natural history of diverticular disease of the colon. Clin Gastroenterol 4:53–69.

Pinczowski D, Ekbom A, Baron J (1994) Risk factors for colorectal cancer in patients with ulcerative colitis: a case-control study. Gastroenterology 107:117–120.

Pohlmann T (1988) Diverticulitis. Gastrointest Clin North Am 17:357–385.

Polacin A, Kalender WA, Brink J, Vannier MA (1994) Measurement of slice sensitivity profiles in spiral CT. Med Phys 21:133–140.

Reilly JM, Ballantyne GH, Fleming FX (1990) Evaluation of the occult blood test in screening colorectal neoplasms. Am Surg 56:119–123.

Rex DK (1998) CT and MR colography (virtual colonoscopy): status report. J Clin Gastroenterol 27:199–203.

Rex DK, Cutler CS, Lemmel GT, et al. (1997) Colonoscopic miss rates of adenomas determined by back-to-back colonscopies. Gastroenterology 112:24–28.

Rex DK, Lehmann GA, Lappas JC, et al. (1986) Sensitivity of double-contrast barium study for left-colon polyps. Radiology 158:69.

Rex DK, Vining D, Kopecky KK (1999) An initial experience with screening for colon polyps using spiral CT with and without CT colography (virtual colonoscopy). Gastrointest Endosc 50:309–313.

Rogalla P, Bender A, Schmidt E, Hamm B (1998) Comparison of virtual colonoscopy and tissue transition projection (TTP) in colorectal cancer. Proceedings of the first international symposium on virtual colonoscopy, Boston, Oct. 1998 :95.

Rogalla P, Mutze S, Hamm B (1996): Body CT: state-of-the-art. Munich: W. Zuckschwerdt, Germany.

Rogalla P, Verdonck B, Truyen R, Hamm B (1999) Efficacy of automatic path tracking for virtual colonoscopy. Radiology 213(P):257–258.

Rogers BHG, Silvis SE, Nebel OT, et al. (1975) Complications of flexible fiberoptic colonoscopy and polypectomy. Gastrointest Endosc 2:73–76.

Romano G, Belli G, Rotondano G (1995) Colorectal cancer. Diagnosis of recurrence. Gastrointest Endosc Clin N Am 5:831–841.

Rooney PS, Hunt L, Clarke PA (1994) Wheat fibre, lactulose and rectal mucosal proliferation in individuals with a family history of colorectal cancer. Br J Surg 81:1792–1794.

Royster AP, Fenlon HM, Clarke PD, Nunes DP, Ferrucci JT (1997) CT colonoscopy of colorectal neoplasms: two-dimensional and three-dimensional virtual-reality techniques with colonoscopic correlation. AJR Am J Roentgenol 169:1237–1242.

Samara Y, Fiebich M, Dachman AH, Kuniyoshi JK, Doi K, Hoffmann KR (1999) Automated calculation of the centerline of the human colon on CT images. Acad Radiol 6:352–359.

Satava RM (1996) Virtual endoscopy: diagnosis using 3-D visualization and virtual representation. Surg Endosc 10:173–174.

Schmieden V, Scheele K (1922): Das Carcinom des Darmes, Vol VI. Berlin Wien: Urban & Schwarzenberg.

Schmutz GR, Hue S, Fournier L, Leproux F, Lepennec A (1999) Contribution of automated path planning in virtual coloscopy. Radiology 213(P):258.

Schoemaker D, Black R, Giles L, Toouli J (1998) Yearly colonoscopy, liver CT, and chest radiography do not influence 5- year survival of colorectal cancer patients. Gastroenterology 114:7–14.

SEER Cancer Statistics Review, 1973–1992 (1995) US Department of Health and Human Services, Public Health Service, NIH.

Selby JV, Friedman GD, Quesenberry CP, et al. (1992) A case control study of screening sigmoidoscopy and mortality from colorectal cancer. N Engl J Med 326:653–657.

Sharma VK, Chockalingham S, Clark V, et al. (1997) Randomized, controlled comparison of two forms of preparation for screening flexible sigmoidoscopy. Am J Gastroenterol 92:809–811.

Shike M, Winawer SJ, Greenwald PH, et al. (1990) Primary prevention of colorectal cancer. Bull WHO 68:377–385.

Silverberg E, Boring CE, Squires TS (1990) Cancer statistics 1990. CA, Cancer J Clin 40:9–26.

Sissons GR, McQueenie A, Mantle M (1991) The ocular effects of hyoscine-n-butylbromide ("Buscopan") in radiological practice. Br J Radiol 64:584–586.

Sonnenberg A, Delco F, Bauerfeind P (1999) Is virtual colonoscopy a cost-effective option to screen for colorectal cancer? Am J Gastroenterol 94:2268–2274.

Tempero M, Brand R, Holdeman K, Matamoros A (1995) New imaging techniques in colorectal cancer. Semin Oncol 22:448–471.

Terwisscha van Scheltinga J, Bosma M, Smit J, Lobregt S (1997) Image quality improvements in volume rendering. Proceedings 4th conf. Visualization in Biomedical Computing, Hamburg, Sept. 22–25 :87–92.

Thoeni RF (1997) Colorectal cancer. Radiologic staging. Radiol Clin North Am 35:457–485.

Thoeni RF, Rogalla P (1994) Current CT/MRI examination of the lower intestinal tract. Baillieres Clin Gastroenterol 8:765–796.

Thoeni RF, Rogalla P (1995) CT for the evaluation of carcinomas in the colon and rectum. Seminars in Ultrasound, CT, and MRI 16:112–126.

Vining DJ (1997) Virtual colonoscopy. Gastrointest Endosc Clin N Am 7:285–291.

Vining DJ (1998) Optimizing bowel preparation. Proceedings of the first international symposium on virtual colonoscopy, Boston, Oct. 1998 :79–80.

Vining DJ, Shifrin RY, Grishaw EK, Liu K, Choplin RH (1994) Virtual colonoscopy. Radiology 1994(P):446.

Von Herbay A, Herfarth C, Otto HF (1994) [Cancer and dysplasia in ulcerative colitis: a histologic study of 301 surgical specimen]. Z Gastroenterol 32:382–388.

Vukasin P, Weston LA, Beart RW (1997) Oral Fleet Phospho-Soda laxative-induced hyperphosphatemia and hypocalcemic tetany in an adult: report of a case. Dis Colon Rectum 40:497–499.

Walter DF, Govil S, Korula A, William RR, Chandy G (1992) Pedunculated colonic polyp diagnosed by colonic sonography. Pediatr Radiol 22:148–149.

Wang G, McFarland EG, Brown BP, Vannier MW (1998) GI tract unraveling with curved cross sections. IEEE Trans Med Imaging 17:318–322.

Wax M, Liang Z, Chiou R, Kaufman A, Viswambharan A (1998) Electronic colon cleansing for virtual colonoscopy. Proceedings of the first international symposium on virtual colonoscopy, Boston, Oct. 1998 :94.

Waye JD, Lwis BS, Frankel A, Geller SA (1988) Small colon polyps. Am J Gastroenterol 83:120–122.

Wess L, Eastwood MA, Wess TJ, Busuttil A, Miller A (1995) Cross linkage of collagen is increased in colonic diverticulosis. Gut 37:91–94.

Wherry DC, Thomas WM (1994) The yield of flexible fibreoptic sigmoidoscopy for the detection of asymptomatic colorectal neoplasia. Surg Endosc 8:279–281.

Whiteway J, Morson BC (1985) Elastosis in diverticular disease of the sigmoid colon. Gut 26:258–266.

Winawer SJ, Fletcher RH, Miller L, et al. (1997) Colorectal cancer screening: clinical guidelines and rationale. Gastroenterology 112:594–642.

Winawer SJ, Zauber A, Diaz B (1987) Temporal sequence of evolving colorectal cancer from the normal colon. Gastrointest Endosc 33:167.

Winawer SJ, Zauber AG, Nah Ho M, et al. (1993) Prevention of colorectal cancer by colonoscopic polypectomy. New Engl J Med 329:1977–1981.

Woolrich AM, DaSilva MD, Korelitz BI (1992) Surveillance in the routine management of ulcerative colitis: the predictive value of low-grade dysplasia. Gastroenterology 103:431–458.

Wyman A, Shorthouse AJ (1996) Familial adenomatous polyposis: an update. J R Soc Med 89:224P-228P.

Yee J, Hung RK, Steinauer-Gebauer AM, Geetanjali A, Wall SD, McQuaid K (1999) Colonic distention and prospective evaluation of colorectal polyp detection with and without Glucagon during CT colonography. Radiology 213(P):256.

Yee J, Thoeni RF, Gorczyka DP, Schrock TR (1994) Value of contrast-enhanced MRI for TNM staging of regional disease in primary and recurrent rectal and rectosigmoid tumors. Am J Roentgenol 162 (S):66.

6.2 A Historical and Clinical Perspective

C. Bartram

The techniques used for colonic imaging have always been dependent on the technology available. The first double-contrast barium enemas (DCBE) may have performed in the early 1920s, but the technique did not become routine until the 1960s. The reason for this is easily understood by anyone who has performed fluoroscopy using a fluorescent screen without intensification. The thin barium layer in double contrast is insufficiently dense radiographically to be visible. The equipment of the day limited radiologists to single-contrast techniques, and it was not until image intensification became available in the late 1950s that the double-contrast technique (Welin 1967) became feasible. For many years the DCBE was the mainstay of radiological investigation of the colon. It has been refined commercially with improvements in barium suspensions, made more tolerable for patients by the use of carbon dioxide, intravenous smooth muscle relaxants and non-washout bowel preparation. Fluoroscopic examination is now entering a new era with digital imaging that has made possible a significant reduction in radiation, and image manipulation to improve perspicuity of the mucosal surface and small lesions.

Over the past decade colonoscopy has had an enormous impact on colonic radiology. In some hospitals a DCBE is now a rare examination, and fluoroscopic skills are generally not being acquired. Although a good case can be made for the cost effectiveness of the DCBE in colorectal cancer (CRC) screening (Glick et al. 1998), the examination has lost both clinical acceptance and the number of radiologists with the skills required to achieve a high standard. CT and MRI are the modalities that radiologists now feel comfortable working with.

The technical developments in CT and computer processing have now made 3D imaging of the colon a reality. Clinicians readily accept virtual colonoscopy as the images are very similar to those that they are used to looking at, to the point where it has been suggested that radiologists should study colonoscopy to improve their interpretation of the virtual images (Fenlon et al. 1998). We are now at the start of an exciting era where radiology has the potential to regain a major role in colonic investigation. To understand how this role may develop we need to consider the nature of the 3D image, its strengths and weaknesses in evaluating colonic pathology.

Most 3D software packages provide a combination of surface or volume rendering techniques with multiplanar 2D imaging. Colouring may be applied to rendered surfaces to simulate an endoscopic view, but of course this is entirely artificial and bears no relationship to the vascularity of the bowel wall. Colour is a very important part of the endoscopic image. It provides an obvious distinguishing feature between a polyp and residue. It is also the key to the early diagnosis of colitis, with mucosal erythema obscuring the normal submucosal vascular plexus, either as a generalised change or discretely in small superficial ulcers. The normal mucosa is relatively transparent, and its surface pattern is not seen endoscopically unless dye spray techniques are used. The smoothing algorithms that are an inherent part of surface rendering prevent recognition of minor surface irregularity. DCBE is more sensitive in surface pattern recognition. The mucosal coating of barium suspension is very thin. The normal mucosa, the innominate groove pattern of the mucosa and lymphoid hyperplasia may be visualised, with mucosal erosions producing characteristic patterns in early colitis. Virtual colonoscopy is less sensitive than DCBE for the diagnosis of early colitis. The exact definition of the mucosal surface in double contrast is also helpful in distinguishing adherent particles of residue from small polyps, although under 5 mm this becomes difficult. Polyps smaller than 5 mm are not diagnosed on DCBE unless characteristic changes are present, to avoid an unacceptably high false-positive rate. Careful interrogation of 2D images may help distinguish residue from small polyps in virtual colonoscopy, but the same constrictions apply as in DCBE radiology, unless faecal tagging has been employed.

Virtual colonoscopy may have some relevance in mural lesions, but little in extra-mural abnormalities where standard axial imaging is more than adequate. Diverticula are easily recognised on virtual colonoscopy, which is important as these are extremely common. Axial 2D imaging clearly differentiates an elevated mucosal lesion, by definition a polyp, from a diverticulum. This is not so with the DCBE, where the "ring shadow" created by a diverticulum may be difficult to distinguish from a polyp, and numerous diverticula create a confusing image that may hide a polyp.

The colon has a large surface area, and unfortunately is not a straight tube. Haustral folds and flexures create more problems for rendering techniques than they do for DCBE. The barium pool may obscure lesions in the same way that retained fluid will on virtual colonoscopy. Fly-through techniques provide a dynamic image that helps the eye recognise a suspicious area, to be interrogated in detail with multiplanar 2D. Fluoroscopy is also a dynamic technique, and most lesions will be recognised during screening by an experienced operator. However, unless the examination was video recorded, all dynamic information is lost when fluoroscopy is finished, whereas the entire data volume is retained with virtual colonoscopy. Repeat fly-through in any direction is possible. This allows a large area of the colon to be reviewed quickly, and repeatedly at will. The overall size of a lesion can be determined accurately, but smoothing techniques limit fine surface detail and the appreciation of minor degrees of wall deformity. The size of a polyp may be the single most important macroscopic feature with regard to risk of malignancy, but other factors should be considered.

Hyperplastic polyps are common in the colon. It is difficult to be certain from the surface pattern of a polyp whether it is hyperplastic or adenomatous, and snare biopsy is usually required for histological confirmation. About 25% of the population aged 50 years have an adenomatous polyp, and the prevalence of adenomas increases with age. Most of these will be small, less than 1 cm. Improvements in virtual colonoscopy, particularly with multislice CT, will improve the detection rates for polyps in the 5–10 mm range. The question will then arise as to what to do with ever increasing numbers of small polyps being diagnosed in low-risk groups. Conventional wisdom would recommend polypectomy for all polyps, but the risk of leaving a small polyp has to be balanced against the risk of intervention. Endoscopic biopsy or hot diathermy may perforate the bowel, and this risk increases for diathermy of small polyps in the proximal colon.

Is it safe to leave small polyps? It is likely that most small adenomas regress spontaneously. In one study (Hofstad et al. 1996) both adenomas and hyperplastic polyps smaller than 5 mm in size tended to grow, those 5–9 mm, to regress. Another study (Ueyama et al. 1995) suggested that only 6% of minute polyps grew 2–3 mm over a 2-year period. There have been very few studies of what happens to larger polyps ≈3 cm in size. One long-term follow-up (Stryker et al. 1987) revealed a cumulative risk of cancer developing at the polyp site of 2.5%, 8% and 25% at 5, 10 and 25 years respectively. This indicates a long "dwell time" for malignant transformation, and a period of 10 years for malignant transformation of a 1-cm adenoma is generally accepted (Glick et al. 1998). It could therefore be argued that it is quite safe to leave a polyp smaller than 1 cm for 3–5 years, and to remove it endoscopically only if significant growth is shown on a repeat examination. However, this probably applies to only about 80% of all CRC. Patients with hereditary non-polyposis colorectal cancer syndromes (HNPCC) may account for 5–10% of all CRC and represent a high-risk group for CRC. Cancers tend to occur at an earlier age and may develop more rapidly than in the non-HNPCC population. Any polyp, however small, in a patient with a family history of cancer should probably be removed immediately.

Not all adenomatous change is related to exophytic mucosal proliferation. The "flat adenoma" described by Muto (Muto et al. 1985) is regarded as relatively uncommon in the West. This may reflect examination technique. Detection of these small lesions requires a meticulous method, searching for a small red spot that marks them out and then using chromoscopy (dye spray) to define the surface topography. Flat adenomas may be more common in HNPCC. The Japanese experience is that these lesions become invasive early on, while still small. Although flat adenomas are found in the West, it has been suggested that they are less invasive (Rubio et al.1995). The true incidence of this type of adenoma and its impact on CRC has yet to be determined.

Flat adenomas may be recognised on DCBE by a contour defect and central depression (Fujiya and Maruyama 1997), but are even more difficult to pick up than on colonoscopy. The contour defect and central depression are below the threshold for recognition by virtual colonoscopy. Localised deformity of the bowel wall might be detectable in favourable circumstances, but it is unlikely that this technique will be of value in this subgroup of CRC.

An endoscopic criticism of CT is the induced cancer rate from ionising radiation. Assuming a risk value of 6% per sievert, the fatal cancer rate for a 10 mSv exposure would be approximately 60 fatal cancers per 100,000 examinations. However, this figure applies to a lifelong risk and needs adjusting for the age of exposure. As most CRC screening would be limited to individuals older than 50 years, the rate would be more than halved, i.e. 30 (personal communication, National Radiological Protection Board, UK). By comparison, the mortality for diagnostic colonoscopy would be at least 20 cases per 100,000, representing a more definite and immediate risk, whereas that for radiation is largely theoretical.

If one assumes that screening for CRC depends on detecting a significant sized polyp of 3 cm, three technologies can compete for its detection: DCBE, virtual colonoscopy and endoscopy. Virtual colonoscopy has many advantages and probably greater patient acceptance than the others, and should reliably detect polyps greater than 6 mm in size (Fenlon et al. 1999). Endoscopists will counter with the argument that to prevent CRC the colon must be cleared of all polyps, irrespective of size. Most studies have done just that, so that the information available to health agencies will be biased towards a policy of total polypectomy. There is evidence to indicate that this is not justified. Apart from the natural history of small adenomas, Swedish studies using DCBE with flexible sigmoidoscopy (Jensen et al. 1990), where polyp detection in the proximal colon would be biased towards larger lesions, have shown that technique to be as effective as total colonoscopy for faecal occult blood positive cases. It is time for major trials and a much greater use of virtual colonoscopy.

References

Fenlon HM, Clarke PD, Ferrucci JT (1998) Virtual colonoscopy: imaging features with colonoscopic correlation. AJR Am J Roentgenol. 170:1303–1309.

Fenlon HM, Nunes DP, Clarke PD, Ferrucci JT (1999) Colorectal neoplasm detection using virtual colonoscopy: a feasibility study. Gut 43, 806–811.

Fujiya M, Maruyama M (1997) Small depressed neoplasms of the large bowel: radiographic visualization and clinical significance. Abdominal Imaging 22:325–331.

Glick SN, Wagner JL, Johnson CD (1998) Cost-effectiveness of double-contrast barium enema in screening for colorectal cancer. AJR Am J Roentgenol 170:629–636.

Hofstad B, Vatn MH, Andersen SN, Huitfeldt HS, Rognum T, Larsen S et al. (1996) Growth of colorectal polyps: redetection and evaluation of unresected polyps for a period of three years. Gut 39:449–456.

Jensen J, Kewenter J, Asztely M, Lycke G, Wojciechowski J (1990) Double contrast barium enema and flexible rectosigmoidoscopy: a reliable diagnostic combination for detection of colorectal neoplasm. Br J Surg 77:270–272.

Muto T, Kamiya J, Sawada T, Konishi F, Sugihara K, Kubota Y et al. (1985) Small "flat adenoma" of the large bowel with special reference to its clinicopathologic features. Dis Colon Rectum 28:847–851.

Rubio CA, Kumagai J, Kanamori T, Yanagisawa A, Nakamura K, Kato Y (1995) Flat adenomas and flat adenocarcinomas of the colorectal mucosa in Japanese and Swedish patients. Comparative histologic study. Dis Colon Rectum 38:1075–1079.

Stryker SJ, Wolff BG, Culp CE, Libbe SD, Ilstrup DM, MacCarty RL (1987) Natural history of untreated colonic polyps. Gastroenterology 93:1009–1013.

Ueyama T, Kawamoto K, Iwashita I, Kitagawa S, Haraguchi Y, Muranaka T et al. (1995) Natural history of minute sessile colonic adenomas based on radiographic findings. Is endoscopic removal of every colonic adenoma necessary? Dis Colon Rectum 38:268–272.

Welin S (1967) Results of the Malmo technique of colon examination. JAMA 199:369.

7 Virtual Cystoscopy

T.R. Fleiter, E.M. Merkle, C. Wisianowsky

CONTENTS

Two out of three malignancies of the urinary tract are located in the bladder, and carcinoma of the urinary bladder makes up nearly 7% of all malignant tumors in men and about 4% in women. It is estimated that, in the United States, about 14,600 women and 38,300 men developed a malignant process involving the bladder in 1996 and that about 3900 women and 7800 men would die as a result of their malignancies (Parker et al. 1996). The incidence of all malignancies of the bladder is still increasing (Lamm et al. 1996). Most of the tumors (80–90%) are macroscopically papillary and only 10–20% are solid. Multifocal development of tumors has been seen in more than 25% of cases. The overwhelming majority (>90%) of the tumors are urothelial carcinomas. As cystoscopy still plays the key role in the diagnosis of malignancies of the urinary bladder, virtual endoscopy or cystoscopy could be the less invasive alternative in the diagnostic workup. The objective still is to ascertain whether virtual cystoscopy based on helical CT scan data sets can deliver viewing and diagnostic capabilities similar to those achieved with fiberoptic cystoscopy. One of the most important parts of the examination is to assure the complete filling and distension of the bladder as a hollow organ, to prevent the appearance of pseudolesions due to incomplete distension (Olcott et al. 1998).

T.R. Fleiter, MD; E.M. Merkle, MD; C. Wisianowsky, MD
Department of Diagnostic Imaging, University Hospital of Ulm, Steinhövelstrasse 9, 89075 Ulm, Germany

7.1 Indications

Although some reports have been published about virtual cystoscopy, the indications are still limited. Fiberoptic cystoscopy plays the key role in the diagnosis of malignancies of the bladder, whereas ultrasound is still the gold standard for preoperative imaging; CT is rarely used by most and is focused on detecting tumor infiltrations and metastasis. However, there are different limits for fiberoptic and virtual cystoscopy, e.g., urethral strictures as a contraindication for the mechanical procedure but not the virtual one. Nevertheless, CT has been described as helpful in detecting anatomical changes of the bladder such as diverticula. Carcinomas arising from these diverticula have a poorer prognosis because of early transmural infiltration. Dondalski et al. (1993) reported that CT and MRI was superior to cystography in the detection of diverticula. Virtual endoscopy, being generated from these examination techniques, might therefore prove an additional diagnostic tool.

The clinical criteria for virtual cystoscopy are almost the same as those for fiberoptic examinations: hematuria and suspected bladder wall thickening on abdominal ultrasonography. Even if virtual cystoscopy could be performed using images acquired during the standard preoperative CT of the abdomen and pelvis, the drawback remains that a guided biopsy cannot be obtained without the fiberoptic endoscope. However, this limitation is not exclusive to virtual cystoscopy, but so far applies to virtual endoscopy in all hollow organs.

7.2 Preparation

Beside the requirement to distend the bladder, it is important to increase the contrast difference between the bladder wall and the lumen in order to optimize the virtual endoscopy independently of the reconstruction technique using surface or volume-rendering algorithms.

There are two different principles for distending the urinary bladder and increasing the intraluminal contrast: retrograde via a Foley catheter with insufflation of air or contrast medium (Vining et al.; Fenlon et al. 1997) or using the excretory function of the urinary system to fill the bladder with intravenously injected contrast material (Merkle et al. 1998). As the second method does not require placement of any tubes it is less invasive and is the preferred one for daily routine work, but it requires detailed preparation and timing. Depending on the speed of the scanner, the injected contrast can be used for at least biphasic display of the bladder. The early arterial phase (Fig. 7.1) must be followed by a delayed scan after a latency period of 30 min (Fig. 7.2). In our experience this delay insures homogeneous filling of the bladder; the distension of the bladder should be checked by ultrasound prior to the scan. Our trials using the urine-filled bladder for virtual endoscopy were unsuccessful because the low contrast attenuation between the urine and the bladder resulted in noisy images that were unusable for diagnostic purposes in 90% of the cases (Fig. 7.3). The scans should be performed during one breath-hold to prevent breathing artifacts. Slice thickness can therefore be as low as 1 mm with multislice scanners at pitch 1 or lower. To prevent additional noise from the contrast-filled bladder, 140 kV is usually used to scan the whole pelvis.

7.3 Reconstruction

Virtual cystoscopy of the bladder is not limited to a specific reconstruction technique if the contrast attenuation between the bladder wall and the contrast-filled lumen is sufficient. Volume and surface rendering can both be used to calculate the internal views of the bladder and possible tumor masses. The first step in achieving virtual cystoscopy of the urinary bladder is to detect the surface of the bladder mucosa in the CT scan data set. This can be done by manual control for a surface rendering or using a specific attenuation class for volume rendering. Unlike virtual colonoscopy, interactive navigation is a must to create complete virtual cystoscopy. The changeable perspective of the virtual camera can be used to generate "fisheye" perspectives of the bladder lumen and this improves orientation compared to fiberoptic examinations (Figs. 7.4, 7.5). Multiplanar images corresponding to the position of the virtual camera are useful to provide the examiner with adequate orientation during the workup. Usually all virtual endoscopy findings are documented using these images.

7.4 Results

In our experience, scan protocols using 1 mm collimation and pitch 1 with dual or multislice CT are neces-

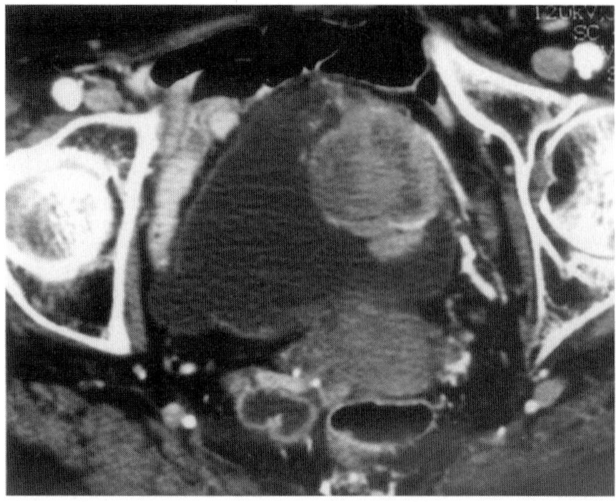

Fig. 7.1. Late arterial phase of contrast injection: inhomogeneous enhancement of a large bladder carcinoma

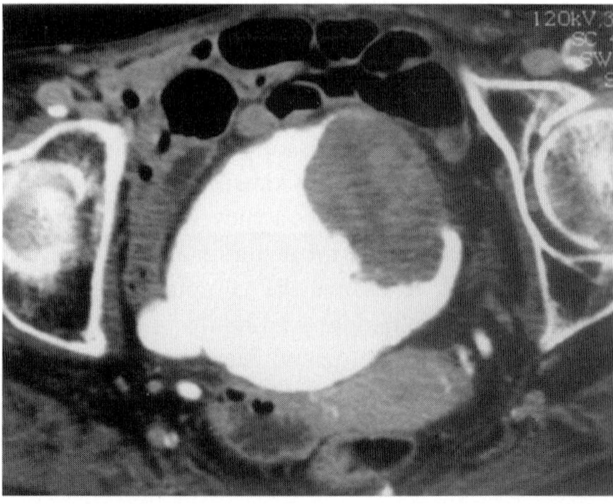

Fig. 7.2. Same tumor as in Fig. 7.1 after a latency period of 30 min. The bladder is homogeneously filled with contrast and fully distended

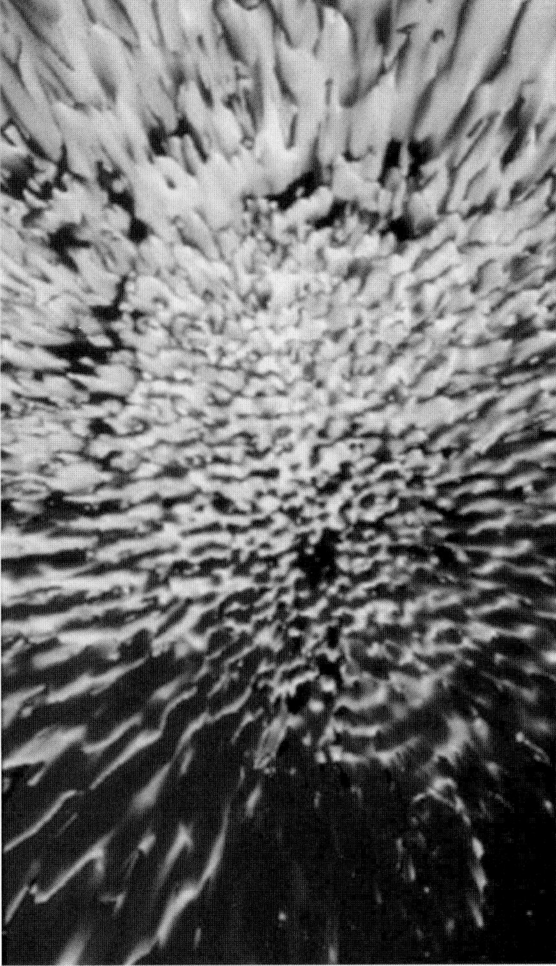

Fig. 7.3. Display of the bladder using the natural contrast of urine: the high noise level and the low contrast difference between the bladder wall and the urine results in unusable virtual cystoscopy images

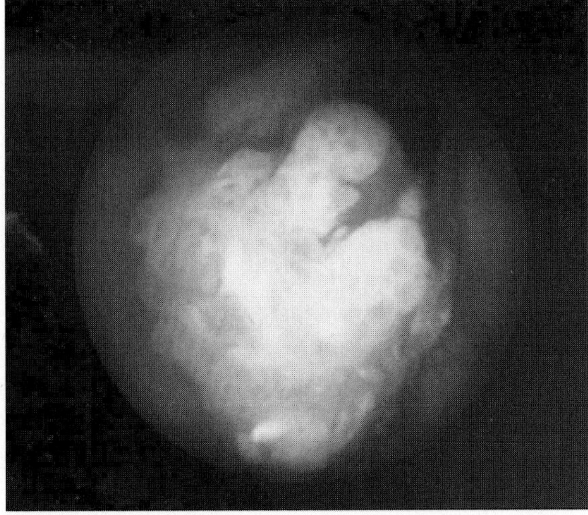

Fig. 7.4. Fiberoptic view of a papillary bladder carcinoma

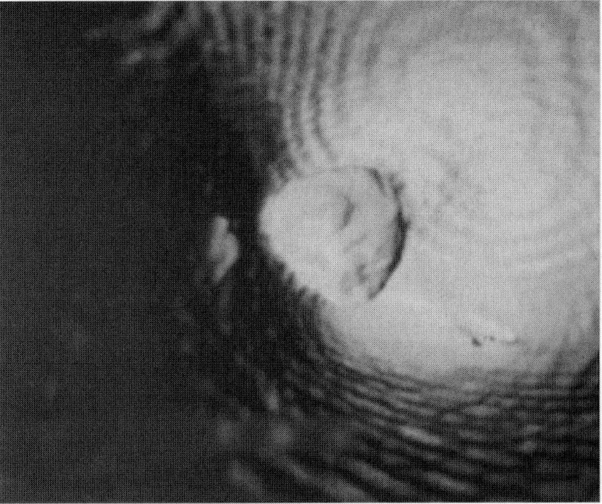

Fig. 7.5. Virtual view of the same tumor as in Fig. 7.4. The bleeding and the area of biopsy are not displayed

sary to provide high spatial resolution and to reduce step artifacts as much as possible. In all cases we were able to achieve contrast attenuation between the bladder lumen and the wall above 100 HU using intravenous contrast injections, which was sufficient for a reliable virtual cystoscopic examination. The difference between the urine-filled bladder and the wall reached a maximum of only 30 HU. Using these data sets it was not possible to generate a smooth display of the mucosa and the tumors. The arterial phase after the contrast injection (average delay: 40 s) showed the uptake within the tumor masses but was not adequate for generating an acceptable virtual cystoscopic study. Nevertheless, these images are most important for diagnostic purposes (Figs. 7.1, 7.2). The best results in generating virtual cystoscopy sequences were obtained using late data sets: here, the bladder was filled with contrast medium, resulting in an excellent attenuation gradient (>100 HU) between the vesical mucosa and urine (Figs. 7.6, 7.7). In immobile, bedridden patients, sedimentation of contrast medium in the bladder was observed, with a resultant minor reduction in the attenuation gradient between bladder wall and urine. However, the attenuation gradient remained high enough to distinguish between vesical mucosa and bladder lumen in all cases. Even using 1 mm collimation the ostia of the ureter could not be delineated by virtual cystoscopy but was delineated by fiberoptic cystoscopy. Tumors with a diameter of at least 0.5 cm could be identified by both virtual and fiberoptic cystoscopy. There was one real drawback of the virtual approach: it was not possible to distinguish between a tumor mass and cystitis.

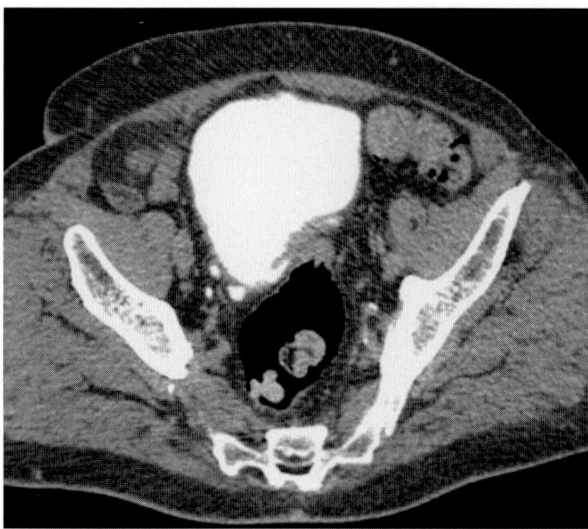

Fig. 7.6. Tumor infiltration of the posterior bladder wall. Delayed scan 30 min after contrast injection

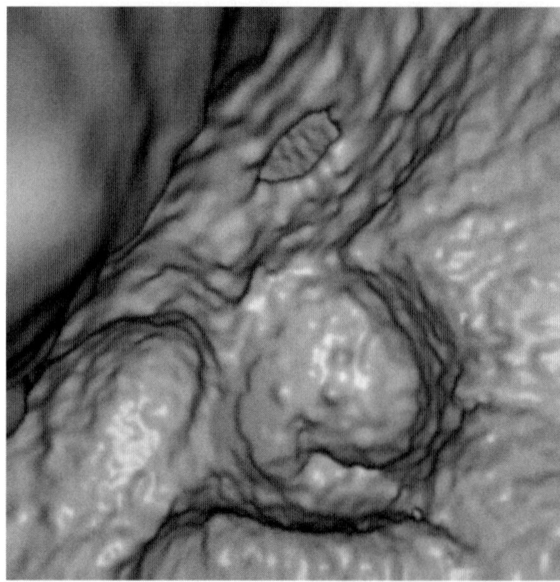

Fig. 7.7. Virtual view of the same tumor as in Fig. 7.1. Note the opening of a pseudodiverticulum at the top

7.5 Summary

The foundation of all forms of virtual endoscopy of hollow organs is still a high "visual gradient" between the visceral lumen and wall structures: this allows differentiation of these structures, depending on the selection of a suitable threshold value or definition of tissue class. Primarily air-filled spaces such as the paranasal sinuses (Rubin et al. 1996), the larynx (Rodenwaldt et al. 1996) and the tracheobronchial tree (Fleiter et al. 1997; Vining et al. 1996; Feretti et al. 1995) offer optimal conditions for CT due to the high attenuation gradient between air and mucosa. Similarly, data sets for virtual colonoscopy are acquired subsequent to transrectal air insufflation (Dachmann et al. 1996; Hara et al. 1996; Vining et al. 1995), both to achieve maximum distension of the large bowel and to obtain a high visual gradient.

Vining et al. (1996) have postulated that virtual cystoscopy is also possible with gas insufflation. They insufflated the bladders of two patients with confirmed carcinoma of the bladder and one healthy volunteer with 300 ml CO_2 via a Foley catheter and obtained views of the tumors similar to those returned by fiberoptic cystoscopy. This method is convenient, for example, in patients with indwelling Foley catheters because they have macrohematuria. On the whole, however, the acceptance of catheterization seems rather low, and the method is associated with a risk of infection.

Virtual cystoscopy on the basis of unenhanced helical CT was almost impossible, since the difference in CT-measured attenuation between the vesical mucosa and urine was in most cases insufficient to obtain a continuous wall structure. The intravenous administration of contrast medium increased the CT attenuation of the mucosa, which, in some cases, proved capable of yielding a sufficiently high degree of contrast. Because individual nontumorous segments of vesical mucosa show only minor contrast medium uptake (Fig. 7.1), it is often very difficult to determine a suitable threshold value. Unfortunately the same happens using volume-rendering techniques.

The best visual gradients are obtained by waiting for the renal elimination of contrast medium (Figs. 7.2, 7.6). With this technique, it is possible to generate virtual cystoscopy in real time and clearly delineate the intravesical tumor. An advantage of this method compared with fiberoptic cystoscopy lies in its noninvasive character, although, in the hands of an experienced examiner, the rate of complications with the fiberoptic examination is very low and serious complications have very rarely been reported (Curley et al. 1995).

Nevertheless, several serious disadvantages of virtual cystoscopy compared with the fiberoptic method remained unchanged. In addition to the radiation exposure (additional scan following the latency period) and the possibility of patient sensitivity to the contrast medium, virtual cystoscopy does not deliver information about the structural relief of the mucosa or any tumors developing flush with the mucosal surface, even when it is based on data sets with thin slices (1 mm collimation). Naturally, virtual cystoscopy does not allow biopsy of suspected lesions. Moreover, the described technique of virtual cystoscopy fails to visualize the ureteral ostia, which is important for preoperative planning in patients with bladder carcinoma. There is even a loss of information compared with axial CT slices, since with the latter the prevesical segment of the ureter is delineated in the great majority of cases.

For these reasons virtual cystoscopy has yet to achieve the quality of the fiberoptic examination and remains restricted to individual cases in which a fiberoptic examination cannot be performed. However, the additional views delivered by virtual cystoscopy can support the primary diagnosis using axial and multiplanar reconstructed images. To date, virtual cystoscopy has not led to a change in the diagnostic workup; fiberoptic cystoscopy still represents the gold standard.

References

Curley P, Ralph D, Scott DJA (1995) Critical limb ischemia – a complication of cystoscopy. Br J Urol 76: 515

Dachman AH, Chen SYJ, Lieberman J, Newmark GM, Hoffmann K, McGill J (1996) Virtual colonoscopy of simulated lesions of pig colon. AJR Am J Roentgenol 166: 83

Dondalski M, White EM, Ghahremani GG, and Patel SK (1993) Carcinoma arising in urinary bladder diverticula: imaging findings in six patients. AJR Am J Roentgenol 161(4):817–820

Fenlon HM, Bell TV, Ahari HK, Hussain S (1997) Virtual endoscopy: early clinical experience. Radiology 205:272–275

Feretti G, Knoplioch J, Coulomb M (1995) Virtual bronchoscopy: multiplanar reformation and 3D shaded surface displays of the tracheobrochial tree. Radiology 197(P): 201

Fleiter T, Merkle EM, Aschoff AJ, Lang G, Stein M, Gorich J, Liewald F, Rilinger N, Sokiranski R (1997) Comparison of real-time virtual and fiberoptic bronchoscopy in patients with bronchial carcinoma: opportunities and limitations. AJR Am J Roentgenol 169:1591–1595

Hara AK, Johnson CD, Reed JE et al. (1996) Feasibility of Colorectal Polyp Detection by 2D and 3D Helical CT (CT Colography). AJR Am J Roentgenol 166: 84

Lamm DL, Torti FM (1996) Bladder cancer, 1996. CA Cancer J Clin 46: 93–112

Merkle EM, Wunderlich A, Aschoff AJ, Rilinger N, Gorich J, Bachor R, Gottfried HW, Sokiranski R, Fleiter TR, Brambs HJ (1998) Virtual cystoscopy based on helical CT scan datasets: perspectives and limitations. Br J Radiol 71:262–267

Olcott EW, Nino Murcia M, Rhee JS (1998) Urinary bladder pseudolesions on contrast-enhanced helical CT: frequency and clinical implications. AJR Am J Roentgenol 171:1349–1354

Parker SL, Tong T, Bolden S, Wingo PA (1996) Cancer statistics, 1996. CA Cancer J Clin 46: 5–27

Rodenwaldt J, Kopka L, Roedel R, Grabbe E (1996) Dreidimensionale Oberflächendarstellung des Larynx und der Trachea mittels Spiral-CT: virtuelle Endoskopie. Fortschr Röntgenstr 165: 80–83

Rubin GD, Beaulieu CF, Argiro V et al. (1996) Perspective volume rendering of ct and mr images: applications for endoscoping imaging. Radiology 199: 321–330

Vining DJ, Liu K, Choplin RH, Haponik EF (1996) Virtual bronchoscopy. Relationships of virtual reality endobronchial simulations to actual bronchoscopic findings. Chest 109: 549–553

Vining DJ, Teigen EL, Stelts D, Vanderwerken B, Kopecky KK, Rex D (1995) Virtual colonoscopy: a 60-second colon examination. Radiology 197(P): 281

Vining DJ, Zagoria RJ, Liu K, Stelts D (1996) CT cystoscopy: an innovation in bladder imaging. Am J Roentgenol 166: 409–410

8 Virtual Endoscopy of the Vessels

T. H. Wiese, P. Rogalla

CONTENTS

8.1 Introduction

Advances in CT and MRI technology enabling the rapid acquisition of volumetric data sets with high-resolution isotropic pixels or voxels have stimulated dramatic developments in three-dimensional (3D) image postprocessing techniques for clinical use (Rubin et al. 1996). Three-dimensional images rendered from two-dimensional (2D) source data sets facilitate the quantitative and qualitative analysis of complex morphologic and pathologic structures (Roelandt et al. 1994). Although the 3D images created by various rendering techniques in general do not contain more information than the original data sets, they often help the reviewer to grasp spatial relationships, for instance when assessing the extent of a pathologic process (Bartolozzi et al. 1998; Remy et al. 1998). Moreover, 3D reconstructions from sectional images provide new tools for teaching anatomy (Remy et al. 1998).

There is an extensive discussion going on at present regarding the diagnostic benefits to be derived from the different postprocessing techniques compared to an analysis of the 2D source images alone. This debate focuses on computer processing capacities and the extra time needed to generate the 3D images (Hany et al. 1998). No clinical data have been published to date showing, for instance, a diagnostic advantage of virtual endoscopy (VE) over other rendering techniques (Jolesz et al. 1997).

8.1.1 Postprocessing Techniques in Vascular Imaging

In vascular imaging, a basic distinction of postprocessing techniques for data sets acquired by computed tomography, i.e., computed tomographic angiography (CTA), or magnetic resonance imaging, i.e., magnetic resonance angiography (MRA), is made between surface-based reconstruction techniques (e.g., shaded surface display) and volume-based techniques (volume rendering technique) (Freund et al. 1995).

The major indications for these rendering techniques in vascular imaging include the following:

1. Evaluation of the thoracic aorta for aneurysm, dissection, or anomalies
2. Stenoses of the carotid artery
3. Aneurysms of the abdominal aorta
4. Stenoses of the renal artery
5. Follow-up after stent placement
6. Acute and chronic pulmonary embolism

Another classification of the postprocessing techniques distinguishes planimetric analysis and volumetric analysis.

T. H. Wiese, MD; P. Rogalla, MD
Department of Radiology, Charité, Campus Charité Mitte, Humboldt-Universität zu Berlin, Schumannstrasse 20/21, 10098 Berlin, Germany

8.1.1.1
Planimetric Analysis

Multiplanar reconstruction (MPR) generates 2D images along axes that differ from the scanning axis used to acquire the volumetric data set. This technique yields different views of target structures that are not located parallel to the scanning plane. State-of-the-art software allows online planning of MPR on the basis of axial – or sagittal and coronal – scout views (Remy et al. 1998). Structures that lie outside the selected multiplanar section are not visualized. A curved structure that does not run in a single scanning plane can be rendered by so-called "curved MPR", which is a depiction along the course of the target structure (Remy et al. 1998).

8.1.1.2
Volumetric Analysis

Volumetric analysis is based on a slab, which is a stack of several axial sections forming a data volume (Remy et al. 1998). Rendering algorithms that can be applied to a slab include shaded surface display, minimum intensity projection, maximum intensity projection, and volume rendering technique. An improvement in reconstructions from volumetric data sets is best attained when the voxel geometry approaches an isotropic geometry, in other words, when the voxel edges are identical in all spatial axes (i.e., x, y, and z) (Remy et al. 1998).

The basic procedure leading from image acquisition to 3D rendering, regardless of the imaging modality used, comprises the following steps (Kay et al. 1996):

1. Initial image acquisition
2. Image transfer and generation of the volumetric data set
3. Image segmentation or classification: thresholding technique/region growth technique
4. Three-dimensional image rendering

8.1.1.3
Maximum Intensity Projection – Minimum Intensity Projection

In maximum intensity projection (MIP) a 2D image from a preselected viewing angle is generated by casting rays through a stack of individual sections (Napel et al. 1993) and selecting for each ray the highest attenuation or intensity value encountered on its way through the volume. In minimum intensity projection (mIP), the image is created analogously by projecting the lowest attenuation or intensity value through which each ray has passed.

The ray-casting techniques do not require thresholding (Remy et al. 1998). Prokop et al. (1997) emphasized the value of MIP renderings for depicting small vessels and simple anatomic structures, for which the problem of overlaying of foreground and background is negligible, and gives the abdominal aorta as an example. Sliding thin-slab MIP (STS-MIP) is a sequence of MIPs with each individual MIP consisting of a small number of individual sections (Napel et al. 1993).

MIP images enable depiction of intraparenchymal vessels but do not always show the actual spatial relationships of extraparenchymal vessels to organs. No 3D assessment of overlapping vessels is possible (Johnson et al. 1998). A 3D impression including depth information can be created by generating a series of MIPs, in different orientations, from the volumetric data set and then viewing these images in a cine loop (Remy et al. 1998).

8.1.1.4
Volume Rendering Technique

The volume rendering technique (VRT) is a 3D reconstruction of a volumetric data set and allows viewing of this volume from any angle (Johnson et al. 1998). VRT displays allow differentiation of calcifications from the vessel lumen, which is often impossible on shaded surface display images (Johnson et al. 1998). Since VRT uses the entire source data set without exclusion of pixels or voxels, this projection technique requires powerful computer hardware and software (Remy et al. 1998). VRT is superior to MIP in the 3D visualization of overlapping vessels and accurately depicts spatial relationships, for instance between liver tumors and intrahepatic vessels (Johnson et al. 1998).

8.1.1.5
Shaded Surface Display

To generate a shaded surface display (SSD), the operator first has to select a threshold value by means of which the pixels of a data set are subdivided into two groups: those above the threshold and those below (Remy et al. 1998). The pixels below the threshold are not used for image generation (Rubin et al. 1993), resulting in a considerable loss of information. For the remaining pixels above the threshold, a virtual surface is computed (surface rendering). In a second step, the surface thus generated is illuminated by a virtual light source from an operator-selected position to cast a virtual shadow on the surface, which is how the 3D effect is created. The displayed gray scale represents the computer-generated shadow and not attenuation levels. The resulting surface display represents only a fraction of the information contained in the original data set. Calcifications are often difficult to separate from the opacified vessel lumen. Circumferential calcifications may be misinterpreted as patent vessels (Rubin et al. 1993).

Three categories of diagnostic pitfalls associated with SSD are known:

1. Pitfalls resulting from thresholding: depending on the selected threshold, vascular stenoses may be overestimated or underestimated. A wrongly selected threshold excludes delicate vessels from being depicted (Remy et al. 1998).
2. Pitfalls associated with the section thickness chosen for acquisition of the source images: partial volume effects and step artifacts.
3. Pitfalls induced by motion artifacts occurring during acquisition of the original data (Remy et al. 1998). More recent SSD techniques use an upper threshold and a second lower one instead of only one threshold and generate the display from the pixels or voxels between these two values.

8.1.1.6 Virtual Endoscopy

Virtual endoscopy (VE) is the computer-generated simulation of actual endoscopic images derived from data sets acquired by CT or MR imaging. The presentations thus created allow the viewer to explore the inner surfaces of anatomic structures (Jolesz et al. 1997) as with a real endoscope (Dessl et al. 1997). In order to create virtual endoscopic views, the target surfaces must contrast sufficiently with surrounding structures or contents (Jolesz et al. 1997). Today the most widely used image processing techniques used for the virtual endoscopy of vessels are based on volume rendering.

Volume rendering techniques are more demanding in terms of computer hardware and software and require much larger storage capacities and much more processing time for reconstruction. Since volume rendering processes the information of all voxels from the initial data set, no information is lost, in contrast to MIP or SSD (Rubin et al. 1996). With volume rendering, it is possible to analyze the reconstructed inner surface simultaneously with the outer surface and adjacent structures. The virtual endoscopist can pass through the wall of the organ he or she is exploring to inspect surrounding structures, for instance, to evaluate the extent of a pathology.

VE based on surface rendering reconstructs surfaces from an initial data set relative to a threshold value to be selected by the operator (Dessl et al. 1997). After selection of the threshold value (given in Hounsfield units in CT) the computer generates the surface using a so-called ray-casting algorithm which displays the visible voxels in a 3D image from the perspective of an imaginary observer. The position of this observer can be freely selected (Dessl 1997). This type of VE requires much less powerful computer hardware and software than VE using volume rendering techniques.

SSD, VRT, and VE all allow perspective presentation of the image information. To create such a perspective effect, the images are altered from a predefined distant viewing point in such a way that objects closer to this point are magnified while objects farther away are made to appear smaller (Rubin et al. 1996).

Since the generation of VE images requires large disk storage capacity and is very time-consuming, the user can select from various interpolation algorithms provided by the computer, ranging from rapidly generated reconstructions with a low resolution for initial orientation to very complex reconstructions with maximal resolution and depiction of detail (Dessl et al. 1997).

Since all VE presentations are created by use of an interpolation algorithm that smoothes the vessel wall, pathologies of the wall such as atherosclerotic changes are more difficult to evaluate (Davis et al. 1996).

The reconstructed images can be viewed either individually or as a moving fly-through endoscopic display in which a consecutive series of individual images is presented (Dessl et al. 1997). In this mode, the reconstructed individual images are stored and displayed in a cine loop (Bartolozzi et al. 1998). Two main options are used for viewing VE reconstructions in the fly-through mode. The first is "manual camera movement," in which the radiologist interactively navigates the virtual endoscope through the target vessel with the mouse of the computer. In the second option, "automatic path planning," the radiologist selects a starting point and endpoint in the vessel, from which the computer calculates the shortest path through the vessel and does not leave the vessel.

An advantage of VE compared to conventional angiography may result from the potential to also examine vessels that are not accessible by conventional angiography (Rubin et al. 1996). Furthermore, unlike digital subtraction angiography (DSA), 3D postprocessing techniques allow retrospective manipulation of the original images and depiction of specific vessel segments in different orientations (Lawrence et al. 1995).

The following parameters are essential for good quality VE of the vessels:

1. Adequate scanning parameters for acquisition of the source data set by CT and MR imaging
2. Selection of suitable threshold values for surface rendering (Dessl et al. 1997; Ladd et al. 1996) and volume rendering

Selection of the proper threshold is the most crucial step in generating the VE presentations.

Today, software is available that enables automated segmentation of pixels or voxels by means of the so-called "region growing technique." The radiologist selects a reference voxel against which the computer checks the tissue densities of adjacent voxels for inclusion in or exclusion from the surface rendering. In regions where the interface between tissues of different attenuations is not clear-cut, even the most sophisticated software will fail to adequately define the surface automatically. Such cases require manual editing by the operator.

Problems arise when surface rendering is done by selecting a single fixed threshold value, above which all pixels are assigned an identical gray-scale value. When this procedure is used, it will be difficult or even impossible to differentiate depositions on the vessel wall from beam-hardening artifacts. Selection of an inadequate threshold value for VE rendering may create apparent stenoses or eliminate structures of interest (Dessl et al. 1997).

To minimize the risk of misinterpretations, it is mandatory to review the reconstructed VE together with the initial sectional scans. This can be done using modern software with so-called multiview or split-screen display for the parallel presentation of VE, original images, and multiplanar reconstructions (Auer et al. 1998) (Fig. 8.1). This type of image display additionally facilitates orientation in the VE presentation. A pointer on the screen indicates the position of the virtual endoscope on the axial images or the multiplanar reconstructions (Jolesz et al. 1997).

When VE was first introduced, the viewing direction of the observer in the fly-through mode was restricted to the direction of flight (Davis et al 1996). More recent software enables the viewer to freely select a viewing direction and thus, for instance, to navigate through the vessel looking back. To change the direction is likewise unproblematic.

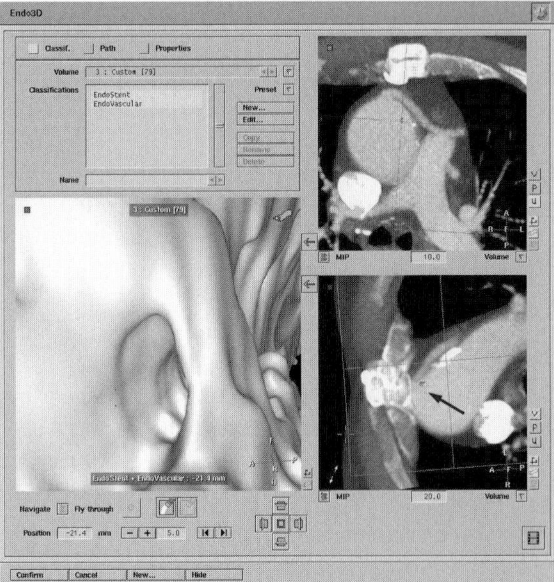

Fig. 8.1. Split-screen display. Parallel presentation of virtual endoscopy (VE) (*lower left*), maximum intensity projection (MIP) (*upper right*), and multiplanar reconstruction (MPR) (*lower right*) of an aortocoronary vein bypass. The *arrow* marks the position of the virtual observer in the MPR to explain the view in the VE

8.2 Angiography Based on Cross-Sectional Imaging

VE presentations are generated from CT or MR imaging data sets consisting of high-resolution volumetric sectional scans (Jolesz et al. 1997).

8.2.1 General Remarks

The advantages of MRA over CTA are as follows:

- Allergic reactions to MRA contrast agents are less frequent and milder.
- Three-dimensional rendering is less time-consuming in MRA since less extensive editing of the initial images is required. For instance, it is not necessary to remove bone-dense structures in MRA.
- No exposure to ionizing radiation.
- Free selection of the scanning plane adjusted to the target structure (Prokop et al. 1997).

CTA has the following advantages over MRA:

- No suppression of tissue signals.
- Shorter overall examination times.
- Superior differentiation of calcified from uncalcified plaques in vascular imaging.

- CTA is an easy to perform examination that is easier to learn than MRA.
- CTA is less expensive than MRA.
- Direct access to the patient and better monitoring make CTA the more suitable procedure for examining critically ill patients, e.g., patients with suspected aortic dissection, pulmonary embolism, or aortic rupture (Prokop et al. 1997).

8.2.2 Spiral Computed Tomography

Spiral CT today allows rapid image acquisition with shorter scanning times and – in comparison to conventional incremental CT – reduced motion artifacts.

In general, spatial resolution increases with the quality of the reconstructed 3D image and is optimal at a small collimation of the roentgen ray, low table feed, maximum overlapping of sections, and a high tube output. However, optimal setting of all of these parameters would result in an unacceptably high radiation exposure for the patient. Limitations result from differences in patient cooperation, e.g., the length of time that individuals can hold their breath, in the quality of the venous access, or from compromised kidney function (Bartolozzi et al. 1998). A middle ground between acceptable image quality and acceptable radiation exposure has to be found on an individual basis before each examination.

The advent of spiral CT has boosted the development of CTA, which is now a routine clinical procedure. Advantages of spiral CT over conventional incremental CT are the volumetric acquisition during a single breath-hold, the reduction of motion artifacts, better enhancement of vessels, and the possibility to reduce the dose of contrast agent (Hopper et al. 1996). A volumetric data set acquired by spiral CT can be reconstructed at different reconstruction intervals, by which means it is possible to improve spatial resolution. Adequate 3D rendering at reduced radiation exposure is achieved by combining overlapping image reconstruction with spiral CT acquisition at a pitch >1 (pitch = ratio of table feed per gantry rotation to collimation).

Typical indications for CTA today are aneurysms, dissections and anomalies of the thoracic aorta, stenoses of the carotid artery, aneurysms of the abdominal aorta, stenoses of the renal arteries, and acute and chronic pulmonary embolism (Bartolozzi et al. 1998). A wealth of other indications, such as diseases of the coronary arteries, are presently being investigated.

Higher collimation results in a decrease in longitudinal resolution and an increase in partial volume effects. CTA of the thoracic and abdominal aorta is typically performed at a collimation ranging between 3 mm and 8 mm. To depict smaller vessels, a lower collimation has to be used (Diederichs et al. 1996). The pitch selected affects both scanning time and longitudinal resolution. Typically, a pitch between 1 and 2 is used, with a pitch smaller than 1.5 being recommended for CTA. In patients with a limited capacity to hold their breath, acquisition time can be shortened by using a pitch between 1.5 and 2 (Bartolozzi et al. 1998). As a rule, higher pitch is associated with poorer image quality of 3D reconstructions and lower resolution along the *z*-axis (Diederichs et al. 1996).

For contrast-enhanced imaging, it is recommended to administer an iodine concentration of at least 300 mg/ml. Determination of circulation time by giving a test bolus allows precise coordination of contrast agent administration and data acquisition, thereby ensuring scanning during the maximal opacification of the target vessels (Bartolozzi et al. 1998). The circulation time is measured over the vascular segment to be examined. The amount of contrast agent and rate of administration are determined in relation to the scanning time. Typically, a flow rate of 3–4 ml/s is used for CTA. Known limitations of CTA include the unreliable depiction of thin vessels and the misrepresentation of high-grade stenoses as vascular occlusions. Further drawbacks may be pitch-related distortions of axial sections, partial volume effects, and beam-hardening artifacts (Diederichs et al. 1996; Marks et al. 1993).

8.2.3 Magnetic Resonance Imaging

Contrast-enhanced 3D MR angiography (CE-MRA) has developed into another alternative to conventional angiography. With high diagnostic accuracy, CE-MRA has certain advantages over CT. The patient is not exposed to ionizing radiation and the administration of potentially nephrotoxic contrast agents is not required. Advances in MRI technology have considerably shortened data acquisition times, thereby providing the means to acquire 3D volumetric data sets during breath-hold and reducing motion artifacts (Hany et al. 1998). For CE-MRA in the abdomen and the chest, a body phased-array coil is used (Bongartz et al. 1997), and the best results are achieved by imaging at 1.5 T.

Contrast agents are administered to shorten the T1 relaxivity of the blood relative to surrounding tissue. A short TR and TE enhance the opacified vasculature while at the same time reducing the signal from surrounding structures (Hany et al. 1998), resulting in maximum contrast between vessels and surrounding tissue. A recent study described advantages of CE-MRA over phase-contrast MRA (PC-MRA) and time-of-flight MRA (TOF-MRA) (Bongartz et al. 1997).

Time-of-flight MRA is primarily used to assess fast, unidirectional flow phenomena. Signal inhomogeneities occur when flow is multidirectional or turbulent. The extent and severity of stenoses may be overestimated by TOF-MRA due to signal losses induced by turbulent flow and dephasing distal to stenotic vessel segments (Bongartz et al. 1997; Marks et al. 1993). Large volumetric data sets cannot be handled by TOF-MRA. Compensating technical variants such as sequential 2D data acquisition prolong imaging times to up to 20–30 min, resulting in the occurrence of motion artifacts in most patients (Bongartz et al. 1997).

Phase-contrast MRA allows acquisition of larger volumetric data sets. This examination technique is independent of saturation effects (Bongartz et al. 1997) but necessitates precise estimation of expected flow velocities. If the velocity encoding of the MRI sequence used does not match actual flow, reduced or turbulent flow signals will occur. As in TOF-MRA, long image acquisition times and the occurrence of background motion artifacts are drawbacks of this technique.

CE-MRA combines the use of ultrafast 3D sequences with the T1-shortening effect of paramagnetic contrast agents. CE-MRA minimizes signal losses and inhomogeneities induced by saturation effects or turbulent flow (Bongartz et al. 1997). Data acquisition times of less than 20 s enable the CE-MRA examination to be performed during a single breath-hold in most patients, thereby considerably reducing the occurrence of motion artifacts compared to CE-MRA with free breathing (Prince 1994). The contrast agents used in CE-MRA are gadolinium compounds, which have an extracellular, but no strictly intravascular, distribution. Thus, the optimal time for image acquisition is the first pass prior to extravasation.

Advances brought about by CE-MRA are extension of the indications to vascular systems not accessible by conventional MRA and improved clinical acceptance of the method as a result of the reduction in examination times in those indications where MRA has already been employed with success (Bongartz et al. 1997). CE-MRA is performed using 3D gradient-echo sequences with a large flip angle (25–50°). The contrast material is administered at a constant flow rate of 1.5–2.5 ml/s by means of an automatic injector with subsequent injection of physiologic saline solution for bolus optimization (Prokop et al. 1997; Rühm and Debatin 1999). Reports in the literature recommend administration of a single dose of 0.1 mmol gadolinium per kilogram body weight for the diagnostic assessment of central and peripheral vessels.

Exact timing of the contrast agent bolus is crucial for data acquisition during the arterial phase and to minimize intervening signals from overlying venous vessels. This is typically done by administering a test bolus to determine the time of contrast agent influx into the target area (Hany et al. 1998). The scan delay is calculated as follows: influx of the contrast material in the middle of the MRA acquisition minus 10% if sequences with sequential K-space ordering are used. Alternatively, repeated 10-s data acquisitions can be performed at defined intervals from the start of contrast agent injection (Bongartz et al. 1997). The latter protocol can be used in all cases where administration of a test bolus is inconclusive, in CE-MRA of the carotid artery, and in patients who are unable to hold their breath long enough. Recent bolus timing methods (e.g., smart prep) allow online determination of contrast agent influx without additional administration of a test bolus (Prokop et al. 1997). For this purpose, the aorta is scanned with a very fast sequence at a high temporal resolution. As soon as this sequence identifies a signal change resulting from influx of the contrast agent into the aorta, the actual examination sequence is started (Rühm and Debatin 1999).

A well-established drawback of 3D MRA is the overestimation of vascular stenoses, which is attributable to intravascular signal inhomogeneities primarily occurring in the presence of turbulent flow (Hany et al. 1998). Advantages of 3D CE-MRA over conventional DSA include the possibility of imaging without administration of nephrotoxic contrast agents, the use of gadolinium-based contrast material with considerably less allergic reactions, and the depiction of a blood vessel from an infinite range of viewing angles (Prince et al. 1997).

The main disadvantages of 3D CE-MRA compared to conventional DSA include the difficulties or even the impossibility of performing the examination in claustrophobic patients or in patients with certain implanted metal devices, such as pacemakers or automated implanted cardioverters (AICD). MRA still remains an imaging technique with limited availability, and the spatial resolution in MRA is considerably lower than that in DSA (Prince et al. 1997).

8.3 Virtual Endoscopy of the Aorta

In the diagnostic assessment of the thoracic aorta, CTA has a significant role in evaluating aortic dissection (Bartolozzi et al. 1998; Prokop et al. 1997), irrespective of whether it originates in the ascending or descending part of the aorta (Stanford type A and B, respectively) and of its extension. In addition to spiral CT, ultrafast electron beam CT has been used for assessing type A aortic dissection (Hamada et al. 1992). In a study of 17 patients, CTA by means of electron beam CT accurately depicted the intimal lesion in 93% of the cases. Only one tear of the intima in the area of the aortic arch was missed (Hamada et al. 1992). In this study, the entire aorta from the aortic arch to the bifurcation was examined in 74 s without breath-hold, and the authors emphasized that this protocol was well-suited for critically ill patients.

Prince reported the use of CE-MRA in 125 patients with suspected disorders of the aorta. In this study, CE-MRA was found to have a sensitivity of 88% with a specificity of 97% in diagnosing stenoses and occlusions of the aorta and was 100% sensitive and specific in depicting aneurysms of the aorta or iliac arteries (Prince 1994).

Zeman et al. compared the usefulness of various reconstruction techniques (MIP and MPR) for CTA data sets in the diagnostic assessment of patients with suspected aortic dissection (Zeman et al. 1995). Analysis of the axial source scans in 23 patients yielded 15 true-negative, seven true-positive, and one false-positive finding. In three of the seven patients with aortic dissection, the intimal tear was difficult to localize. Visualization of the intimal flap was found to be poorest on the MIP images. The authors conclude that review of the axial scans alone is sufficient for the diagnostic assessment of aortic dissection in the majority of patients and recommend use of the MPR technique in cases where these findings are inconclusive.

MPR enables visualization of the aorta with optimal slice orientation including depiction of the spatial relationship of the aortic dissection to the supra-aortic branches (Bartolozzi et al. 1998; Prokop et al. 1997). SSD is useful for depicting aneurysms of the aortic arch and of the proximal descending aorta. VE offers an intraluminal view of the aorta including the orifices of the supra-aortic branches and, in the presence of dissection, allows inspection of the false lumen through the entry of the dissection (Bartolozzi et al. 1998). Vessels originating from the true and the false lumen can be differentiated (Prokop et al. 1997) (Fig. 8.2a–c).

Kimura et al. found the virtual endoscopic views to be useful in the diagnostic assessment of aneurysms of the distal aortic arch for depicting the relationship of the aneurysm to vessels originating in the aortic arch. They examined 12 patients with aneurysms located in the distal aortic arch using spiral CT. In 42% of these cases, the relationship between the aneurysm and the origin of the left subclavian artery was established using the axial CT scans alone. With additional virtual endoscopic views, the diagnostic accuracy increased significantly to 92% (Kimura et al. 1996). No diagnostic gain resulting from VE was found for the assessment of aortic dissection. In ten patients with aortic dissection, no significant differences were seen between the 2D source scans and virtual endoscopic views in depicting the relationship between the origins of the aortic branches and the intimal flap. Both procedures allowed the correct diagnosis to be established in all patients but correctly identified the entry site in only two-thirds of the cases (Kimura et al. 1996). The 2D source images allowed differentiation of the entry site from calcification, which is not depicted by VE.

Neri et al. also investigated the virtual endoscopic display of aortic dissection based on CTA data sets. VE depicted the intimal flap and the entry site of aortic dissection in all nine cases investigated (Neri et al. 1997). The site of rupture was identified in seven out of eight patients with aortic rupture. With VE, calcified plaques and dilatations of the aorta were reliably diagnosed. The authors described two types of artifacts that occurred in VE of the aorta: pierced surfaces and floating shapes. The severity of these artifacts was found to be dependent on threshold selection.

Davis et al. evaluated VE generated from CE-MRA data sets of the aorta. They employed VE in 21 patients with the following indications: four cases each of stenosis of the aortic isthmus and aortic dissection, seven instances of follow-up of aortic prosthesis, and one case each of congenital double aortic arch, abdominal aortic aneurysm, and Leriche's syndrome. CE-MRA was performed at 1.5 T. The total postprocessing time required to generate the VE presentations was 10–20 min. The quality of the VE images was a direct result of the homogeneous opacification of the blood, which was severely impaired in areas of turbulent flow. Performed by an experienced radiologist, VE is able to differentiate the vessel wall from

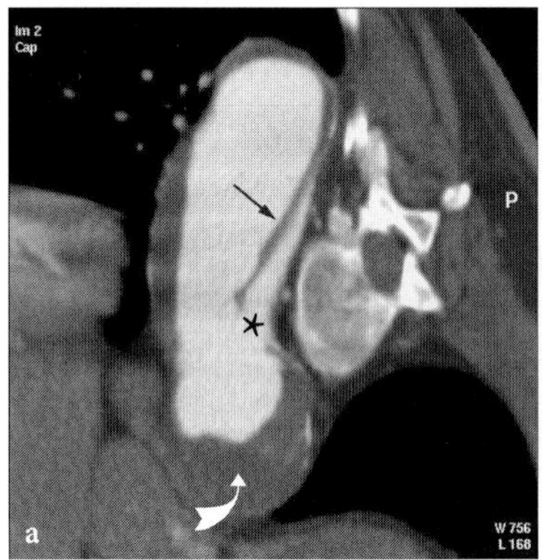

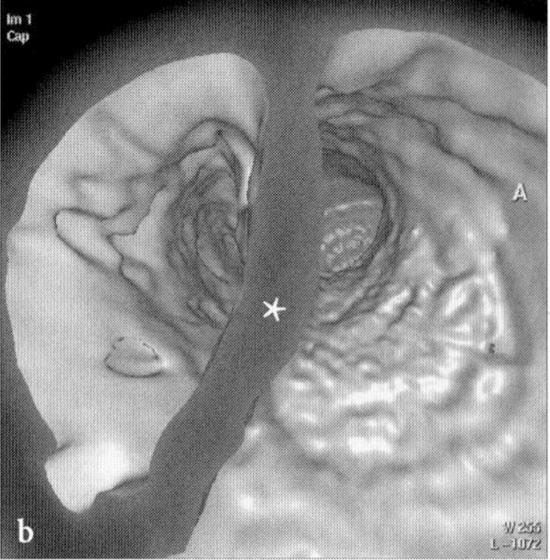

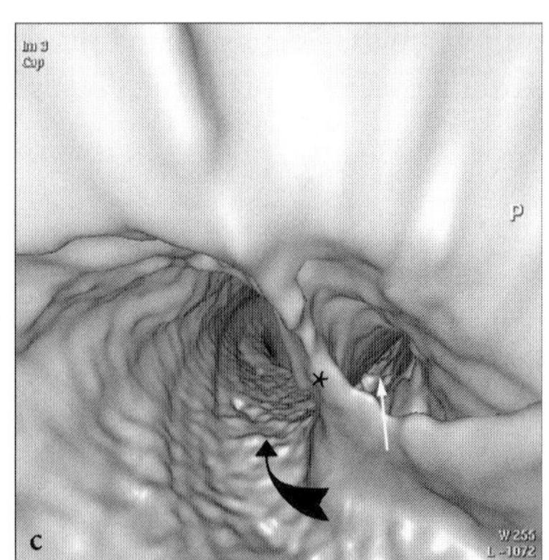

Fig. 8.2a–d. De Bakey type III aortic dissection in a 55-year-old man. CT angiography (CTA). **a** MPR shows the intimal tear (*star*), intimal flap (*arrow*), and an aortic thrombus (*curved arrow*). **b** Virtual fly-through in the same patient. The *star* marks the intimal flap between the true lumen on the *left* and the false lumen on the *right* of the image. **c** VE at the position of the intimal tear. The virtual observer is looking in a retrograde direction into the true lumen on the right (*arrow*) and the false lumen on the *left* (*curved arrow*). **d** Digital subtraction aortography (DSA)

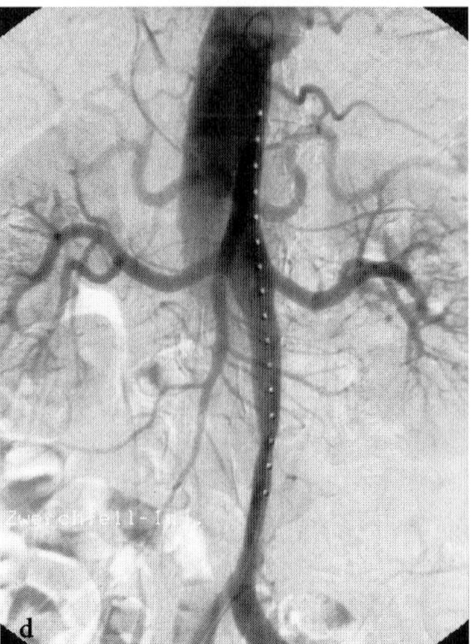

wall-bound thrombi. The authors found VE to be of potential benefit for the following indications: follow-up after balloon angioplasty with assessment of vascular dissection and follow-up after stent placement for the occurrence of restenosis and development of neointima (Davis et al. 1996).

In patients with abdominal aortic aneurysm (AAA), CTA and CE-MRA allow diagnostic assessment of the extent of an aneurysm and its spatial relationship to branches of the aorta (e.g., renal arteries, celiac trunk, mesenteric arteries, and iliac vessels), which is crucial for planning the surgical approach (Jolesz et al. 1997; Bartolozzi et al. 1998; Prokop et al. 1997). CE-MRA depicts the lumen only when flow is present. To assess thrombotic portions of an aneurysm, an additional T1-weighted sequence (fast gradient-echo sequence) is used (Rühm and Debatin 1999) (Fig. 8.3). CTA and CE-MRA reliably diagnose Leriche's syndrome and other occlusions of the aorta. Both procedures depict the vessels proximal to the occlusion as well as the subsequent distal vessels and collaterals (Fig. 8.4). A useful indication for CE-MRA is the assessment of developmental abnormalities of the aorta in children. The extent of a stenosis of the aortic isthmus may be depicted by CE-MRA, and VE can be used to assess the stenosis from an intraluminal perspective (Prokop et al. 1997).

Wildermuth et al. developed a system for virtual planning of the placement of endoluminal aortic stents. With this software, it is possible to review different multiplanar reconstructions from 3D MRA data sets simultaneously with VE. The endoluminal

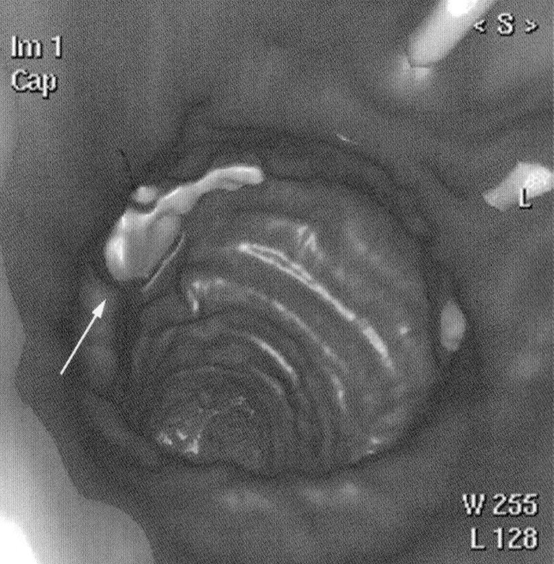

Fig. 8.3. VE from the neck of an abdominal aortic aneurysm. CTA. Using two different classifications for the vessel lumen and for calcifications, calcified plaques (*arrow*) are depicted on VE

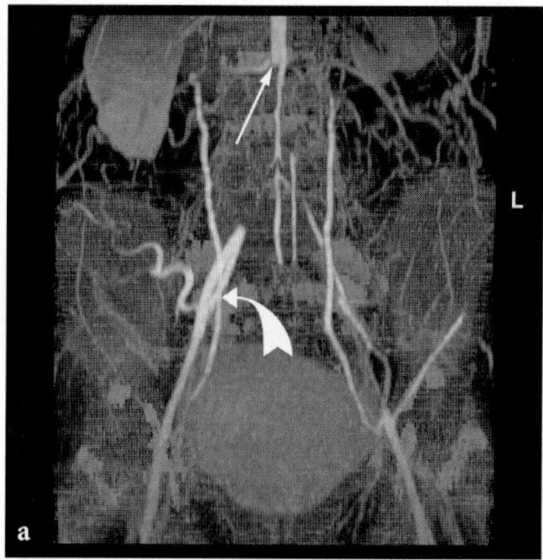

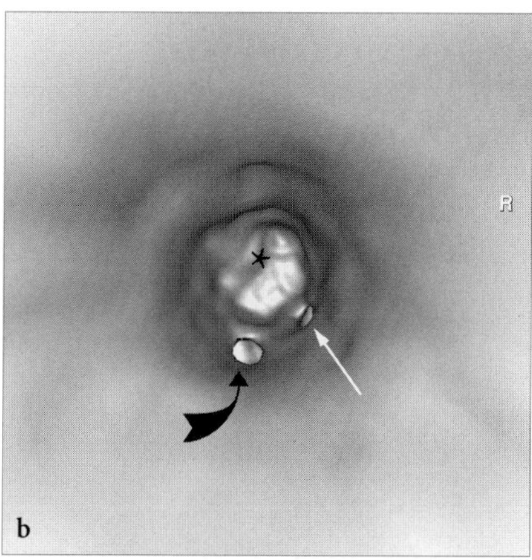

Fig. 8.4a, b. Leriche's syndrome with infrarenal occlusion of the abdominal aorta. CTA. **a** MIP with clear depiction of the aortic occlusion below the origins of the renal arteries (*arrow*). Iliac arteries (*curved arrow*) show perfusion via collaterals. **b** VE adds no significant additional information. Occlusion of the abdominal aorta (*star*) and the origins of the right renal artery (*arrow*) and the superior mesenteric artery (*curved arrow*) are seen

VE views allow easy determination of vessel diameters and virtual planning of stent positioning. The system was successfully used in 12 cases of abdominal aortic aneurysm (Wildermuth et al. 1998/1999).

Rodenwaldt et al. investigated the clinical potential of VE in depicting implanted vascular stents in an in vitro model. The following protocol for acquisition of the CT scans was developed using this model:

- 1 mm slice thickness at a pitch of 2.5 to 3, or
- 3 mm slice thickness with a pitch of 1 to 1.5

Virtual endoscopic views generated from these data sets correctly detected and assessed all stenoses artificially created in a phantom study. In ten patients who had undergone implantation of an endovascular vessel prosthesis, the stents were reliably localized by VE in all cases. The intima was also depicted by VE (Rodenwaldt et al. 1997).

Rogalla and Rückert examined patients before and after transfemoral stent placement for nondissecting AAA by helical CT and used VE and MIP reconstructions of the initial data sets. In 27 patients CTA was performed using the following scanning parameters:

- 3 mm collimation
- 5 mm table feed
- 2 mm reconstruction interval
- 120 kV, 200–250 mA
- 512×512 image matrix at a field of view of 180–220 mm

The authors found VE to yield useful additional diagnostic information in the follow-up of stent implantation for AAA. Depiction of the entire stent was best on MIP images, while VE most clearly showed the spatial relationship between the stent and the renal arteries and was the only procedure that demonstrated extension of the implanted stent into a renal artery ostium. However, Rogalla et al. (1998) also emphasized that neither VE nor MIP can replace interpretation of the axial source scans (Figs. 8.5–8.9). Rilinger investigated the use of VE generated using

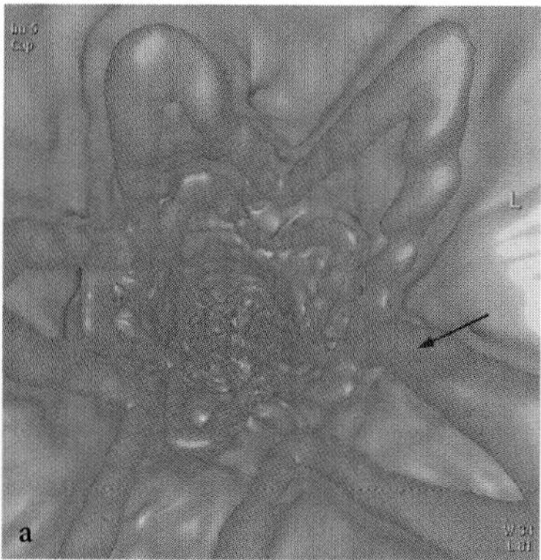

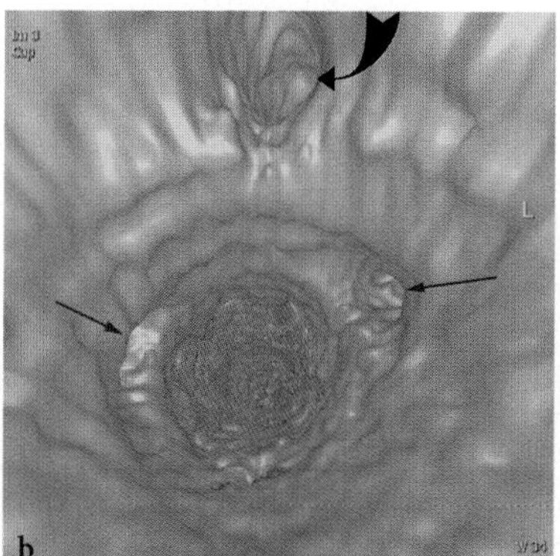

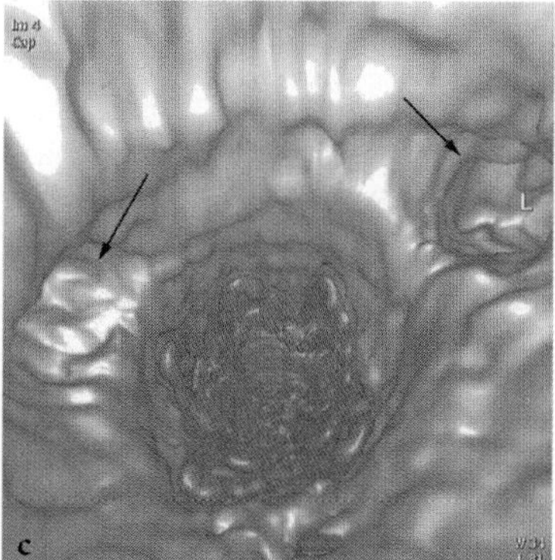

Fig. 8.5a–c. VE after placement of an intraluminal stent (Talent) in an infrarenal abdominal aortic aneurysm. CTA. **a** Using different thresholds for the stent and the aortic lumen, VE allows a clear depiction of the stent (*orange*, *arrow*) and its position in the aorta. **b, c** VE confirms exact stent position with free origins of the renal arteries (*arrows*) and the superior mesenteric artery (*curved arrow*)

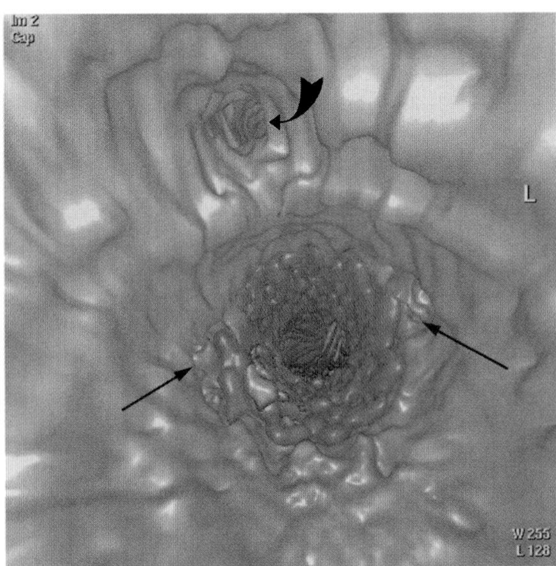

Fig. 8.6. VE after placement of an intraluminal stent in an infrarenal abdominal aortic aneurysm. CTA. The VE demonstrates a proximal stent position with the stent (*orange*) overlying the origin of the renal arteries (*arrows*). Free origin of the superior mesenteric artery (*curved arrow*)

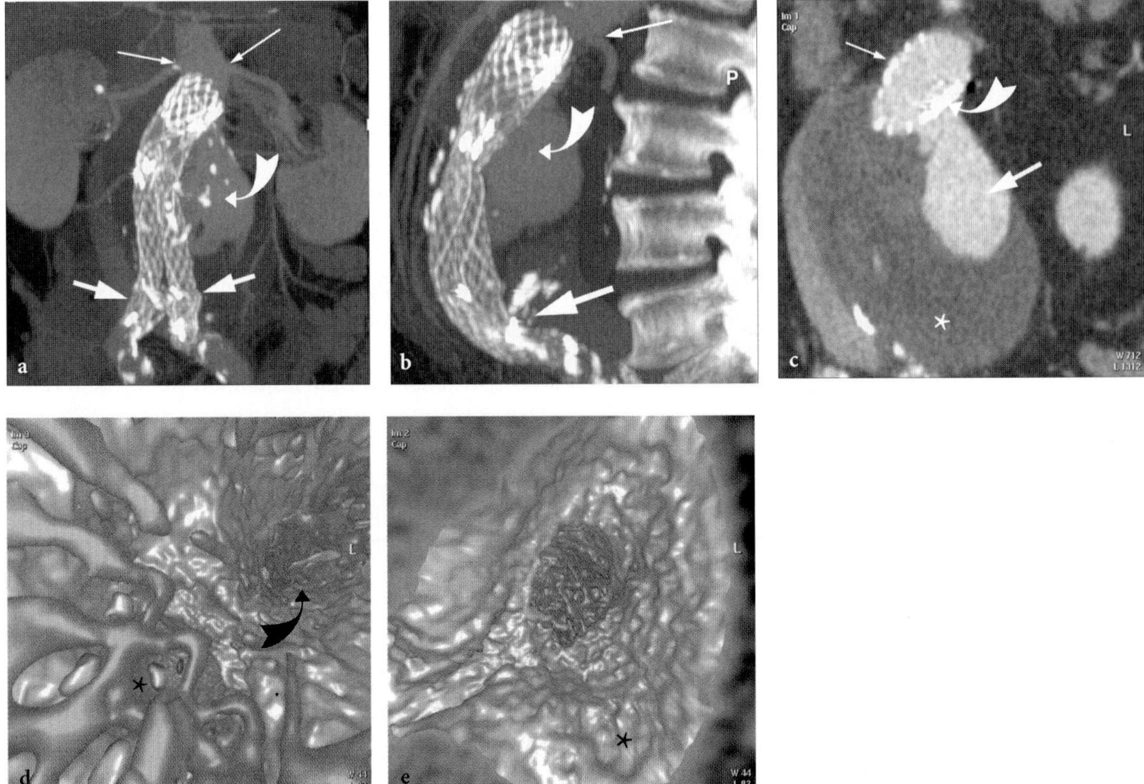

Fig. 8.7a–e. Endoleak after placement of an intraluminal stent in an infrarenal abdominal aortic aneurysm. CTA. **a, b** MIP in coronal (**a**) and sagittal planes (**b**) provides an excellent overview of the stent, its extension into both common iliac arteries (*thick arrow*), and its position relative to the origin of the renal arteries (*thin arrow*). The aneurysm sac (*curved arrow*) is clearly depicted, while the endoleak cannot be seen in the chosen perspectives. **c** MPR with a paraaxial plane chosen demonstrates the endoleak into the aneurysmal sac with its entry at the proximal part of the stent (*curved arrow*). Contrast material perfusing the aneurysmal sac can be seen (*thick arrow*). *Star*, thrombus in the aneurysmal sac, *thin arrow* stent. **d** Virtual endoscopic view through the mesh of the stent (*orange*) into the perfused part of the aneurysmal sac (*star*). *Arrow*, lumen of the abdominal aorta with the stent in situ. **e** The virtual observer positioned in the endoleak in the front (*star*) looking back onto the aortic stent (*orange*) crossing the view

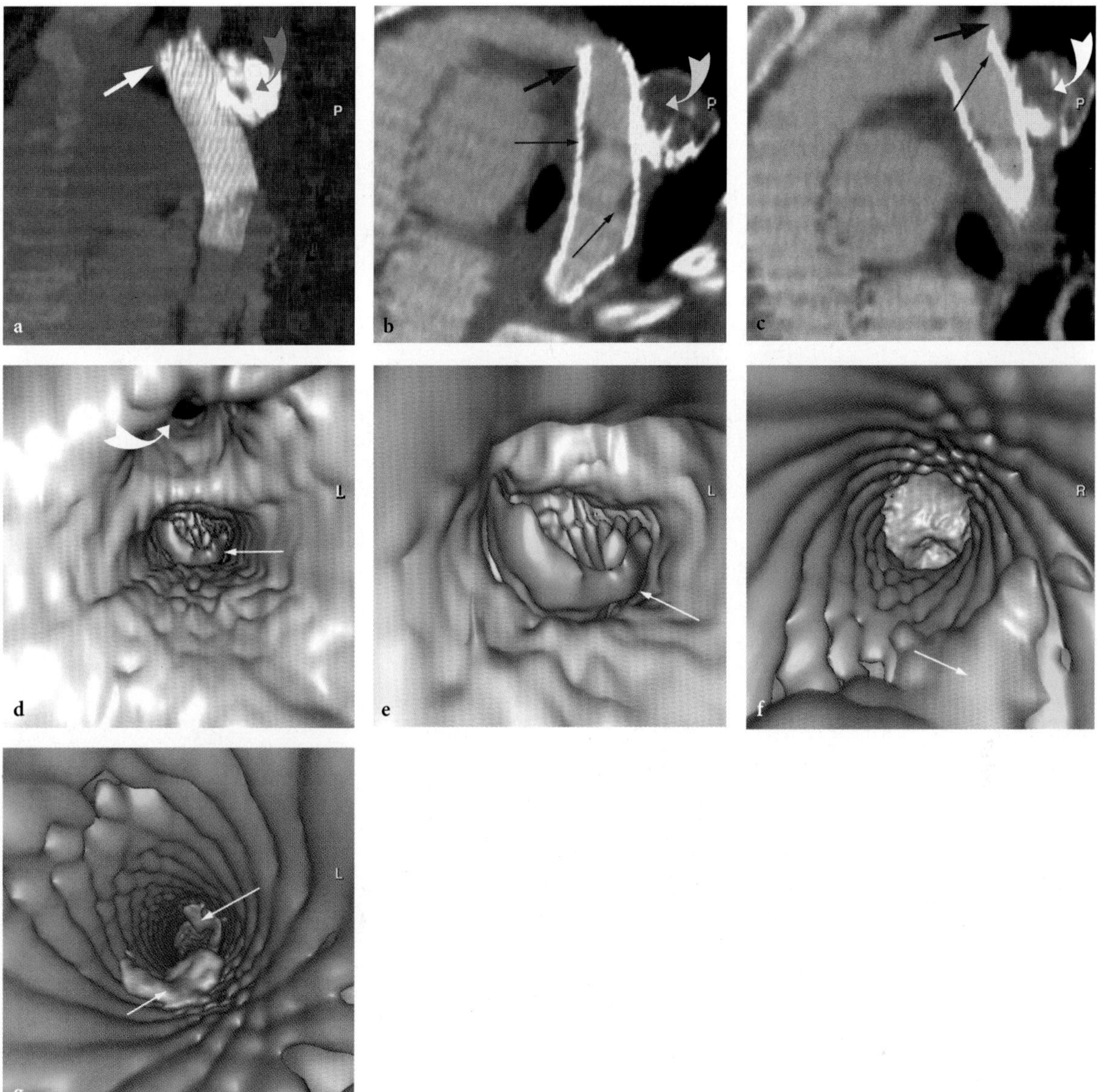

Fig. 8.8a–g. An 18-year-old patient with an aneurysm of the proximal descending aorta after implantation of an intraluminal aortic stent. CTA. **a** MIP and **b** MPR demonstrate the full length of the intraluminal stent and its extension into the distal aortic arch (*thick arrow*), showing successful exclusion of the aortic aneurysm (*curved arrow*). **c** MPR in a plane axial to the aortic arch reveals the relation between the implanted stent (*thin arrow*) and the origin of the left subclavian artery (*thick arrow*). *Curved arrow*, excluded aneurysm. **d, e** VE with the virtual observer in the proximal aortic arch looking into the distal parts of the arch. The stent (*orange, arrow*) extending too far into the aortic arch is clearly seen. The origins of the supraaortic branches (*curved arrow* in **d**, brachiocephalic trunk) are depicted. **f, g** VE of the implanted stent (*orange*) with the virtual observer in the stent looking in a retrograde direction into the aortic arch in **f** and into the descending aorta in **g**. When different thresholds are used, thrombotic material in the stent (*arrows*) – as marked in **b** by *thin arrows* – can be visualized

spiral CT data sets from patients with pathologies of the aorta (see also Fig. 8.10), the carotid artery, and the iliac arteries. VE posed no problem in differentiating calcified plaques and radiodense endovascular stents in the vascular lumen and allowed reliable assessment of stenotic vessel segments and endoleaks. The authors emphasized the simplicity of presenting the findings interactively (Rilinger 1998).

"Thoracic outlet syndrome" is the term used to describe neurovascular compression at the level of the upper thoracic aperture resulting from the natural narrowness of this anatomic region. CTA in com-

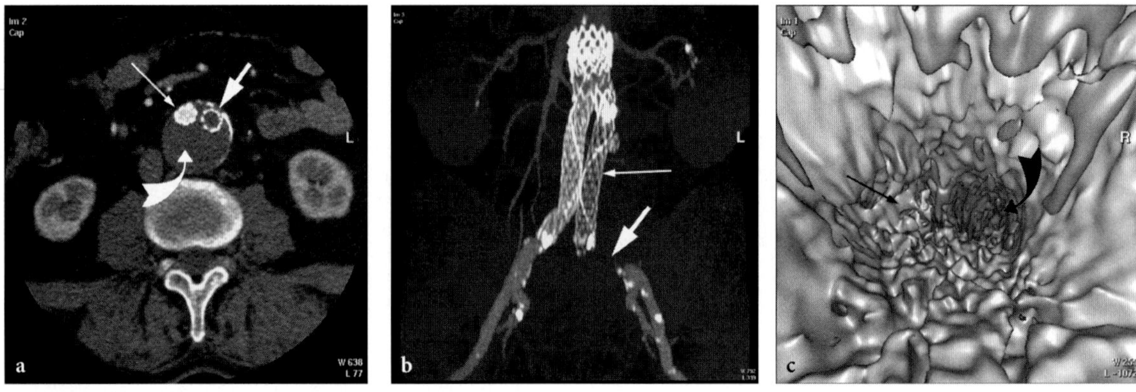

Fig. 8.9a–c. Occlusion of an intraluminal aorto-biiliac stent. CTA. **a** Axial source images reveal the occlusion of the left iliac part of the Y-stent (*thick arrow*). The left iliac part of the stent (*thin arrow*) shows normal perfusion with contrast enhancement after intravenous administration of contrast material. *Curved arrow*, thrombus in the aneurysm sac. **b** MIP provides an excellent overview over the entire length of the stent. The aneurysm sac is less well depicted. Occlusion of the left iliac part of the stent (*thin arrow*) can be identified. Lack of contrast enhancement of the common iliac artery distal to the stent on the left side. **c** VE of the implanted stent with the virtual observer in front of the stent bifurcation looking distally, with clear depiction of the stent occlusion on the left side (*thin arrow*). *Curved arrow*, normal perfusion of the right iliac part of the stent

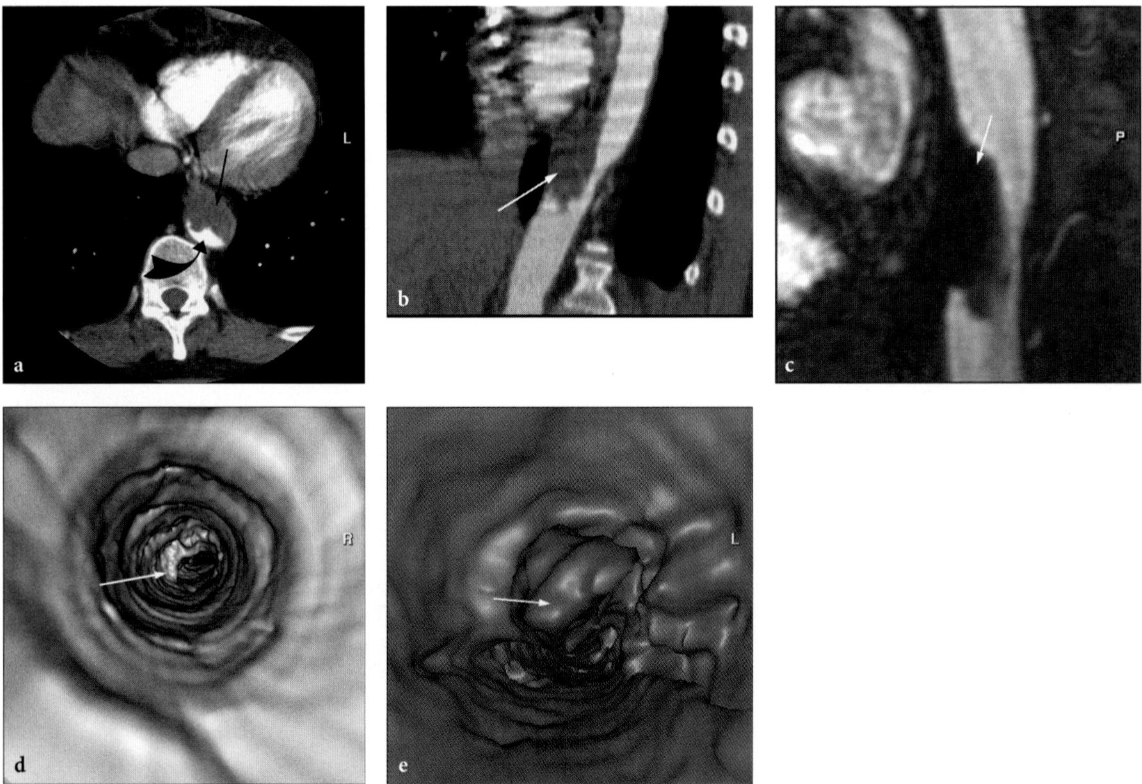

Fig. 8.10a–e. A 64-year-old with a rare case of primary aortic sarcoma. CTA. **a** Axial source images show a extended hypodense mass in the descending aorta (*arrow*). *Curved arrow*, perfused remainder of the aortic lumen. **b, c** MPR in a plane along the axis of the descending aorta reveals the craniocaudad extension of the tumor (*arrow*) by the narrowing of the perfused aortic lumen. **d, e** VE fly-through through the aorta. The tumor growth (*arrow*) into the aortic lumen is well depicted with the virtual observer's point of view above (**d**) and below (**e**) the tumor

bination with MPR and SSD allows assessment of this syndrome even without administration of intravenous contrast material and accurately depicts the spatial relationships of bones, vascular bundles, and muscles. VRT precisely depicts the subclavian artery in the costoclavicular space and its spatial relationship to the anterior scalene muscle (REMY et al. 1998). There are as yet no published reports on the use of VE in the diagnostic assessment of the thoracic outlet syndrome.

8.4 Virtual Endoscopy of the Pulmonary Vessels

In the assessment of acute and chronic pulmonary embolism, CTA demonstrates emboli in the pulmonary arteries down to the segmental level (BARTOLOZZI et al. 1998) and questionably also at the subsegmental level and allows differentiation of intramural thrombi from intraluminal ones (PROKOP et al. 1997). Diagnostic assessment of pulmonary embolism by CTA necessitates determination of the contrast agent circulation time through the pulmonary arterial system. Several studies have demonstrated the accuracy of spiral CT and electron beam CT with sensitivities and specificities of over 90% in the diagnostic evaluation of central pulmonary artery embolism (Fig. 8.11). Emboli in lobar arteries, segmental arteries, and subsegmental arteries are demonstrated by CTA with decreasing sensitivity; thus, reliable depiction of emboli in subsegmental pulmonary arteries by CTA is not possible (REMY-JARDIN et al. 1997). REMY-JARDIN et al. have shown that depiction of segmental and subsegmental pulmonary arteries by CTA can be achieved by reducing collimation from the typical 5 mm to 3 mm (table feed 5 mm, pitch 1.7) or 2 mm (table feed 4 mm, pitch 2). Reduction of collimation to 2 mm resulted in adequate visualization of 61% of the subsegmental arteries as opposed to only 37% at 3 mm collimation.

The diagnostic assessment of pulmonary artery embolism is hampered by the diagonal course of the pulmonary arteries. This problem is well known for both anterior upper lobe segments, the right middle lobe, the left lingula, and both apical lower lobe segments (REMY et al. 1998). A problem for MRA of the pulmonary arteries is the rapid superimposition of arterial and venous vessels (BONGARTZ et al. 1998; WIEPOLOWSKI et al. 1992), which can be overcome by employing CE-MRA in the fastest mode available. Many patients undergoing diagnostic assessment for acute pulmonary embolism are severely ill and require close monitoring, which is difficult during an MRI examination and may limit its general use in these patients; however, typical indications for CE-MRA are chronic and postoperative alterations of the pulmonary vascular system (BONGARTZ et al. 1997). Due to the relatively open scanner design in CT, monitoring of the patient poses no problem in CTA, making the latter a suitable modality for critically ill patients (PROKOP et al. 1997).

REMY-JARDIN et al. demonstrated the value of MPR from data sets acquired by spiral CT. They found MPR images to improve the diagnostic assessment of pulmonary embolism in all cases where the

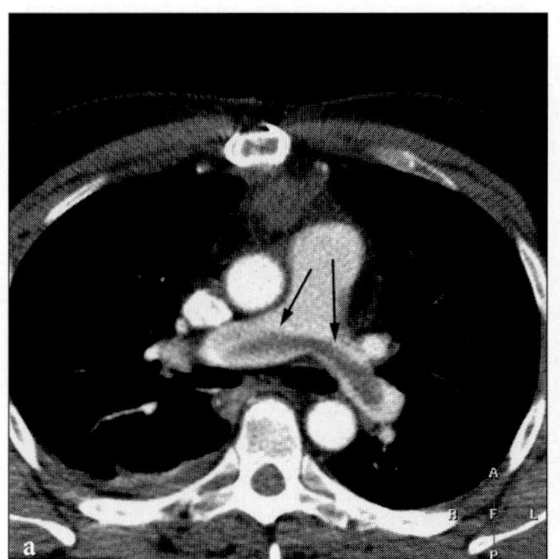
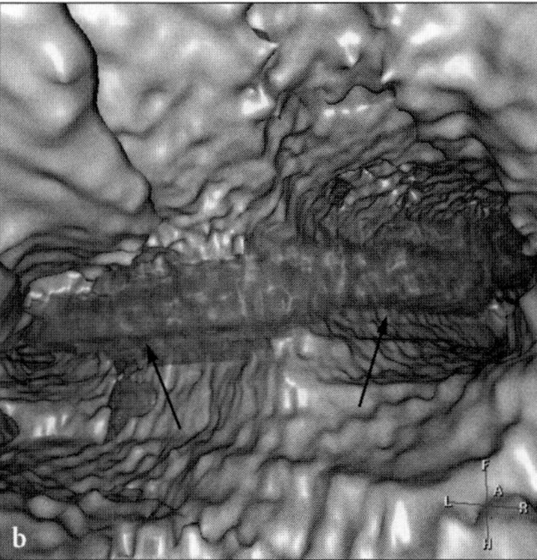

Fig. 8.11a, b. Acute pulmonary embolism in a 53-year-old patient. Electron beam CT angiography. **a** Axial slices show a pulmonary embolus extending into both pulmonary arteries (saddle embolus, *arrows*). A small pleural effusion is seen. **b** VE of the central pulmonary arteries with the virtual observer in the pulmonary trunk looking at the bifurcation into the right and left pulmonary arteries. Using different thresholds, VE provides a 3D impression of the embolus (*arrows*) descending bilaterally into the pulmonary arteries

axial source scans were inconclusive with regard to segmental pulmonary arteries. MPR allows reconstruction of the pulmonary arteries along their main axis (Remy-Jardin et al. 1995) and is well suited to determine the extent of a thrombus. In those cases where viewing of the axial source scans allowed reliable assessment of pulmonary embolism, no gain in diagnostic accuracy resulted from evaluation of the MPR images. The authors concluded that MPR should be used only when the axial images yield no clear-cut findings.

In pulmonary artery embolism, MIP is unable to visualize an embolus as a filling defect in an otherwise opacified vessel, unless the embolus is located in the immediate vicinity of the vessel wall. Ladd et al. evaluated virtual endoscopic views generated from CE-MRA images obtained in a healthy volunteer and in a patient with known pulmonary artery embolism. They performed CE-MRA during breathhold with an acquisition time of 24 s using the following protocol:

- 1.5-T scanner
- TE 1.6 ms
- TR 3.4 ms
- Flip angle 40°
- In-plane resolution 1.7↔1.7 mm
- Slice thickness 2 mm

Even subsegmental arteries with diameters of less than 3 mm could be explored by VE. In the patient with pulmonary embolism virtual endoscopic views depicted the occluding embolus. A second, smaller embolus that was missed on the MIP images could be identified by VE and VRT. Again, the authors emphasized that selection of a proper threshold is of the utmost importance for VE of the pulmonary arteries. Inhomogeneous opacification of the vessels may lead to misrepresentations in the vessel lumen and subsequent errors in interpreting the endoscopic presentation (Ladd et al. 1996). The time needed to generate a virtual presentation was found to be between 10 and 40 min, depending on the length of the vessel segment to be rendered.

VE of the pulmonary arteries also has been ascribed a potential role in the diagnostic assessment of rare malignant tumors of the pulmonary arteries (Remy et al. 1998). When used in CTA data sets, VE allows the direct representation of the location and extent of an embolus (Fishman and Heath 1997) from an angioscopic perspective, demonstrates the patency of the vessel lumen (Bartolozzi et al. 1998), and identifies mural emboli (Prokop et al. 1997). Fishman and Heath (1997) conclude that VE based on CTA is a suitable diagnostic tool for assessing pulmonary artery embolism but concede that the diagnostic gain is limited compared with the information already provided by the axial source images.

Preoperative evaluation of the pulmonary vessels to determine operability prior to surgical resection in patients with bronchial cancer can be done by CTA supplemented by MPR and SSD (Remy et al. 1998), which also seems to be a suitable procedure for postoperative monitoring. Lung transplants can likewise be assessed for pulmonary vessel stenoses by CTA, and 3D rendering techniques yield additional information since stenotic segments and vessel kinking rarely run parallel to the axial section orientation of the source scans (Remy et al. 1998). Pulmonary arteriovenous malformations (PAVMs) are visualized by spiral CT with an accuracy of 95% (Remy et al. 1994). For PAVM assessment alone, no intravenous contrast agent is needed. The best results in the diagnostic assessment of PAVMs were achieved by analyzing SSD 3D reconstructions in combination with the axial source scans. The SSD images were found to be particularly helpful for preoperative planning and postoperative follow-up (Remy-Jardin et al. 1997). Selection of a suitable threshold is important to prevent underestimation of small vessels feeding the PAVM. Remy et al. (1998) also reported their experience with use of STS-MIP reconstructions, which enable diagnostic assessment of PAVMs without the need to administer an intravenous contrast agent. They were able to demonstrate PAVMs with a size of less than 1 mm by means of STS-MIP. The tortuous course of the vessels in PAVMs impairs accurate assessment by MPR; however, definitive data on this problem are not available.

Silverman et al. (1994) studied the use of MRI to assess pulmonary vascular malformations in eight patients with PAVM. Besides spin-echo and gradient-echo sequences, they used phase-contrast imaging to determine blood flow in the PAVM and found the latter to be the most suitable MRI sequence in the diagnosis of PAVM.

Dillon et al. (1993) investigated the usefulness of spiral CT in differentiating duplication of the superior vena cava from partial anomalous pulmonary venous return (PAPVR) from the left upper lobe into the left brachiocephalic vein. The authors used SSD reconstructions in seven patients (five patients with double superior vena cava, two patients with PAPVR) but did not discuss the potential diagnostic gain of the reconstructed 3D images compared with reviewing the axial scans alone. No published reports are available in the literature on the use of VE in the diagnostic assessment of PAVM or PAPVR.

Assessment of the superior vena cava by CTA in combination with 2D renderings prior to vessel stenting is able to distinguish external compression from infiltration by a tumorous process (REMY et al. 1998). This is a potential indication for assessing the vessel wall of the superior vena cava by VE on the basis of contrast-enhanced CTA. However, no publication has as yet described this use of VE.

8.5 Virtual Endoscopy of the Renal Artery

Renal arterial stenosis induced by atherosclerosis is the most frequent cause of secondary hypertension. The prevalence of renal arterial stenosis in hypertensive subjects is 3–5% (KAATEE et al. 1997). Early detection and treatment of the stenosis can prevent progressive renal failure in some patients. Today, digital subtraction angiography (DSA) is the widely accepted standard diagnostic modality for demonstrating renal arterial stenosis, but its invasiveness challenges the radiologist to find a less invasive procedure for diagnosing the condition (PRINCE et al. 1997). Excellent results achieved with CTA in diagnosing renal arterial stenosis have been reported by PROKOP et al. (1997). CTA not only demonstrates the grade of renal arterial stenosis but also identifies the presence of vascular plaques and of accessory renal arteries. Normal findings on CTA of the renal arteries practically exclude the presence of any relevant renal arterial stenosis (PROKOP et al. 1997). KAATEE et al. (1997) found CTA to have a sensitivity and specificity of 96% in diagnosing renal arterial stenosis. They recommend using a collimation of 2 mm to achieve optimal depiction of the renal arteries.

In vitro studies by BRINK et al. (1995) identified a collimation of 2 mm, a pitch of 1–2, and a reconstruction interval of 1 mm as the optimal technical parameters for CTA of the renal arteries. Reducing collimation to 1 mm was associated with a pronounced increase in image noise, unless the X-ray energy (mAs) was correspondingly increased, resulting in increased radiation exposure of the patient. In obese patients, image noise is less pronounced when collimation is increased to 3 mm (GALANSKI et al. 1993). When the pitch is increased from 1:1 to 2:1, twice the volume can be acquired, which markedly improves the diagnostic assessment of accessory renal arteries (RUBIN et al. 1997).

Using CE-MRA, the renal arteries can be imaged without administration of a contrast agent, which may potentially be nephrotoxic (PROKOP et al. 1997). To successfully perform MRA of the renal arteries, image acquisition has to take place during breath-hold (RÜHM and DEBATIN 1999). PRINCE et al. (1997) recommend a combination of a T1-weighted spin-echo sequence, 3D CE-MRA, and 3D PC-MRA. The advent of contrast-enhanced 3D gradient-echo MRA has made it possible to also depict the peripheral segments of the renal arteries, which is of special importance when examining patients with fibromuscular dysplasia (DAVIS et al. 1996). Scanning times of less than 30 s for acquisition of an entire data set allow the examination to be performed during a breath-hold, thus improving image quality.

PRINCE (1994) found sensitivity of 85% and specificity of 93% in the demonstration of renal artery stenoses by CE-MRA with MIP reconstructions and MPR. HANY et al. (1998) assessed various rendering techniques for data sets acquired by 3D CE-MRA in the diagnostic assessment of stenoses of the abdominal aorta, renal arteries, and iliac arteries and compared these with conventional angiography. They obtained the best results with a combination of MIP and MPR, which had sensitivity of 96% and specificity of 97% in depicting significant stenoses. These results could not be improved by additional use of SSD and VE. On the contrary, these additional rendering techniques actually decreased specificity to 95% (MIP, MPR plus SSD) or 96% (MIP, MPR plus VE) while the sensitivity remained constant.

The time needed to generate virtual endoscopic views was found to be much longer than that needed for MIP or SSD reconstructions; an average of 40 min has been reported for VE of the renal arteries as well as for VE of the aorta and of the iliac vessels, compared with 8 min for MIP, 9 min for MPR, and 15 min for SSD (HANY et al. 1998). Hany et al. conclude that the diagnostic gain does not justify the time-consuming generation of virtual endoscopic images of the renal arteries on a routine basis, but they suggest using VE as an additional rendering technique in specific settings, for example in patients with fibromuscular dysplasia (HANY et al. 1998; PROKOP et al. 1997) (Figs. 8.12–8.14). BARTOLOZZI et al. (1998), on the other hand, described a diagnostic gain resulting from the combination of MPR and VE. This gain was due to the possibility of viewing a stenotic area from an angioscopic perspective and of assessing the relationship of atherosclerotic plaques to the ostium of the renal artery.

Following stenting of a renal artery stenosis, CTA allows non-invasive follow-up to assess stent patency and re-stenosis and check the position of the

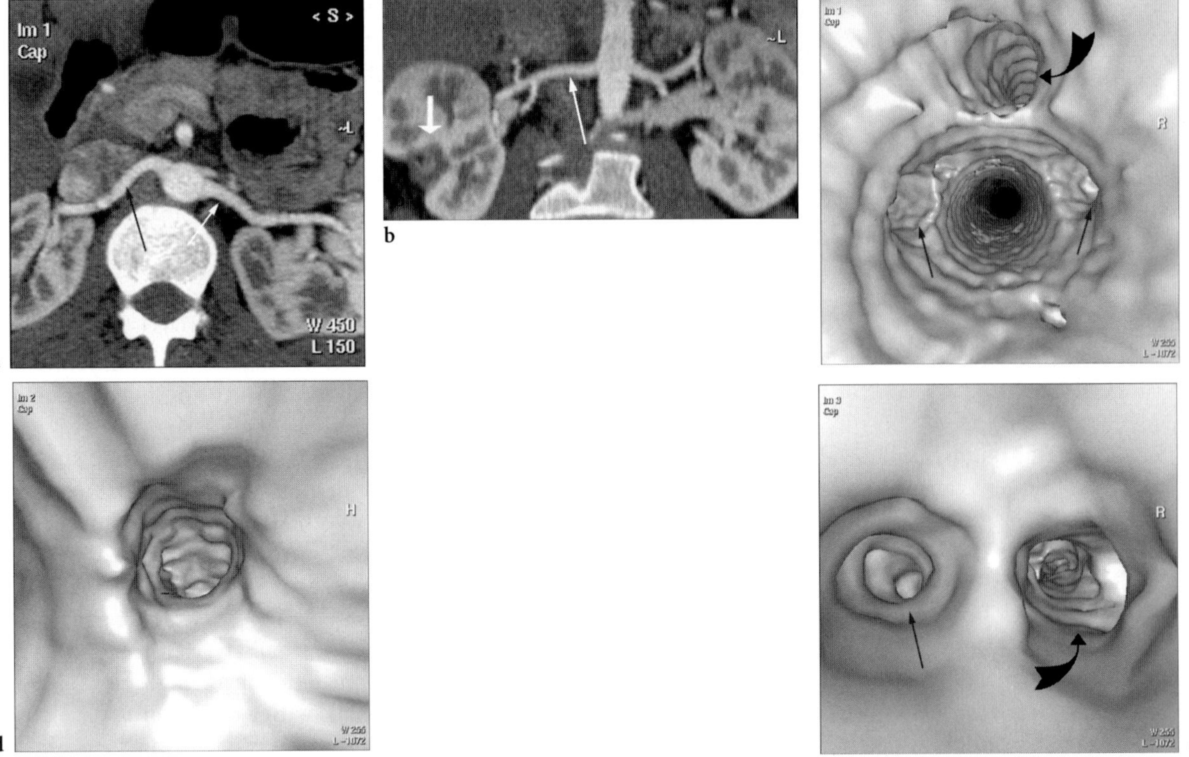

Fig. 8.12a–e. Normal renal arteries. CTA. **a, b** Axial slices (**a**) and MPR (coronal, **b**) show normal renal arteries (*thin arrow*) without the presence of significant stenoses (side finding: angliomyolipoma, *thick arrow*). **c** VE with the virtual observer in the abdominal aorta. Normal origins of the renal arteries are depicted (*arrows*). *Curved arrow*, origin of the superior mesenteric artery. **d** VE with the virtual observer in the aortic lumen looking into the origin of the right renal artery. No stenosis. **e** VE of the origin of the left renal artery (*arrow*). *Curved arrow*, abdominal aorta

stent. This information is reliably provided by MPR and SSD. Additional information may be provided by VE resulting from the direct depiction of the stent from an endoluminal position (Bartolozzi et al. 1998); however, its clinical value has to be judged critically. Neri et al. (1999) evaluated virtual endoscopic displays based on CTA in the follow-up of renal artery stents in 25 patients. VE using the volume rendering technique enabled viewing of the stent from within the lumen and assessment of its position relative to the ostium of the renal artery. The authors regard VE as a useful procedure for this kind of follow-up.

Davis et al. (1996) reported the time required to generate a virtual endoscopic presentation of the renal arteries as ranging from 10 to 20 min. In fibromuscular dysplasia, VE can depict the beaded dilatations of the vascular lumen (Davis et al. 1996). In a case of renal artery aneurysm, VE demonstrated the pathologic process as a dilatation of the lumen with subsequent tapering of the vessel at the end of the aneurysm. Intrarenally located aneurysms in panarteritis nodosa could not be differentiated from surrounding renal parenchyma in the virtual endoscopic displays (Davis et al. 1996) (Fig. 8.15). Neri et al. (1999) described the depiction of accessory renal arteries by means of VE, which was successful in all seven patients investigated.

8.6 Virtual Endoscopy of the Carotid Artery

Stenosis of the carotid artery secondary to atherosclerosis is a major cause of cerebrovascular disorders (Takahashi et al. 1997; Schwartz et al. 1992). The gold standard for diagnosing carotid artery stenosis is conventional angiography (DSA). The aims of imaging in the preoperative assessment of the carotid artery prior to endarterectomy are to precisely determine the degree of stenosis, to differentiate high-grade stenosis from vascular occlusion, and to identify associated vascular anomalies that

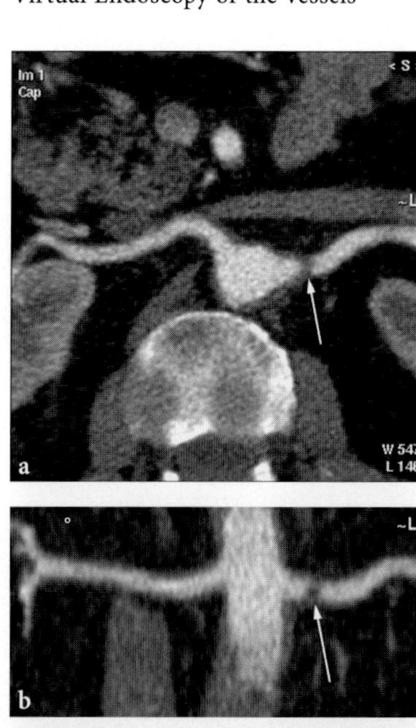
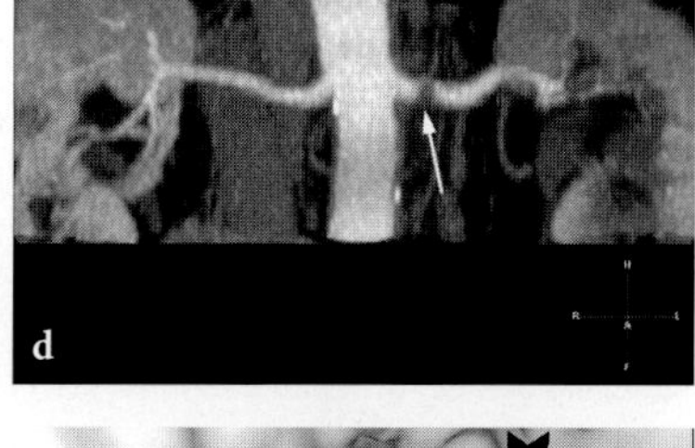
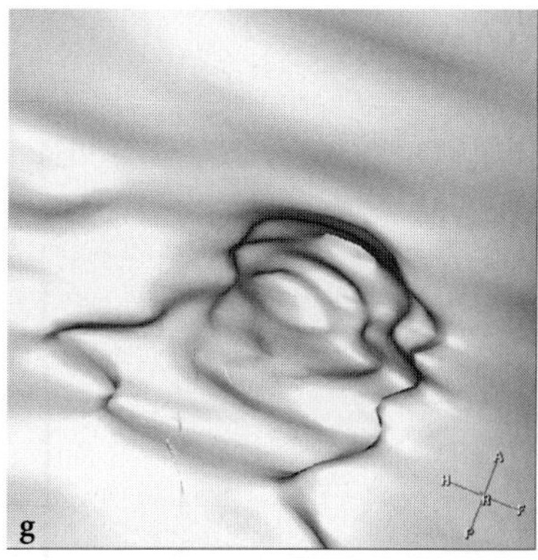
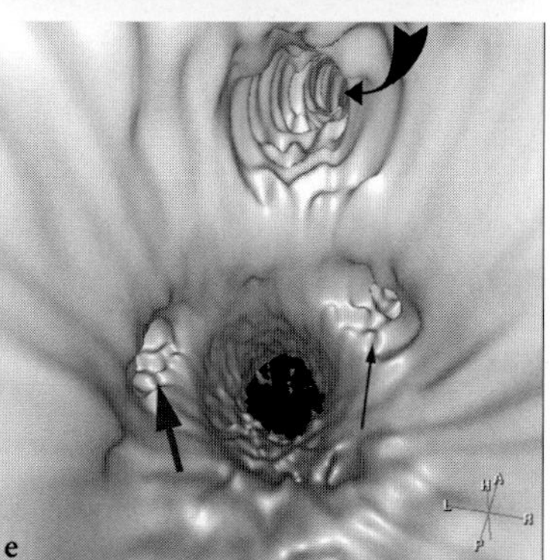
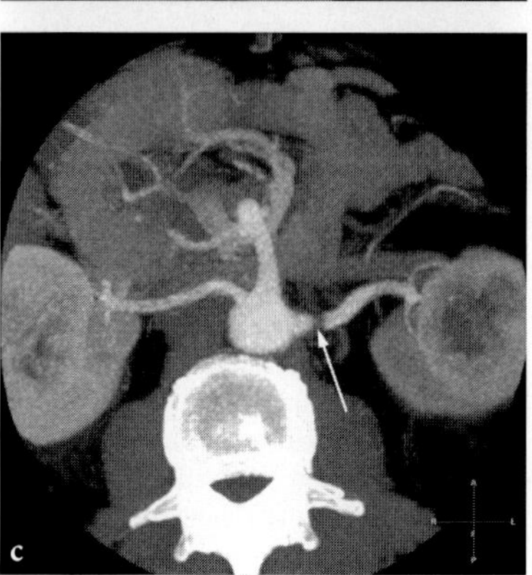
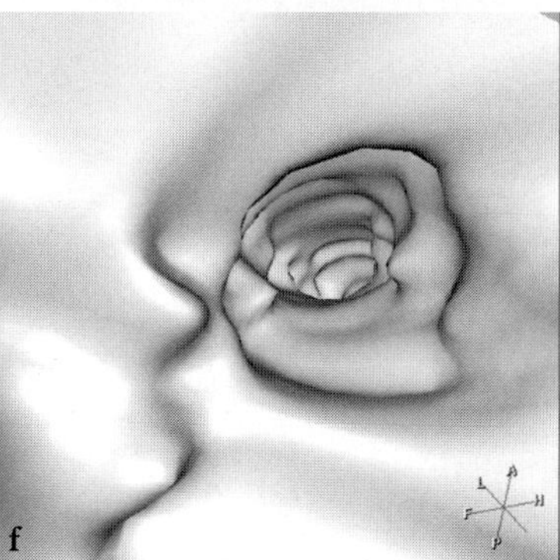

Fig. 8.13a–g. Renal artery stenosis in the proximal left renal artery. CTA. **a, b** MPR (**a** paraaxial, **b** paracoronal) reveals significant stenosis (*arrows*) of the left renal artery. Stenosis of the right artery can be ruled out. **c, d** MIP provides a better anatomic overview by depicting adjacent structures without weakening the diagnostic quality. Renal arterial stenosis can be clearly seen (*arrows*). **e** VE with the virtual observer in the abdominal aorta. From this angle the stenosis in the left renal artery would be missed. *Thick* and *thin arrows*, origin of the left and right renal arteries; *curved arrow*, origin of the superior mesenteric artery. **f** VE with the virtual observer in the lumen of the aorta looking at the origin of the right renal artery. No stenosis. **g** VE of the origin of the left renal artery from the aortic lumen. With the threshold chosen here the significant stenosis can be misinterpreted as total arterial occlusion

affect surgical planning, such as tandem stenosis. These aims are to be achieved with a maximum of diagnostic accuracy and a minimum of risk to the patient at an acceptable cost (Dillon et al. 1993).

A general problem in depicting the carotid artery by cross-sectional imaging is the risk of artifacts induced by patient movement, especially swallowing (Takahashi et al. 1997). Artifacts resulting from vessel pulsation become fewer as the distance to the aortic arch increases and completely disappear beyond the bifurcation.

Suspected stenosis is the main indication for CTA of the carotid artery (Bartolozzi et al. 1998). In the assessment of significant stenoses of the carotid artery (greater than 70%), in different studies full agreement (100%) was found between angiography and CTA, and agreement ranging between 50% and 97% for stenoses smaller than 70% (Bartolozzi et al. 1997; Marks et al. 1993).

Using a CTA protocol with a collimation of 2 mm and a pitch of 1, Link et al. (1995) found a correlation of 80% between DSA and CTA in the diagnosis of stenoses of the carotid artery. Difficulties occurred in assessing mild stenoses, but there was excellent assessment of high-grade stenoses and vessel occlusions. Simultaneous CTA of the carotid artery from the aortic arch to the intracranial carotid segments does not seem to be feasible at present (Prokop et al. 1997; Link et al. 1995). New, faster techniques of CTA with ultrafast acquisition (electron beam CT) or multislice CT will in the future allow depiction of the entire carotid artery.

CTA is limited in depicting the collateral supply of the carotid artery and in identifying tandem stenoses, although these findings are crucial for therapeutic decision-making (Link et al. 1995). Typical protocols for CTA of the carotid artery comprise cranial spiral acquisition starting at the level of C6/C7 using

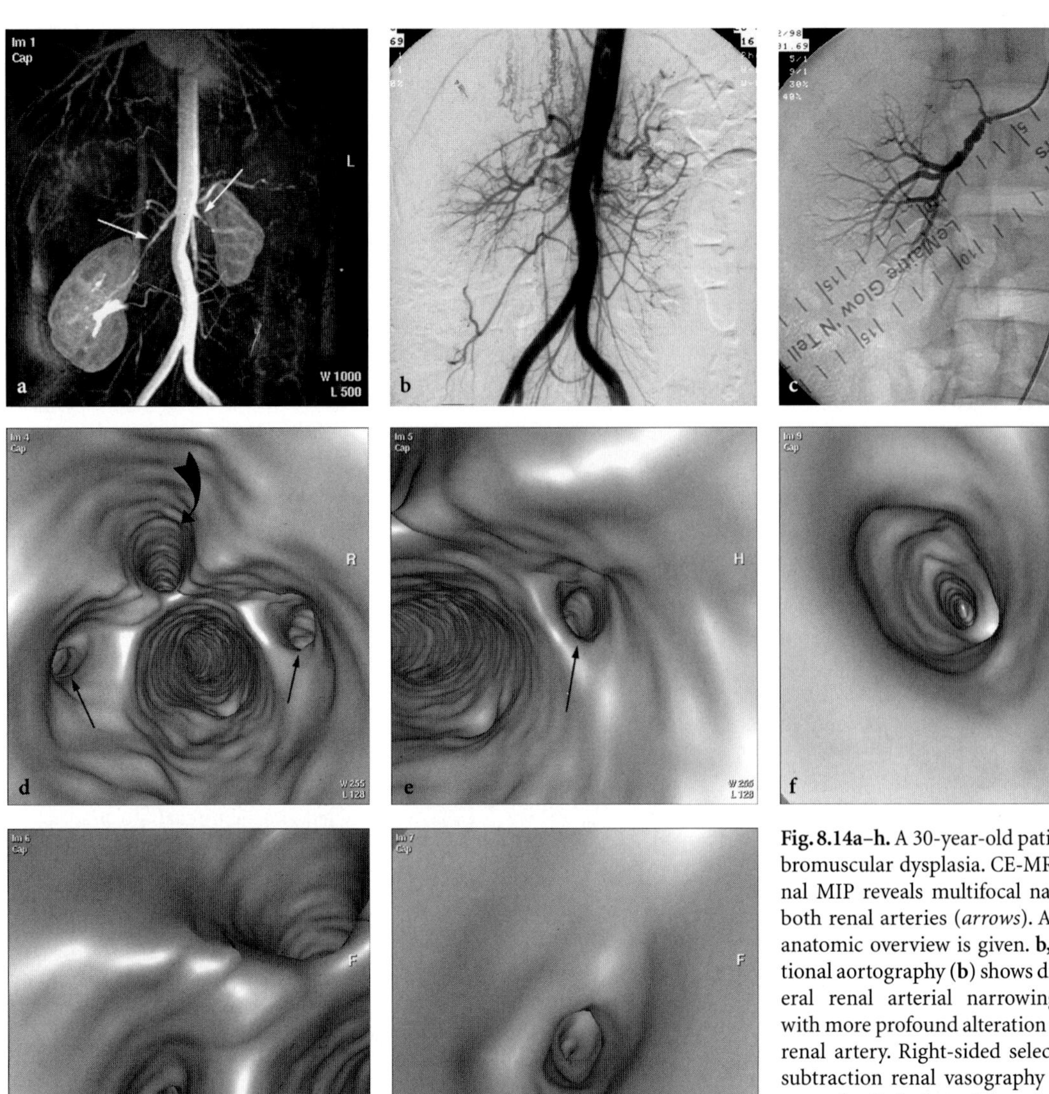

Fig. 8.14a–h. A 30-year-old patient with fibromuscular dysplasia. CE-MRA. **a** Coronal MIP reveals multifocal narrowing of both renal arteries (*arrows*). An excellent anatomic overview is given. **b, c** Conventional aortography (**b**) shows diffuse bilateral renal arterial narrowing (*arrows*) with more profound alteration of the right renal artery. Right-sided selective digital subtraction renal vasography (**c**) gives a more detailed view of the selected artery (*arrow*). **d** VE with the virtual observer in the abdominal aorta. Relatively normal depiction of the right renal artery origin with a narrowed left renal artery (*arrows*). *Curved arrow,* origin of the superior mesenteric artery. **e, f** VE of the right renal artery (*arrow* in **e**). Only mild narrowing of the arterial lumen is seen. VE does not provide a sufficient overview over the pathology as seen in **a–c**. **g, h** VE of the left renal artery (*arrow* in **g**). Extensive narrowing of the artery. With the threshold chosen, pseudo-occlusion of the artery is visualized in **h**

the following scanning parameters (Marks et al. 1993; Takahashi et al. 1997):

- 2 or 3 mm beam collimation
- 2 or 3 mm table increment (pitch 1:1)
- 1 mm reconstruction interval

Selection of the contrast agent bolus should ensure optimal opacification of the carotid artery with minimal superimposition of the jugular vein (Castillo 1993). Artifacts resulting from inhomogeneous vessel opacification can be reduced by automatic administration of the contrast material (Takahashi et al. 1997). When a large slice thickness is used, a stenosis shorter than the slice thickness will be underestimated due to partial volume effects. It is therefore advisable to use the smallest slice thickness possible (Takahashi et al. 1997).

CE-MRA of the carotid artery is performed with a neck Helmholtz coil. Imaging in the area of the carotid artery is mostly done by TOF-MRA (Bongartz et al. 1997). This technique depicts even small vascular changes such as ulcerations, as well as intra-

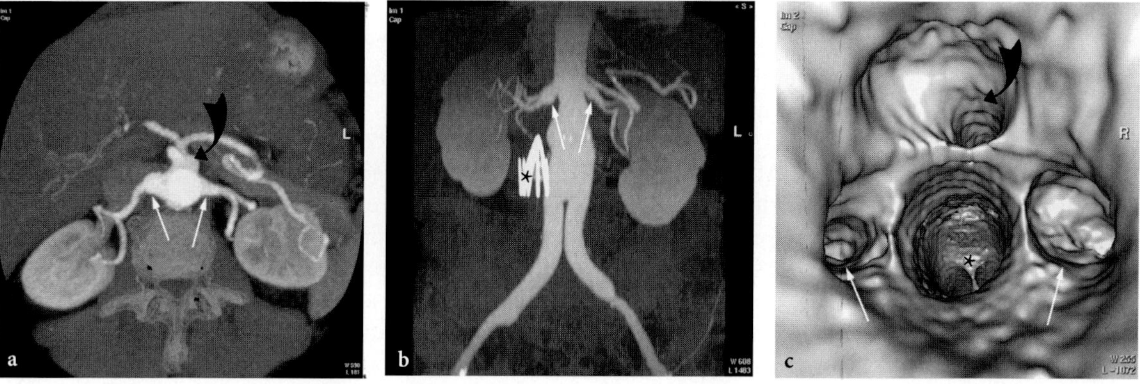

Fig. 8.15a–c. Aneurysmal dilatation of the proximal renal arteries and the superior mesenteric artery. CTA. **a, b** MIP provides an excellent overview of the pathology (**a** axial, **b** coronal). *Arrows*, aneurysmal dilatation of the proximal renal arteries; *curved arrow* (**a**), dilated superior mesenteric artery; *asterisk* (**b**), stent in the inferior vena cava. **c** VE depicts the pathology from the lumen of the aorta with dilatation of the origins of the renal arteries (*arrows*) and the superior mesenteric artery. The entire infrarenal abdominal aorta as far as the aortic bifurcation (*asterisk*) can be seen

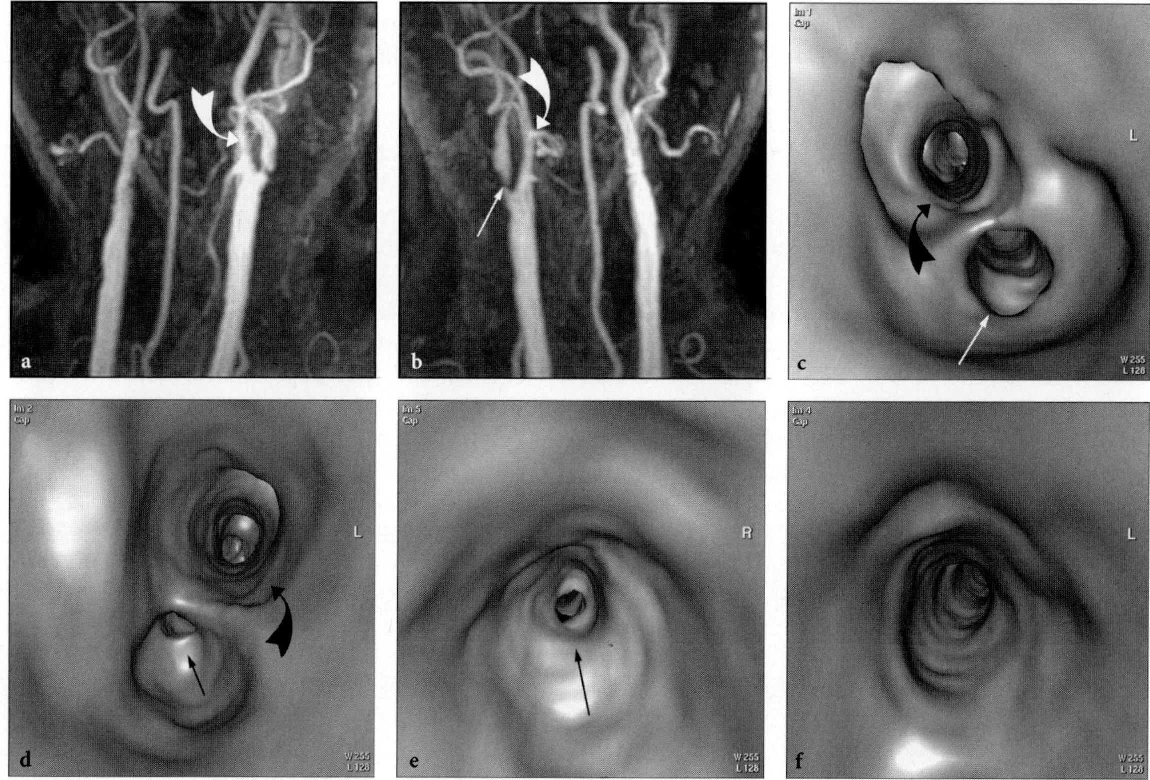

Fig. 8.16a–f. Bilateral stenosis of the internal carotid artery in a 63-year-old patient. CE-MRA. **a, b** MIP reveals significant stenosis of the proximal internal carotid artery (*arrows*, *right* in **a** and *left* in **b**). *Curved arrow*, external carotid artery. **c** VE with the virtual observer in the right common carotid artery looking at the carotid bifurcation. Moderate narrowing of the proximal internal carotid artery can be seen (*arrow*). External carotid artery without stenosis (*curved arrow*). **d** VE from the same position as in **c** on the left side. High-grade stenosis of the proximal carotid artery is depicted. Stenosis of the external artery can be ruled out (*curved arrow*). **e** ICA stenosis on the right side as a virtual view in a retrograde direction from the distal internal artery (*arrow*). **f** VE in an antegrade direction with the virtual observer looking through the ICA stenosis. Normal depiction of the distal ICA without further stenoses

mural atheromas and vascular stenoses. Modern MRI techniques for assessing the carotid artery use 3D CE-MRA, which depicts the entire length of the carotid artery and reliably identifies dissections (Bongartz et al. 1997) (Fig. 8.16).

The well-known tendency of MRA to overestimate narrowing results in a rather low negative predictive value of only 39% for the presence of high-grade stenoses (Dillon et al. 1993). Heisermann reported an accuracy of 100% in differentiating high-grade stenosis from vascular occlusion. Direct comparison of CTA and MRA of the carotid artery showed MRA to be superior in assessing the origins of the vessel in the aortic arch or brachiocephalic trunk because of their direct coronal visualization (Bongartz et al. 1997). However, the plaque contour in carotid stenosis is depicted less reliably by TOF-MRA than by CTA (Marks et al. 1993).

Among the 3D rendering techniques, MIP was found to reliably depict atherosclerotic plaques (Bartolozzi et al. 1998). SSD was less suitable for assessing carotid stenoses since the surface reconstruction of the vessel does not allow reliable differentiation between the opacified lumen and atherosclerotic plaques. VE, on the other hand, shows the extent of atherosclerotic plaques and their relationship to the carotid bifurcation (Jolesz et al. 1997).

When SSD rendering is used for assessing the carotid artery, selection of a proper threshold value again plays a crucial role. A higher threshold results in narrowing of the vessel, while a lower value makes the vessel appear wider (Takahashi et al. 1997). Thresholds have to be determined on an individual basis for each examination. In CTA, the edges of calcified plaques have density values similar to the opacified vessel lumen due to partial volume effects. This similarity may lead to mistakes in segmentation for SSD renderings (Takahashi et al. 1997).

8.7 Virtual Endoscopy of Intraabdominal Vessels

When using MRA to assess abdominal vessels, it is important to specifically adjust bolus timing to the target vasculature (Bongartz et al. 1997). CE-MRA is highly accurate in depicting stenoses and occlusions of the proximal mesenteric vessels (Rühm and Debatin 1999) and in identifying embolic complications in their typical locations at the origin of the middle colic artery, whereas small peripheral mesenteric vessels cannot be assessed (Rühm and Debatin 1999). Data acquisition in CE-MRA is 25–30 s, which is too long to be performed during breath-hold in patients with acute mesenteric ischemia. MIP reconstructions are superior to SSD in depicting intrahepatic and intrasplenic vessels (Rubin et al. 1993). Figures 8.17 and 8.18 show the use of the VE in patients with stenosis and occlusion of the coeliac trunk.

Soyer et al. (1996) described the role of SSD images generated from CT data sets acquired during arterial portography (CT-AP) and found the 3D renderings of the intrahepatic venous system to be significantly better than the 2D source images in the subsegmental assignment of hepatic tumors. SSD renderings based on CT-AP requires individual adjustment of a threshold level that will maximize vessel depiction while at the same time minimizing overlying liver parenchyma. Comparison of MIP, SSD, and VRT images reconstructed from CT-AP data for depiction of the venous and portal venous systems showed that step artifacts were least pronounced in the MIP reconstructions. The latter also showed the best overall quality. The 3D depiction of fifth-order portal branches was achieved in the MIP and VRT reconstructions but rarely on the SSD images (Soyer et al. 1996). Three-dimensional render-

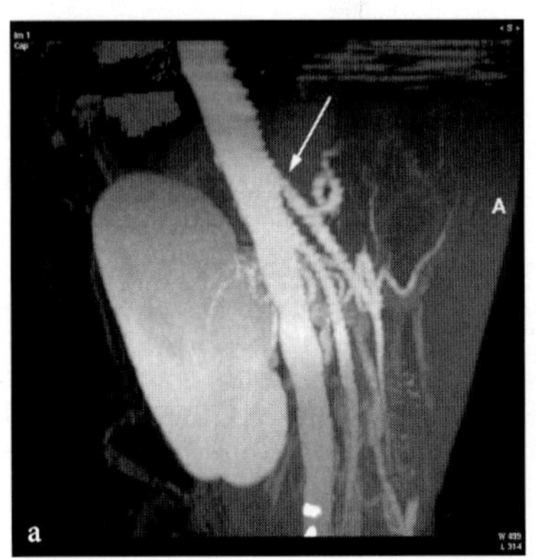

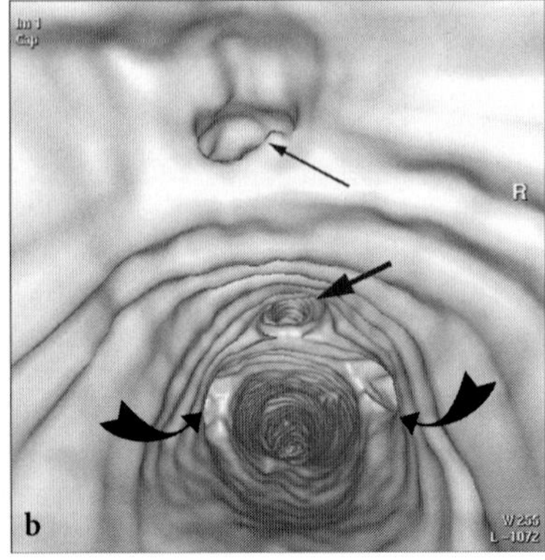

Fig. 8.17a,b. Stenosis of the coeliac trunk in a 34-year-old patient. CTA. **a** MIP provides a good overview of the pathology, depicting a stenosis of the coeliac trunk at its origin (*arrow*). **b** VE of the proximal stenosis of the coeliac trunk as seen from the aortic lumen (*arrow*). The superior mesenteric artery (*thick arrow*) and the origins of the renal arteries (*curved arrows*) are depicted

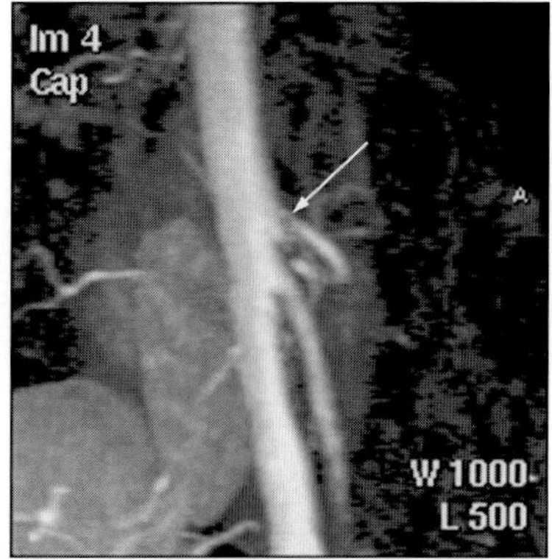

a

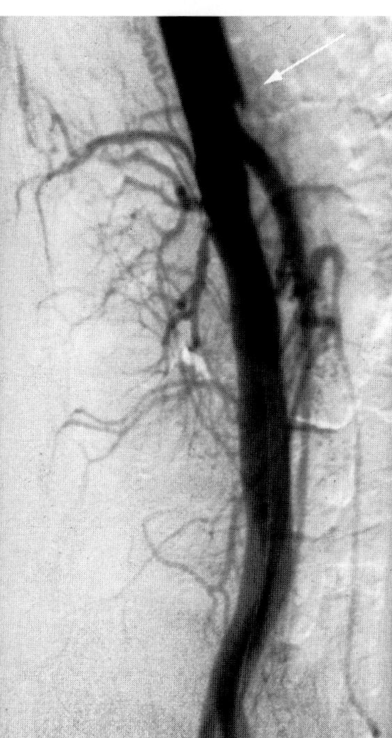

b

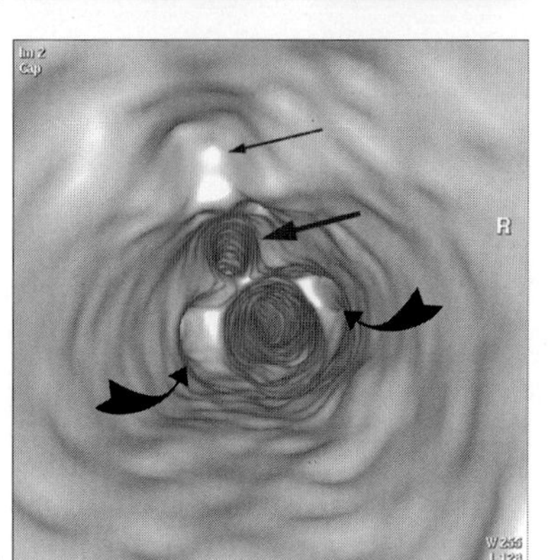

c

Fig. 8.18a–c. Proximal occlusion of the coeliac trunk in the 30-year-old patient from Fig. 8.14 with fibromuscular dysplasia. CE-MRA. **a** In this MIP the occlusion of the coeliac trunk can be missed due to the presence of overlying vessels. **b** Digital subtraction aortography clearly shows the proximal coeliac trunk occlusion (*arrow*). **c** VE from the aortic lumen with excellent demonstration of the proximal coeliac trunk occlusion (*arrow*). *Thick arrow,* superior mesenteric artery; *curved arrows,* origins of the renal arteries

ing of the liver anatomy, which has a special role in locating intrahepatic lesions for surgical planning, was best on the MIP images, which showed lower interobserver variability. Despite the good depiction of the venous system in the MIP reconstruction, the latter was unreliable in visualizing a liver tumor involving intrahepatic venous structures (Soyer et al. 1996).

Toda et al. (1997) evaluated VE of the portal vein generated from spiral CT data sets obtained in 62 patients. They found good visualization of peripheral branches and stenoses of the portal vein. However, assessment of tumor involvement of the portal vein was poor. VE was limited by threshold artifacts and problems of orientation within the portal vein. Figure 8.19 shows an example of the use of VE in thrombotic disease of the superior vena cava.

8.8 Virtual Endoscopy of Peripheral Vessels

CTA of the peripheral arteries has substantial limitations. The stretch of vessel to be scanned (i.e., extension along the z-axis) is too long for adequate resolution for the identification of stenoses to be achieved (Prokop et al. 1997). These limitations will probably be overcome – as early clinical results indicate – by the development of subsecond and multislice CT technology. However, no experience using these techniques has been published to date.

2D TOF-MRA has by now become an established procedure in the diagnostic assessment of the peripheral arteries. Drawbacks of this technique are the time-consuming examination and postprocessing, the occurrence of saturation effects, and poor resolution (Prokop et al. 1997). Compared to TOF- and PC-MRA, CE-MRA offers the advantage of a shorter scanning time, which allows examination of longer vessel segments (Bongartz et al. 1998; Prokop et al. 1997). Possible indications for CE-MRA are evaluation of peripheral vascular occlusive disease, postoperative monitoring of peripheral bypasses, and diagnosis of arteriovenous malformations and fistulas (Prokop et al. 1997). With the aid of table-shifting techniques, which enable the table to be moved during continuous administration of the contrast agent, it becomes possible to scan the entire course of the vessels throughout a limb. This is done by reducing the contrast flow to 0.5–0.7 ml/s (Rühm and Debatin 1999).

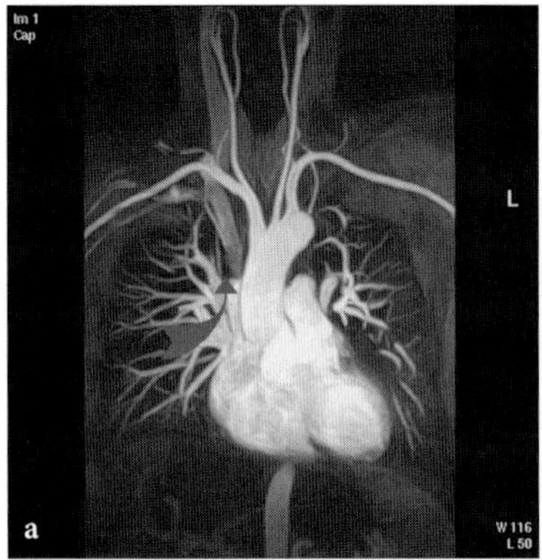

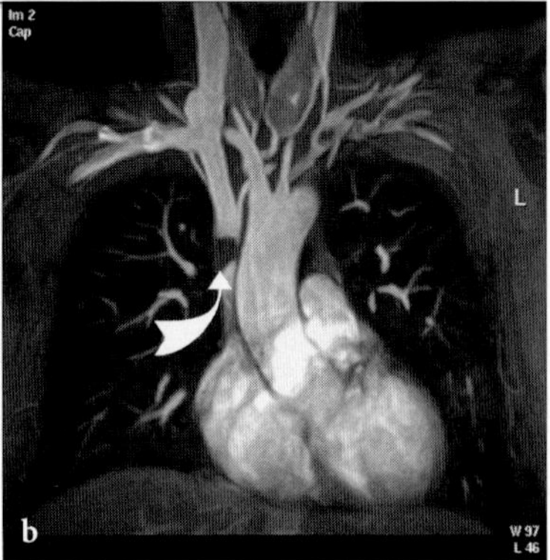

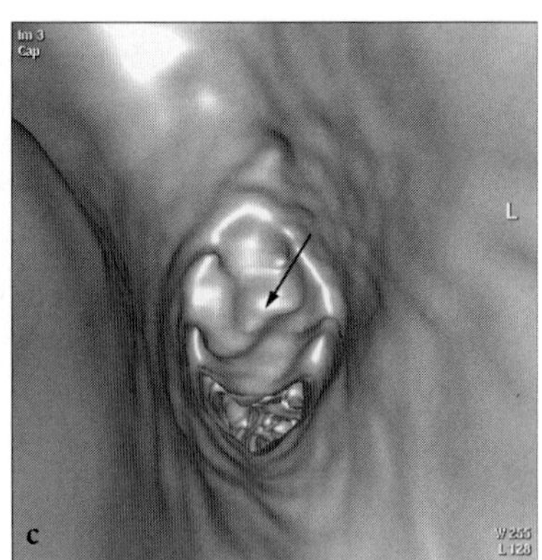

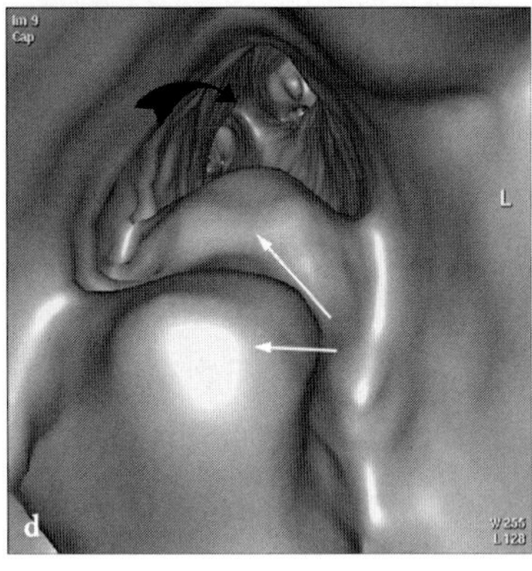

Fig. 8.19a–d. Thrombus in the superior vena cava in a 50-year-old patient. CE-MRA. **a, b** Thrombus is clearly depicted in the MIP of the venous phase (*arrow*, **b**). A remaining lumen of the vein is difficult to demonstrate. Thrombus can be missed on the MIP of the arterial phase (*arrow*, **a**). **c** VE with the virtual observer in the superior vena cava clearly depicts the thrombus (*arrow*). The remaining venous lumen can be seen. **d** VE from the superior vena cava with the virtual observer looking in a cranial direction. Behind the thrombus (*arrows*) the confluence of the brachiocephalic veins is depicted (*curved arrow*)

Freund et al. compared CTA and DSA after placement of iliac stents in 32 patients. They used MIP and SSD reconstructions in addition to the axial scans and found MIP images to be suitable for determining whether a stent was patent or stenotic (Freund et al. 1995). Lawrence et al. also favor MIP reconstructions in assessing peripheral arterial occlusive disease. SSD tends to overestimate or underestimate vascular stenoses depending on the threshold selected. Calcifications are another limiting factor of SSD, which often does not allow differentiation of the opacified vessel lumen from calcified areas (Lawrence et al. 1995).

Freund et al. (1995) compared CTA with DSA and Doppler ultrasonography relative to the walking distance of patients with stenoses in the area of the pelvic arteries and patients who had undergone stent placement in the iliac vessels. Overall, the authors found MIP and SSD to be complementary procedures. In general, MIP images alone are sufficient to determine the location and patency of stents. With the study design used here, the SSD images displayed the stents as well, in contrast to other studies, in which SSD was found to be unreliable in depicting intravascular stents (Freund et al. 1995). In-stent stenoses cannot be assessed on SSD reconstructions.

Rodenwaldt et al. (1997) evaluated VE generated from spiral CT scans for diagnosing intimal hyperplasia and stenosis in 15 patients with a total of 20 stents in the iliac artery. This investigation was performed after optimization of the scanning protocol in a phantom study. The authors found VE to be more suitable for assessing intimal hyperplasia after stent placement in the iliac artery than were SSD and MIP images. Clinically relevant stenoses were not depicted by VE.

8.9 Virtual Endoscopy of Cardiac Vessels

Nakanishi et al. (1998) described the use of VE on the basis of source data sets acquired by ECG-triggered electron beam CT in 22 patients after optimization of the scanning parameters in an animal model. VE of the three major coronary branches was not possible in 14% of the patients owing to the presence of calcifications near the origins or small vessel caliber. In the remaining 19 patients, VE could be done of the origin of the right coronary artery in 89%, and of the left anterior descending coronary artery and RCX in 94%

of the cases. The mean penetration depth of VE was 23.5 mm for the right coronary artery, 29.4 mm for the left anterior descending coronary artery, and 22.5 mm for the RCX. The authors concluded that VE yields additional information for those areas accessible by this procedure (NAKANISHI et al. 1998).

No reports have been published as yet on the use of virtual angioscopy in the diagnostic assessment of aortocoronary venous bypasses (Figs. 8.20–8.24).

8.10 Summary

Virtual endoscopy (VE) of the vessels represents a new tool for displaying the vessels from within. A prerequisite is sufficient contrast between the vascular lumen and the surroundings, on which the ensuing reconstruction depends. In computer tomography, the contrast is produced by intravenous administration of a contrast agent. In MRI, apart from contrast agent

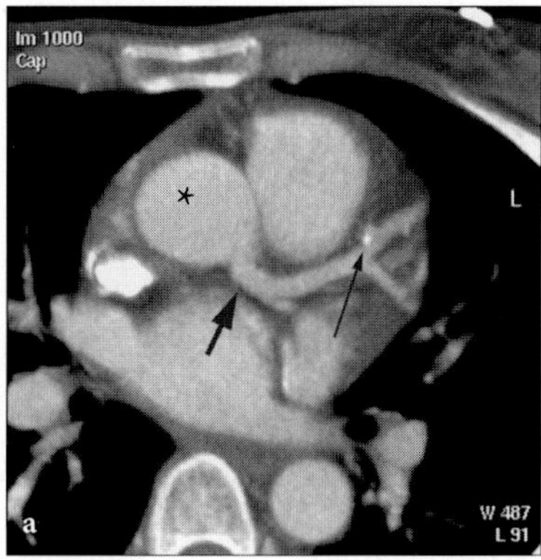

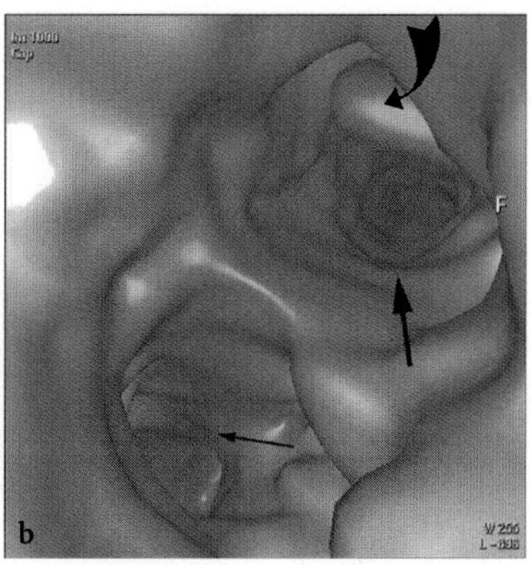

Fig. 8.20a, b. Normal coronary artery. Electron beam CT angiography. **a** MIP of parts of the left coronary artery. The main stem is well depicted (*thick arrow*). The proximal and middle parts of the left anterior descending coronary artery (LAD) as well as the origin of the first diagonal branch can be seen. *Star*, ascending aorta. **b** VE with the observer "flying" through the LAD (*thick arrow*). *Arrow*, origin of the first diagonal branch, *curved arrow*, calcification in the LAD; no significant stenosis can be seen

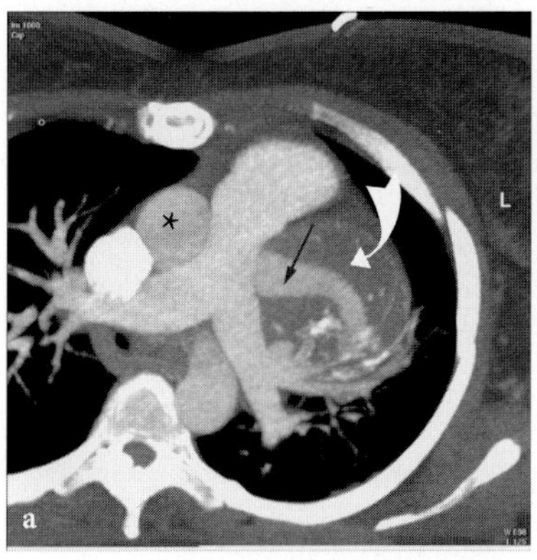

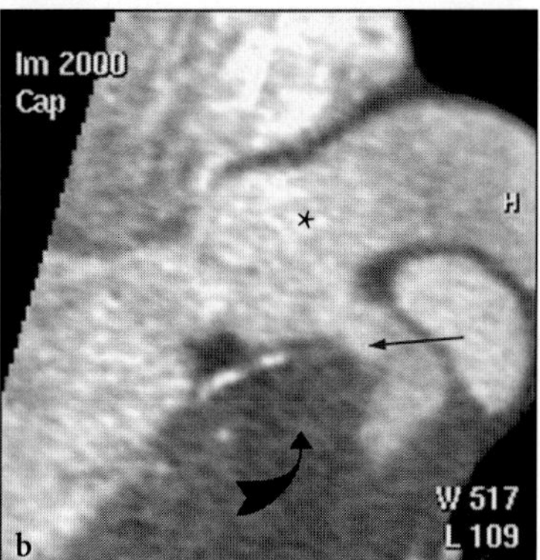

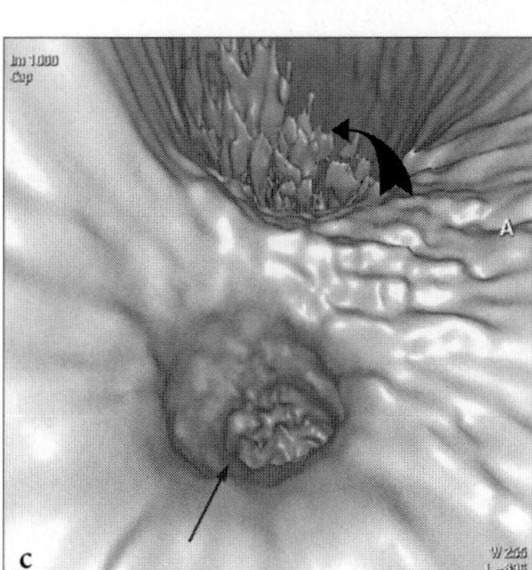

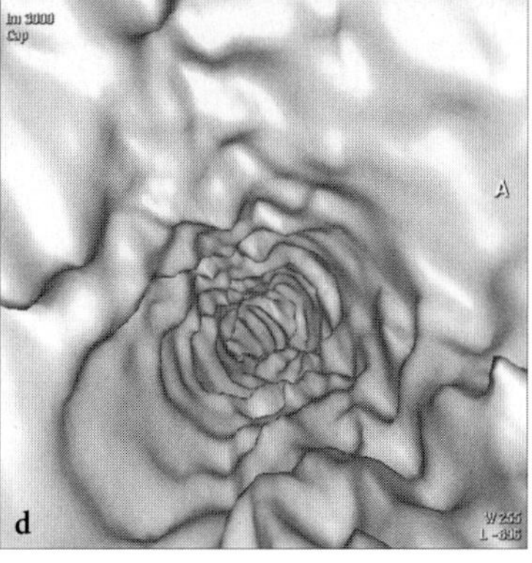

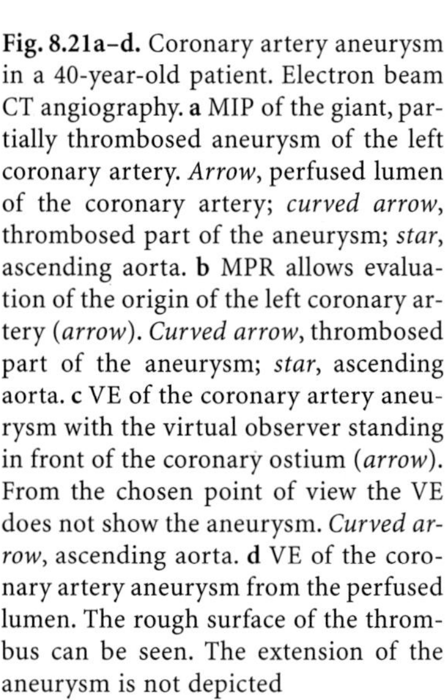

Fig. 8.21a–d. Coronary artery aneurysm in a 40-year-old patient. Electron beam CT angiography. **a** MIP of the giant, partially thrombosed aneurysm of the left coronary artery. *Arrow*, perfused lumen of the coronary artery; *curved arrow*, thrombosed part of the aneurysm; *star*, ascending aorta. **b** MPR allows evaluation of the origin of the left coronary artery (*arrow*). *Curved arrow*, thrombosed part of the aneurysm; *star*, ascending aorta. **c** VE of the coronary artery aneurysm with the virtual observer standing in front of the coronary ostium (*arrow*). From the chosen point of view the VE does not show the aneurysm. *Curved arrow*, ascending aorta. **d** VE of the coronary artery aneurysm from the perfused lumen. The rough surface of the thrombus can be seen. The extension of the aneurysm is not depicted

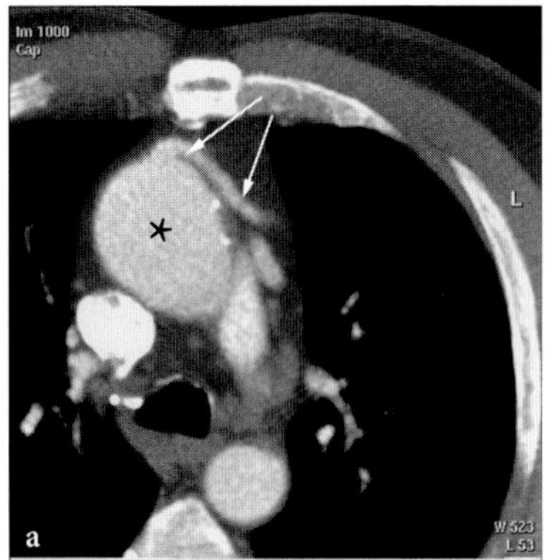
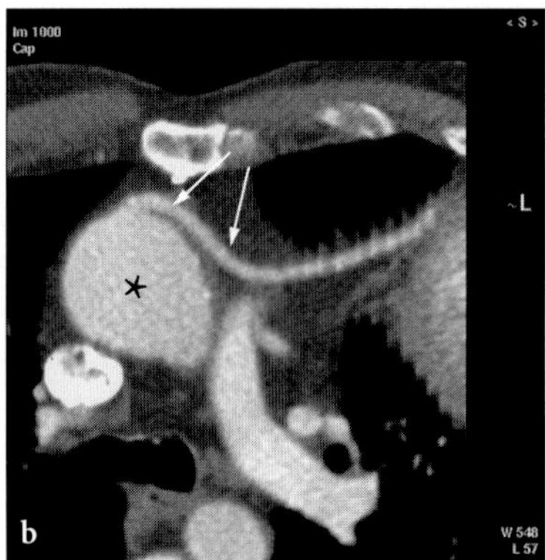
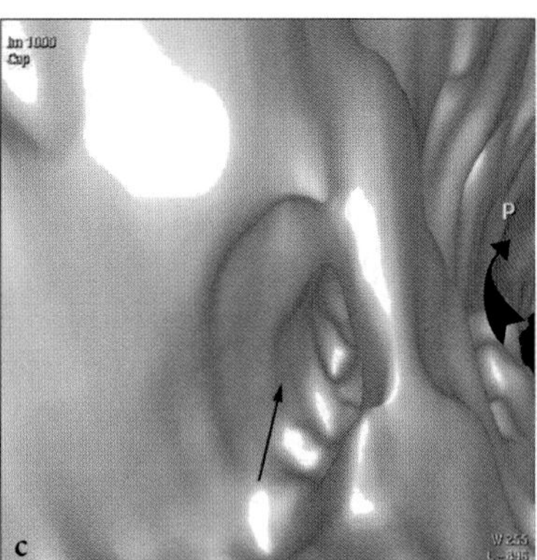
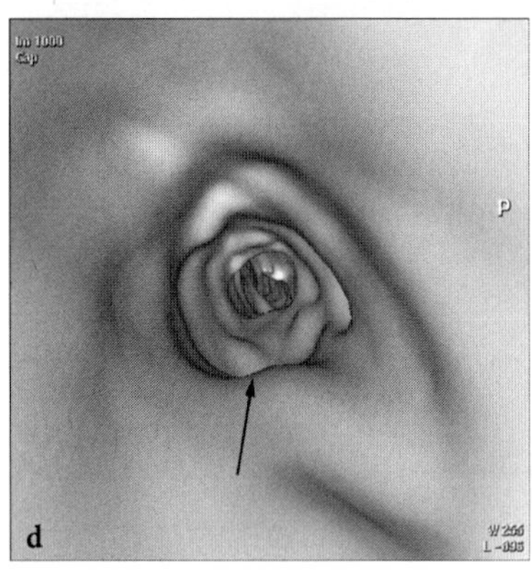

Fig. 8.22a–d. Normal aortocoronary bypass to the LAD. Electron beam CT angiography. **a, b** MPR of a normal aortocoronary bypass without visible stenosis (*arrows*). Curved MPR in **b** depicts the entire bypass from the proximal to the distal anastomosis. *Star*, ascending aorta. **c** Proximal anastomosis of the bypass (*arrow*) in the VE from the aortic lumen (*curved arrow*). Some aortic calcification is detected (*orange*). **d** VE of the bypass (*arrow*). No stenosis can be seen

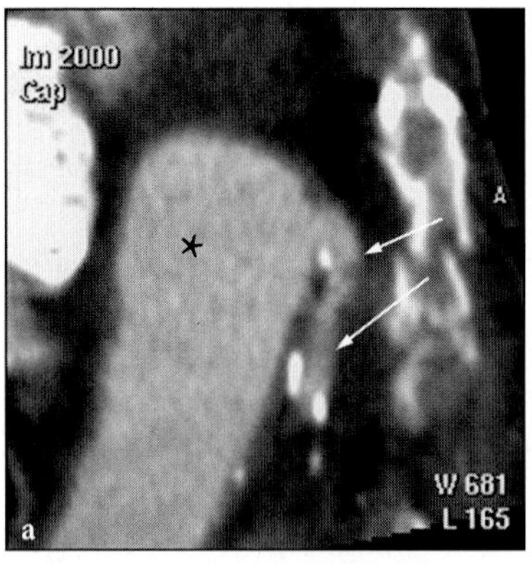

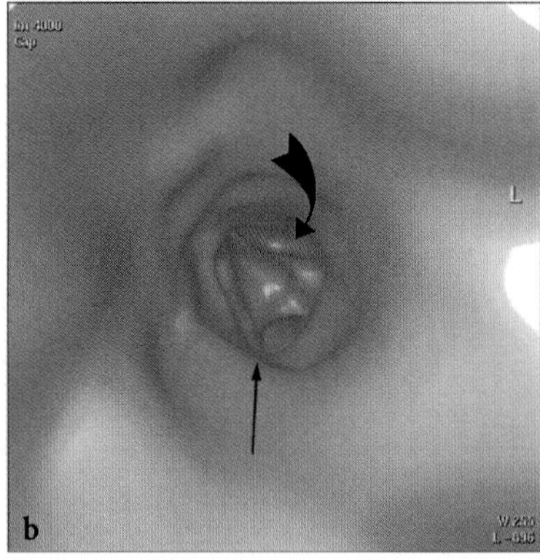

Fig. 8.23a, b. Aortocoronary bypass with calcifications. Electron beam CT angiography. **a** MPR of the aortocoronary bypass shows calcifications, but no high-grade stenosis (*arrow*). *Star*, ascending aorta. **b** VE of the proximal part of the bypass (*arrow*) from the ascending aorta. Calcifications (*curved arrow, orange*) can be seen

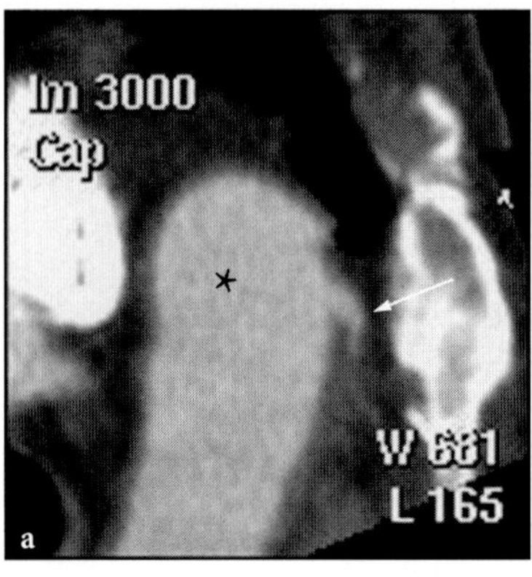

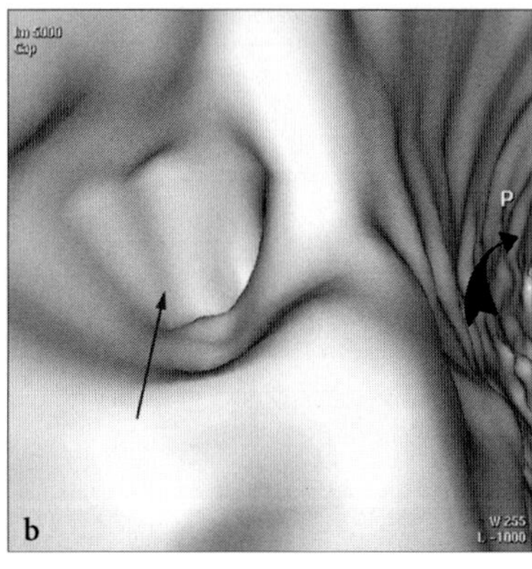

Fig. 8.24a, b. Occlusion of a aortocoronary bypass. Electron beam CT angiography. **a** MPR of the aortocoronary bypass shows proximal bypass occlusion (*arrow*). *Star*, ascending aorta. **b** Virtual observer in the ascending aorta (*curved arrow*) in front of the proximal anastomosis. Occlusion is clearly depicted

administration, both the time-of-flight (TOF) and the phase-contrast (PC) techniques can be used. Homogeneous vascular contrast in the entire region under examination is essential for high-quality virtual reconstruction. This is a problem that, excepting the field heterogeneities in MRI, has been practically eliminated with the advent of multislice CT and the new ultrafast MRI sequences. The main problem in VE of vessels, commonly termed "virtual angioscopy," is the lack of comparison to true endoscopy, as is possible, for example, for the trachea or the colon. For this reason, at present only conventional angiography can be used as the diagnostic gold standard.

Notwithstanding its ability to generate color images with high detail resolution, the clinical value of virtual angioscopy needs critical evaluation. In essence, a perspective that does not allow precise measurement of distances is being incorporated into a distortion-free image. Despite reports to the contrary in the literature, virtual angioscopy as a valuable tool appears to be in the early phases of its development, delayed by more than the relatively high computation times required despite the use of advanced computer technology. However, with the rapid developments in hard- and software, it is highly probable that the clinical value of virtual angioscopy will expand when workstations are capable of generating virtual images automatically.

Acknowledgements. We are grateful to Thomas Kröncke, MD, for providing the MRA data (for Figs. 8.14, 8.16, 8.18 and 8.19) and Dietmar Kivelitz, MD, for reviewing parts of the manuscript.

References

1. Auer LM, Auer DP. Virtual endoscopy for planning and simulation of minimally invasive neurosurgery. Neurosurgery 1998, 43:529–48
2. Bartolozzi C, Neri E, Caramella D. CT in vascular pathologies. Eur Radiol 1998; 8:679–84
3. Beaulieu CF, Baker ME, Chotas HG, McCann R, Kurylo WC, Johnson GA. Volume rendering for 3D helical CT of abdominal aorta. Radiology 1993; 198(P):173
4. Bongartz GM, Boos M, Winter K, Ott HW, Scheffler K, Steinbrich W. Clinical utility of contrast-enhacend MR angiography. Eur Radiol 1997; 7:S178–86
5. Brink JA, Lim JT, Wang G, Heiken JP, Deyoe LA, Vannier MW. Technical optimization of spiral CT for depiction of renal arterial stenosis: in vitro analysis. Radiology 1995; 194:157–63
6. Castillo M. Diagnosis of disease of the common carotid artery bifurcation: CT angiography vs catheter angiography. AJR 1993; 161:395–8
7. Davis CP, Ladd ME, Göhde SC, Pfammatter T, Fass L, Debatin JF. Virtual intravascular endoscopy in the renal arteries: a new way of reading 3-D MR-angiography datasets. RöFo 1996; 165,3:257–63
8. Davis CP, Ladd ME, Romanowski BJ, Wildermuth S, Knoplioch JF, Debatin JF. Human aorta: preliminary results with virtual endoscopy based on three-dimensional MR imaging data sets. Radiology 1996; 199:37–40
9. Debatin JF, Spritzer CE, Grist TM, Beam C, Svetkey LP, Newman GE, Sostman HD. Imaging of the renal arteries: value of MR angiography. AJR 1991; 157:981–90
10. Dessl A, Giacomuzzi SM, Springer P, Stoeger A, Pototschnig C, Völklein C, Schreder SG, Jaschke W. Virtual endoscopy by post-processing of helical CT data sets. Akt Radiol 1997; 7:216–21
11. Diederichs CG, Keating DP, Glatting G, Oestman JW. Blurring of vessels in spiral CT angiography: effects of collimation width, pitch, viewing plane, and windowing in maximum intensity projection. J Comput Assist Tomogr 1996; 20:965–74
12. Dillon EH, Camputaro C. Partial anomalous pulmonary venous drainage of the left upper lobe vs duplication of the superior vena cava: distinction based on CT findings. AJR 1993; 160:375–9
13. Dillon EH, VanLeeuwwen MS, Fernandez MA, Eikelboom BC, Mali WP. CT angiography: application to the evaluation of carotid artery stenosis. Radiology 1993; 189:211–9
14. Fishman EK, Heath DG. Three-dimensional 'virtual angioscopy' of spiral CT data for vascular applications in the thorax: is it of value ? Radiology 1997; 205(P):1573
15. Freund M, Palmié S, Wesner F, Heller M. Spiral-CT angiography after intra-arterial iliac stent placement. RöFo 1995; 163:310–5
16. Galanski M, Prokop M, Chavan A, Schäfer CM, Jandeleit K, Nischelsky JE. Renal artery stenoses: spiral CT angiography. Radiology 1993; 189:185–92
17. Hamada S, Takamiya M, Kimura K, et al. Type A aortic dissection: evaluation with ultrafast CT. Radiology 1992; 183:155–8
18. Hany TF, Schmidt M, Davis CP, Göhde SC, Debatin JF. Diagnostic impact of four postprocessing techniques in evaluating contrast-enhanced three-dimensional MR angiography. AJR 1998; 170:907–12
19. Heath DG, Beauchamp NJ, Fishman EK. Virtual Imaging for Volume Rendered Helical CT Angiography. Radiology 1997; 205(P):262
20. Hopper KD, Pierantozzi D, Potok PS, Kasales CJ, TenHave TR, Meilstrup JW, VanSlyke MA, Mahraj R, Westacott S, Hartzel JS. The quality of 3D reconstructions from 1.0 and 1.5 pitch helical and conventional CT. J Comput Assist Tomogr 1996; 20:841–7
21. Igel BJ, Durham NC, McDermott VG, Nelson RC. Abdominal aortic aneurysms from the inside out: applications and limitatinos of virtual endoscopy. Radiology 1996; 201(P): 467
22. Johnson CD, Hara AK, Reed JE. Virtual endoscopy: what's in a name? AJR 1998; 171:1201–2
23. Johnson PT, Heath DG, Kuszyk BS, Fishman EK. CT angiography with interactive volume rendering: advantages and applications in splanchnic vascular imaging. Radiology 1996; 200:564–8
24. Johnson PT, Heath DG, Kuszyk BS, Fishman EK. CT angiography: thoracic vascular imaging with interactive volume rendering technique. J Comput Assist Tomgr 1997; 21:110–4

25. Jolesz FA, Boston MA, Lorensen WE, Kikinis R, Saiviroonporn P, Phillips MD, Silverman SG. Virtual endoscopy: three-dimensional rendering of cross-sectional images for endoluminal visualization. Radiology 1994; 193(P):469
26. Jolesz FA, Lorensen WE, Shinmoto H, Atsumi H, Nakajima S, Kavanaugh P, Saiviroonporn P, Seltzer SE, Silverman SG, Phillips M, Kikinis R. Interactive virtual endoscopy. AJR 1997; 169:1229–35
27. Kaatee R, Beek FJ, Lange EE, et al. Renal artery stenosis: detection and quantification with spiral CT angiography versus optimized digital subtraction angiography. Radiology 1997; 205:121–7
28. Kay CL, Evangelou HA. A review of the technical and clinical aspects of virtual endoscopy. Endoscopy 1996; 28:768–75
29. Kimura F, Shen Y, Date S, Azemoto S, Mochizuchi T. Three-dimensional CT display of the aorta with the use of the new endoscopic mode: clinical utility for thoracic aortic aneurysm and aortic dissection. Radiology 1994; 193:352
30. Kimura F, Shen Y, Date S, Azemoto S, Mochizuki T. Thoracic aortic aneurysm and aortic dissection: new endoscopic mode for three-dimensional CT display of aorta. Radiology 1996; 198:573–8
31. Komohara Y, Ogata I, Mitsuzaki K, Yamashita Y, Tsuchigame T, Takahashi M. Clinical value of 3D-CT virtual endoscopy. Radiology 1997; 205(P):722
32. Ladd ME, Göhde SC, Steiner P, Pfammatter T, McKinnon GC, Debatin JF. Technical note: virtual MR angioscopy of the pulmonary artery tree. J Comput Assist Tomogr 1996; 20(5):782–5
33. Lawrence JA, Kim D, Kent KC, Stehling MK, Rosen MP, Raptopoulos V. Lower extremity spiral CT angiography versus catheter angiography. Radiology 1995; 194:903–8
34. Link J, Müller-Hülsbeck S, Brossmann J, Grabener M, Voss C, Heller M. First results of spiral CT angiography in the evaluation of carotid artery stenosis. RöFo 1995; 162:204–8
35. Marks MP, Napel S, Jordan JE, Enzmann DR. Diagnosis of carotid artery disease: preliminary experience with maximum-intensity-projection spiral CT angiography. AJR 1993; 160:1267–71
36. Nakanishi T, Yumura A, Fukami K, Ikeda M, Fukuoka H, Ito K. virtual endoscopy of coronary arteries using contrast-enhanced ECG triggered electron-beam CT data sets. Radiology 1998; 209(P):306
37. Napel S, Rubin GD, Jeffrey RB. STS-MIP: a new reconstruction technique for CT of the chest. J Comput Assist Tomogr 1993; 17:832–8
38. Neri E, Caramella D, Falaschi F, Sbragia P, Laiolo E, Bartolozzi C. Virtual endoscopy of the aorta: role of segmentation artefacts in the visualization of detected findings. Radiology 1997; 205(P): 623
39. Neri E, Caramella D, Falaschi F, Sbragia P, Vignali C, Bartolozzi C. Virtual endoscopy of the aorta: segmentation artefacts with perspective surface rendering of spiral CT data sets. Radiology 1997; 205(P):262
40. Neri E, Cioni R, Vignalli C, Bisogni C, Petruzzi P, Trincavelli F, Laiolo E, Bartolozzi C. Renal stents follow-up with real-time volume rendering and virtual endoscopy. Eur Radiol 1999; 9:S475
41. Prince MR. Gadolinium-enhanced MR aortography. Radiology 1994; 191:155–64
42. Prince MR, Schoenberg SO, Ward JS, Londy FJ, Wakefield TW, Stanley JC. Hemodynamically significant atherosclerotic renal artery stenosis: MR angiographic features. Radiology 1997; 205:128–36
43. Prince MR, Yucel EK, Kaufman JA, Harrison DC, Geller SC. Dynamic gadolinium-enhanced three-dimensional abdominal MR arteriography. J Magn Res Imag 1993; 3:877–81
44. Prokop M, Debatin JF. MRI contrast media – new developments and trends. Eur Radiol 1997; 7(Suppl.5):S299–306
45. Prokop M, OhShin H, Schanz A, Schaefer-Prokop CM. Use of maximum intensity projections in CT angiography: a basic review. Radiographics 1997; 17:433–51
46. Remy J, Remy-Jardin M, Artaud D, Fribourg M. Multiplanar and three-dimensional reconstruction techniques in CT: impact on chest diseases. Eur Radiol 1998; 8:335–51
47. Remy J, Remy-Jardin M, Giraud F, Wattinne L. Angioarchitecture of pulmonary arteriovenous malformations: clinical utility of three-dimensional helical CT. Radiology 1994; 191:657–64
48. Remy-Jardin M, Remy J, Artaud D, Deschildre F, Duhamel A. Peripheral pulmonary arteries: optimization of the spiral CT acquisition protocol. Radiology 1997; 204:157–63
49. Remy-Jardin M, Remy J, Cauvain O, Petyt L, Wannebroucq J, Beregi JP. Diagnosis of central pulmonary embolism with helical CT: role of two-dimensional multiplanar reformations. AJR 1995; 165:1131–8
50. Rilinger N, Görich J, Fleiter T, Seifarth H, Sokiranski R, Krämer S, Liewald F, Tomczak R, Brambs HJ. Virtuelle Echtzeit-CT-Angioskopie: Klinische Ergebnisse in verschiedenen Gefäßprovinzen. RöFo 1998; 168:S128
51. Rodenwaldt J, Kopka L, Grabbe E. Intima Hyperplasia and Endoluminal Stenosis after Iliac Stent Implantation Diagnosed by Computed Tomographic Virtual Intraarterial Endoscopy: Facilities and Limitations of a New Postprocessing Technique. Radiology 1997; 205(P): 513
52. Rodenwaldt J, Kopka L, Grabbe E. Diagnosis of intima hyperplasia and endoluminal stenosis after iliac stent implantation with CT-virtual intraarterial endoscopy. Radiology 1997, 205(P): 565
53. Rodenwaldt J, Kopka L, Lotfi S, Grabbe E. Computed tomographic virtual intraarterial endoscopy after intravascular stent implantation: phantom study and clinical assessment. RöFo 1997; 166,3:180–4
54. Roelandt JR, diMario C, Pandian NG, Wenguang L, Keane D, Slager CJ, deFeyter PJ, Serruys PW. Three-dimensional reconstruction of intracoronary ultrasound images. Rationale, approaches, problems, and directions. Circulation 1994; 90:1044–55
55. Rogalla P, Rückert RJ, Gottschalk S, Hamm B. Virtuelle Angioskopie der Aorta nach transfemoraler Stentimplantation bei abdominellem Aortenaneurysma (AAA). RöFo 1998; 168:128
56. Rubin GD, Beaulieu CF, Argiro V, Ringl H, Norbash AM, Feller JF, Dake MD, Jeffrey RB, Napel S. Perspective volume rendering of CT and MR images: applications for endoscopic imaging. Radiology 1996; 199:321–30
57. Rubin GD, Dake MD, Napel S, Jeffrey RB, McDonnell CH, Sommer FG, Wexler L, Williams DM. Spiral CT of renal artery stenosis: comparison of three-dimensional rendering techniques. Radiology 1994; 190:181–9
58. Rubin GD, Dake MD, Napel SA, et al. Three-dimensional spiral CT angiography of the abdomen: initial clinical experience. Radiology 1993; 186:147–52
59. Rubin GD, Napel SA. Helical CT angiography of renal artery stenosis. AJR 1997; 168:1109–11

60. Rubin GD, Napel SA, Beaulieu CF, Dake MD, Jeffrey RB. Virtual angioscopy with volume-rendered CT angiograms: three-dimensional rendering without editing or thresholding. Radiology 1995; 197(P):144
61. Rühm SG, Debatin JF. Contrast-enhanced 3D MR angiography in the chest, anbdomen and lower extremities. Radiologe 1999, 39:100–9
62. Schwartz RB, Jones KM, Chernoff DM, et al. Common carotid artery bifurcation: evaluation with spiral CT - work in progress. Radiology 1992; 185: 513–9
63. Silverman JM, Julien PJ, Herfkens RJ, Pelc NJ. Magnetic Resonance imaging evaluation of pulmonary vascular malformations. Chest 1994; 106:1333–8
64. Soyer P, Heath D, Bluemke DA, Choti MA, Kuhlmann JE, Reichle R, Fishman EK. Three-dimensional helical CT of intrahepatic venous structures: comparison of three rendering techniques. J Comput Assist Tomogr 1996; 20:122–7
65. Takahashi M, Ashtari M, Papp Z, Patel M, Goldstein J, Maguire WM, Eacobacci T, Khan A, Herman PG. CT angiography of carotid bifurcation: artifacts and pitfalls in shaded-surface display. AJR 1997; 168:813–7
66. Toda J, Ueno E, Sakai F, Suzuki K, Okawa T, Isobe Y. Virtual CT endoscopy of portal vein. Radiology 1997; 205(P):566
67. Wielopolski PA, Haacke ME, Adler LP. Three-dimensional MR imaging of the pulmonary vasculature: preliminary experience. Radiology 1992; 183:465–72
68. Wildermuth S, Stern CH, Hilfiker PR, Pfammatter T, Debatin JF. Interactive definition of endoluminal aortic stent size and morphology based on virtual angioscopic rendering of 3D MRA. Radiology 1998; 209(P):362
69. Wildermuth S, Stern CH, Pfammatter T, Marincek B, Debatin JF. Virtuelles Planungssystem basierend auf 3D MR-Angiographien zur Bestimmung von Größe und Morphologie endoluminaler Aortenstents. RöFo 1999; 170:S232
70. Zeman RK, Berman PM, et al. Diagnosis of aortic dissection: value of helical CT with multiplanar reformation and three-dimensional rendering. AJR 1995; 164:1375–80

9 Virtual Neuroscopy

S. Gottschalk

CONTENTS

9.1 Introduction: Virtual Endoscopy of the Central Nervous System

Three-dimensional acquisition techniques for magnetic resonance imaging and computed tomography enable anatomic structures of the central nervous system to be displayed with high resolution of detail. Recently developed postprocessing algorithms generate virtual endoscopic views of the ventricular system, the basal cisterns, and the posterior cranial fossa. Intracranial vessels can be displayed with a virtual angioscopic view or with an extraluminal view that simulates an outside view onto the vessels from within the basal cisterns. Virtual neuroendoscopy yields vivid three-dimensional displays that can serve as teaching aids in the anatomic training of neurosurgeons and improve the planning of endoscope-assisted operations. Neuroradiologists will likewise benefit from optimized three-dimensional reconstructions of the intracranial vessels in planning endovascular interventions.

With advances in the development of microinstruments and very small endoscopes with excellent light sources, endoscopic techniques are being more and more widely employed in neurosurgery (Harris 1994). These reliable and fast surgical techniques involve minimal tissue damage, and thus patients benefit from early postoperative recovery. Important potential indications for endoscopic neurosurgery include the treatment of obstructive hydrocephalus, arachnoid cysts, colloid cysts, and intraventricular tumors (Gaab and Schroeder 1997; Gangemi et al. 1998). The concept of endoscope-assisted microsurgery can also be employed in the performance of minimally invasive surgery of tumors in other locations, especially intratentorial and intrasellar lesions, and aneurysms and neurovascular compression syndromes (Fries and Perneczky 1998; Perneczky and Fries 1998). The wider use of neuroendoscopic procedures also represents a challenge for diagnostic neuroradiology. Neuroradiologists are expected not only to provide a detailed anatomic display and precise characterization of a pathologic process but also to attempt to include the best possible display in relation to the neurosurgeon's specific operative approach. Using rapidly acquired data sets, state-of-the-art three-dimensional rendering techniques generate images of anatomic structures with high resolution of detail and have already been used successfully for computer-assisted neuronavigation (Wirtz et al. 1997). The most recent postprocessing techniques such as perspective volume rendering generate virtual endoscopic images from high-resolution three-dimensional data sets. These volume-rendered displays vividly depict the topographic anatomy of the central nervous system and thus offer ideal material for the training and education of neurosurgeons and for facilitating the planning of neuroendoscopic interventions. Relevant anatomic regions to be considered for virtual endoscopy are the ventricular system, the posterior cranial fossa, and the basal cisterns together with the nerves and

S. Gottschalk, MD
Department of Radiology, Charité Hospital, Humboldt Universität zu Berlin, Schuhmannstrasse 20/21, 10117 Berlin, Germany
Medizinische Universität Lübeck, Institut für Radiologie, Neuroradiologie, Ratzeburger Allee 160, 23538 Lübeck, Germany

vessels coursing through them. No approaches have as yet been developed for the preoperative diagnostic assessment by virtual endoscopy prior to endoscopic surgical interventions in peripheral nerve compression syndromes or minimally invasive surgery of the spinal column and vertebral disks. This is primarily due to the poor soft-tissue contrast in these regions.

9.2 Outline of the Technique of Virtual Endoscopy

Virtual endoscopy is the simulation of endoscopic procedures by means of images generated by the computer from high-resolution anatomic data sets. Such three-dimensional data sets are acquired by computed tomography or magnetic resonance imaging and are then transferred to a workstation for postprocessing with commercially available software packages, which can be purchased from various manufacturers of medical equipment (Philips Medical Systems, Siemens Medical Systems, General Electric Medical Systems, Marconi Medical Systems, and others). Basically, two methods are available for the generation of virtual images. With the first, a so-called shaded surface display (SSD) is generated by performing a surface reconstruction on the basis of a specified, operator-selected threshold. The perception of depth is created by the computer, which retrospectively adds light and shade effects to the surface rendering (Magnusson et al. 1991). The second technique, the volume rendering technique, requires more computation for reconstruction of voxels from a defined volumetric data set. The operator can randomly select a threshold value of minimum or maximum intensity by means of which areas of different intensities can be classified. Thus, one may for instance separate cerebrospinal fluid and brain tissue and then make one classification (e.g., the cerebrospinal fluid) appear transparent. In so-called perspective volume rendering (Rubin et al. 1996), volume elements are reconstructed for each view relative to a target point. A three-dimensional effect in a given view is created by displaying structures in the foreground larger than those that are farther away. The threshold value can be changed interactively and the final image can be smoothly rotated, so that it may be viewed from any orientation. During processing, multiplanar reconstructions in three planes are displayed on the screen in synchrony with the virtual endoscopic image. For better orientation, the operator can follow the viewing angle and the chosen volume on the cross-sectional images. Because of the complexity of the anatomy, it is generally advisable to calculate images for individually selected viewing angles rather than use a fly-through option. The size of the structures on display can be determined from the original data set. The excellent three-dimensional appearance generated with the perspective volume rendering technique yields impressive virtual endoscopic views.

9.3 Virtual Endoscopy of the Intracranial Cerebrospinal Fluid Spaces

9.3.1 Imaging Protocols

State-of-the-art magnetic resonance imaging systems operating at a field strength of 1.5 T and using a conventional circularly polarized head coil allow acquisition of three-dimensional data sets with a voxel size below 1 mm, contiguous scanning, and a high signal-to-noise ratio within an acquisition time of only a few minutes. The sequences to be used for virtual endoscopy of the subarachnoid spaces must yield not only high anatomic resolution with nearly isotropic voxels but also a strong contrast between cerebrospinal fluid and the anatomic structures of interest within the subarachnoid spaces.

Shigematsu et al. (1998a) and Boor et al. (1998) presented a protocol using a constructive interference in steady state (CISS) 3D Fourier transform (3DFT) sequence. The CISS sequence is a gradient-echo sequence with high T2* contrast (Stehling et al. 1995). Flow-related signal voids are reduced by employing flow compensation. Cerebrospinal fluid shows a relatively homogeneous and high signal intensity, whereas all structures within the ventricular system and the cisterns are of low signal intensity. Delicate arachnoid membranes are not visualized. With a 512 matrix and a minimal slice thickness of about 0.5 mm, a voxel size of approximately 0.5 mm can be attained. The acquisition time is about 4–8 min. Clinical studies have shown that this sequence is especially useful for the depiction of acoustic neurinomas and the assessment of inner ear structures (Held et al. 1997; Benoudiba et al. 1998). The high T2* contrast of this sequence facilitates the selection of a threshold, which is a prerequisite for successful classification and reconstruction of virtual endoscopic displays. Near the base of the skull, distortions induced by susceptibility artifacts that are typical for T2*-weighted gradient-echo sequences may occur and they pose a problem especially in assessing the sellar region. Since the overall size of the scanning volume is limited by the slice thickness used, it may become necessary to specifically scan the target volume containing those structures from which virtual endoscopic displays are to be created. The alternative is to perform additional acquisitions that can then be recombined with the other data sets.

A technical alternative has been reported by Auer and Auer (1998), who used an inversion-recovery prepped spoiled gradient-echo sequence, which is a T1-weighted gradient-echo sequence. T1 weighting has the advantage that the entire brain can be scanned in an acquisition time of less than 10 min and at a voxel size below 1 mm. This sequence is less prone to pulsation artifacts, and susceptibility artifacts near the skull base are less pronounced. A disadvantage is the lower contrast between cerebrospinal fluid and brain tissue or nerves, which makes threshold-based reconstruction more difficult. Major advantages of both protocols are the noninvasiveness and the absence of radiation exposure. The acquisition can easily be done within a reasonable time span as part of a clinical examination. Feasible alternative protocols for virtual endoscopy of the cerebrospinal fluid spaces using computed tomography are not available.

Protocols based on CT angiography and MR angiography are discussed in connection with virtual endoscopy of the intracranial vessels in Sect. 9.4.

9.3.2 Applications and Clinical Relevance in Neurosurgery

High-quality virtual endoscopic images of human anatomical structures can be rendered for those tissues that have a high contrast relative to surrounding elements. Excellent examples of virtual endoscopy based on computed tomography with maximum contrast between air and soft tissue have been generated for the tracheobronchial system (McAdams et al. 1998), the nose and paranasal sinuses (Rogalla et al. 1998), and the colon (Fenlon et al. 1999).

In the central nervous system, virtual endoscopy is of primary interest for evaluating the subarachnoid spaces, but the latter also pose technical problems for virtual endoscopy. These spaces are in part very narrow, are septated by arachnoids, they contain very small and anatomically complex structures and are susceptible to pulsation. Manipulation of these spaces for an examination is of course contraindicated. For these reasons, the raw data that are used for reconstruction must be of especially high quality despite the limitations resulting from the problems associated with their acquisition.

An important initial step in creating a virtual endoscopic portrayal is to determine whether the most important anatomic structures are visible on the reconstructed image. These comprise the characteristic features of the topography of the brain surface, the cranial nerves and arterial vessels as well as venous vessels to the extent that they may serve as endoscopic landmarks for the neurosurgeon.

Auer and Auer (1998) studied virtual anatomy in a large series of subjects. The optic chiasm and tract together with the pituitary stalk can be depicted very clearly (Fig. 9.1). The rather large oculomotor and trigeminal nerves are always reliably identified before they enter the cavernous sinus (Fig. 9.2). The visualization of the smaller seventh and eighth cranial nerves largely depends on the quality of the raw data yielded by the three-dimensional sequence. Identification may be difficult when a T1-weighted

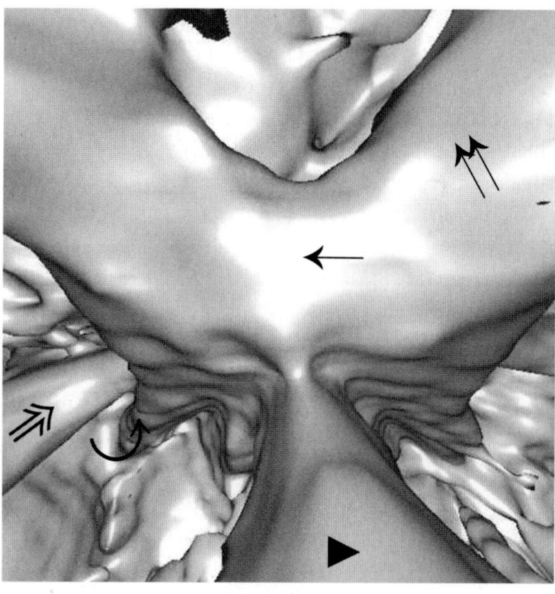

Fig. 9.1. Optic chiasm, suprasellar region. Virtual endoscopic image. Note the excellent depiction of the optic nerve, chiasm, and tract and of the pituitary stalk. *Plain arrow*, optic chiasm; *double arrow*, optic nerve; *curved arrow*, optic tract; *arrowhead*, pituitary stalk; *open arrow* anterior cerebral artery (A1 segment)

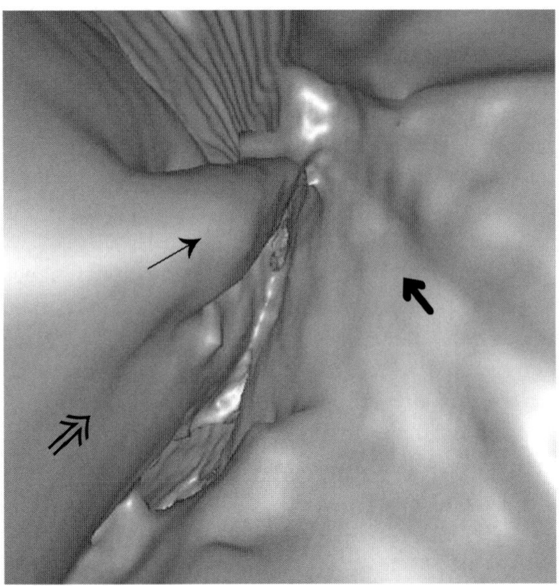

Fig. 9.2. Trigeminal nerve. View onto the trigeminal nerve before entering the cavernous sinus. *Thin arrow*, trigeminal nerve; *open arrow*, brainstem; *thick arrow*, petrous apex

sequence is used, and reconstruction is easier from a T2*-weighted sequence due to the higher contrast. Figure 9.3 shows reconstructions based on a CISS sequence.

Visualization of the abducent nerve might be possible, but no author has as yet reported good visualization of the trochlear nerve and the inferior cranial nerves. This is in accordance with the daily experience of neuroradiologists since the identification of these rather small cranial nerves is already difficult on classical scans.

Solid structures at the margin of the ventricular system can be recognized when they have a characteristic surface. Auer and Auer (1998) reported clear depiction of the quadrigeminal plate, the mamillary bodies, the pons, the cerebral peduncles and the interpeduncular fossa, the pineal gland, and the infundibular recess, as well as adequate visualization of the margin of the caudate nucleus and the fornix.

Intraventricularly, the choroid plexus is clearly delineated (Fig. 9.4). The foramina of Monro are depicted and their size can be measured; the aqueduct and the surrounding anatomy are also clearly visualized (Fig. 9.5). The position of the foramina of Monro may vary, and it is therefore of great practical relevance to know the angle relative to the passage along which an endoscope is to be inserted (Grunert et al. 1994).

Since the protocols for virtual endoscopy discussed here are not based on sequences optimized for MR angiography, visualization of the intracranial vessels is difficult. Using a CISS 3DFT sequence, Shigematsu et al. (1998a) demonstrated that the large basal cranial arteries could be identified around the circle of Willis and that the posterior communicating artery was likewise visible when it was strong enough. Figure 9.6 shows a view of the prepontine cistern looking onto a basilar dolichoectasia. However, veins and small arteries usually cannot be depicted. The thalamostriate vein and the vein of septum pellucidum are anatomic landmarks for neuroendoscopy (Resch et al. 1994). Neither of them can be identified on the wall of the lateral ventricle in the virtual image. This is illustrated by Fig. 9.7, which shows a virtual and a true endoscopic image of the lateral ventricle looking into the foramen of Monro. Visualization of the smaller vessels in the basal cisterns is likewise inadequate.

Boor et al. (1998), Fellner et al. (1998), and Shigematsu et al. (1998b) rendered endoscopic images from the data sets acquired by CT angiography and MR angiography in patients with aneurysms and neurovascular compression syndromes. These approaches are conceptually different from the techniques of virtual endoscopy of the subarachnoid spaces presented here and are therefore discussed in Sect. 9.4 under the heading "Virtual Endoscopy of the Intracranial Vessels."

In addition to a thorough study of the normal virtual endoscopic anatomy in healthy subjects, both Auer and Auer (1998) and Shigematsu et al. (1998a) also investigated whether pathologic changes can be detected by virtual endoscopy and whether this technique can be used to simulate and plan endoscopic surgical interventions. Shigematsu et al. (1998a) presented the successfully reconstructed endoscopic anatomy of suprasellar mass lesions and acoustic neurinomas (Fig. 9.8). However, a small acoustic neurinoma in the internal acoustic meatus was not depicted although it was seen on the original scans acquired by the CISS sequence. Auer and Auer (1998) simulated well-established endoscopic approaches as they are used in minimally invasive neurosurgery: the frontal approach to the foramen of Monro and the third ventricle, the parieto-occipital approach to the posterior horn, pulvinar thalami and temporal horn, the suboccipital approach to the fourth ventricle, and the transseptal, transsphenoidal approach to the sellar region. With respect to the frontal approach, the surgeon especially benefited from the depiction of the foramina of Monro and of

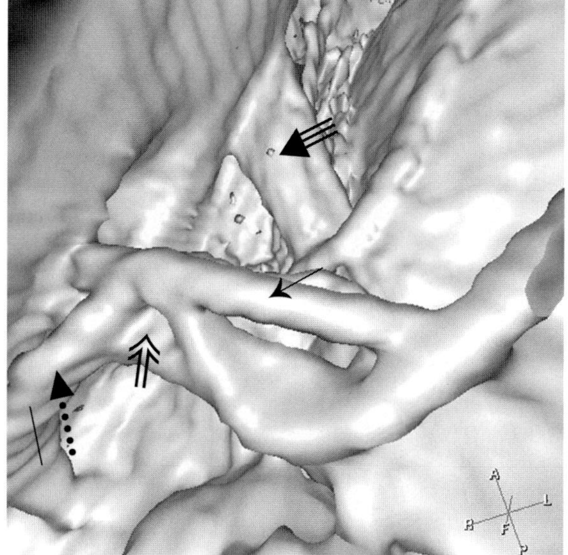

a

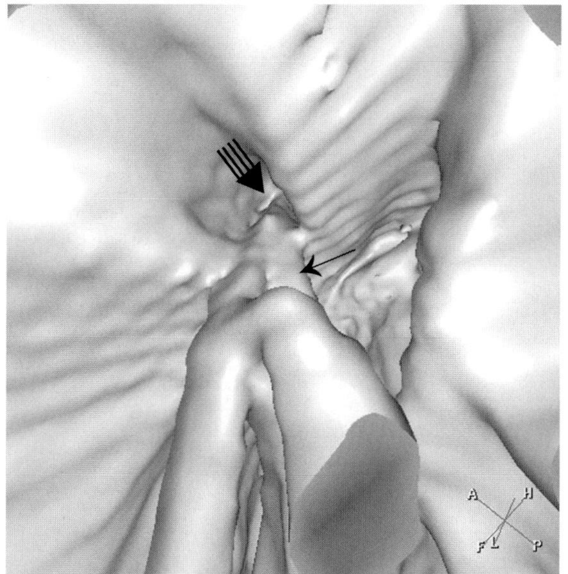

b

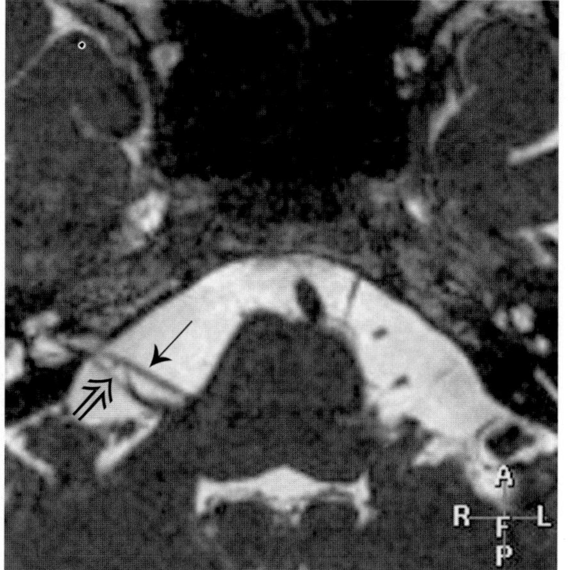

c

Fig. 9.3a–c. Cerebellopontine angle. Depiction of the seventh and eighth cranial nerves and the typical tortuous course of the anterior inferior cerebellar artery. **a** Virtual endoscopic image. View from the bottom of the cerebellopontine cistern looking cranially. **b** Virtual endoscopic image. View from medial looking into internal acoustic meatus. **c** Axial scan acquired with a CISS (3DFT) sequence at the level of the cerebellopontine angle. *Plain arrow*, facial nerve; *open arrow*, vestibulocochlear nerve; *heavy-pointed arrow*, anterior inferior cerebellar artery; *triple-stemmed arrow* trigeminal nerve; *four-stemmed arrow*, internal acoustic meatus

their angle relative to the passage through which the endoscope had to be advanced, as well as from the ability to measure the size of the foramina perpendicular to the endoscope. The simulation of the transsphenoidal approach was praised for its very vivid depiction of the anatomy (Fig. 9.1). Virtual endoscopy of the parieto-occipital access offered an advantage when small lesions were present that were hidden by the choroid plexus.

From a surgical perspective, virtual endoscopy of the cerebrospinal fluid spaces was considered to be helpful in answering specific questions for planning the surgical approach, in particular in patients with intraventricular tumors. Only those pathologies that are readily identifiable by their shape can be depicted. Here again, the failure to visualize small vessels that serve as anatomic landmarks is discussed as a relevant drawback by the authors.

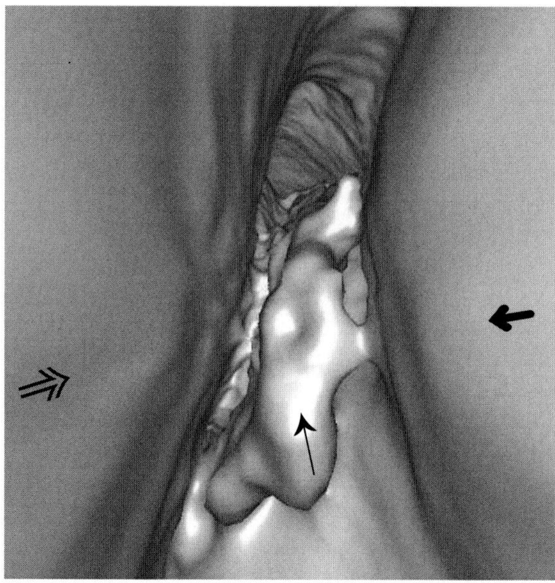

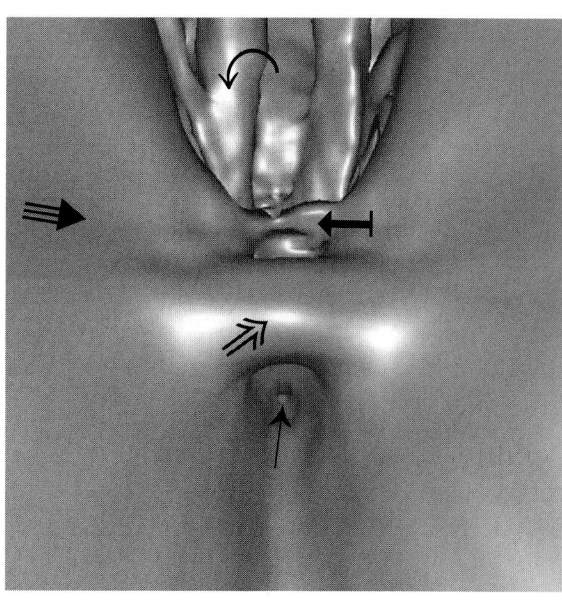

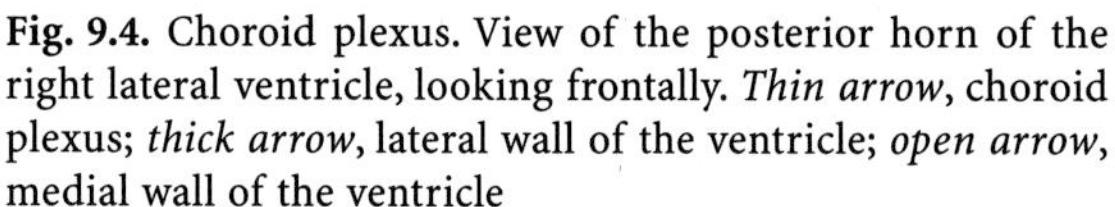

Fig. 9.4. Choroid plexus. View of the posterior horn of the right lateral ventricle, looking frontally. *Thin arrow*, choroid plexus; *thick arrow*, lateral wall of the ventricle; *open arrow*, medial wall of the ventricle

Fig. 9.5. View into the third ventricle, looking dorsally to the aqueduct and posterior commissure. Note also the clear depiction of the habenular commissure; *Thin arrow*, aqueduct; *double arrow*, posterior commissure; *arrow with base*, habenular commissure; *triple arrow*, thalamus; *curved arrow*, internal cerebral vein

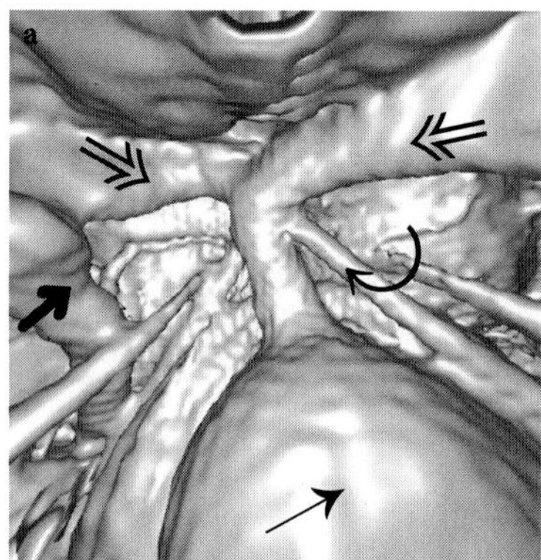

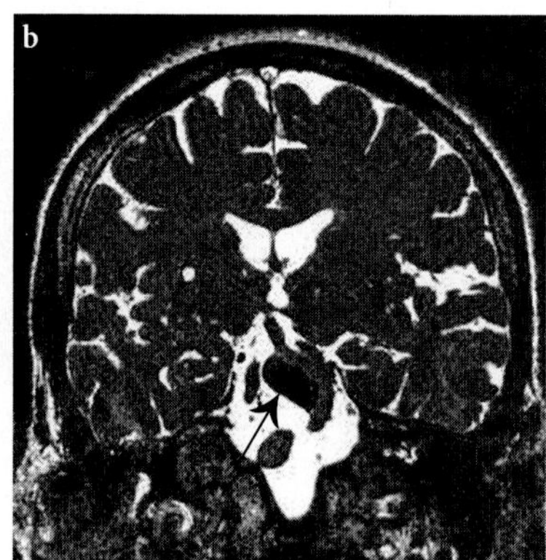

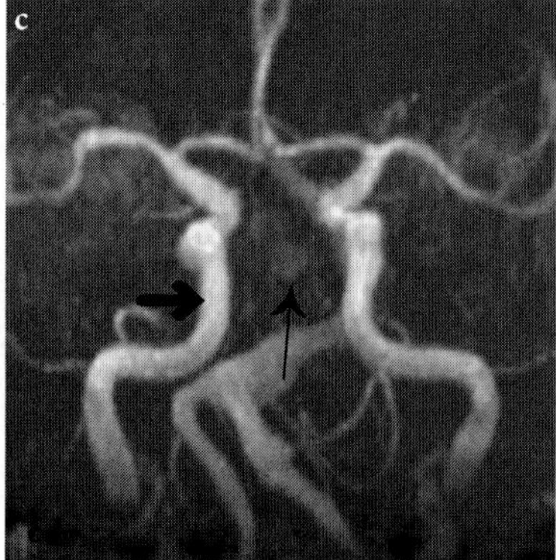

Fig. 9.6a–c. Basilar dolichoectasia. View of the prepontine cistern looking onto a basilar dolichoectasia with a fusiform aneurysm containing an intraluminal clot. **a** Virtual endoscopic image using a CISS (3DFT) sequence. **b** Coronal scan acquired with a CISS (3DFT) sequence. **c** MR angiography, maximum intensity projection (MIP). Note the depiction of the outer rim of the basilar artery including an intraluminal clot using the CISS (3DFT) sequence in contrast to the depiction by MR angiography. *Thin arrow*, basilar dolichoectasia; *open arrow*, posterior cerebral artery; *thick arrow*, internal carotid artery; *curved arrow*, oculomotor nerve

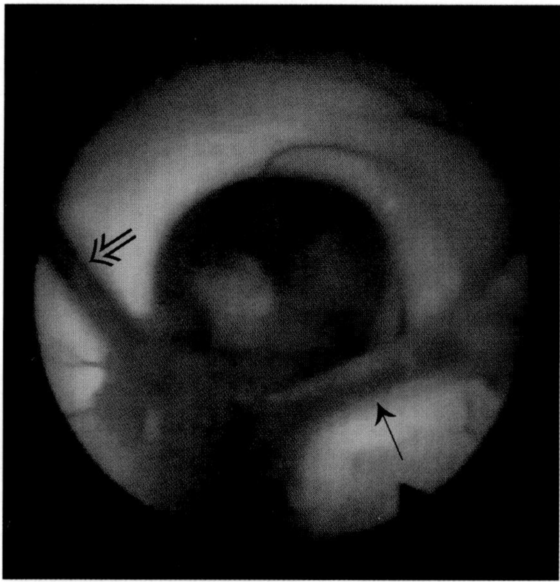

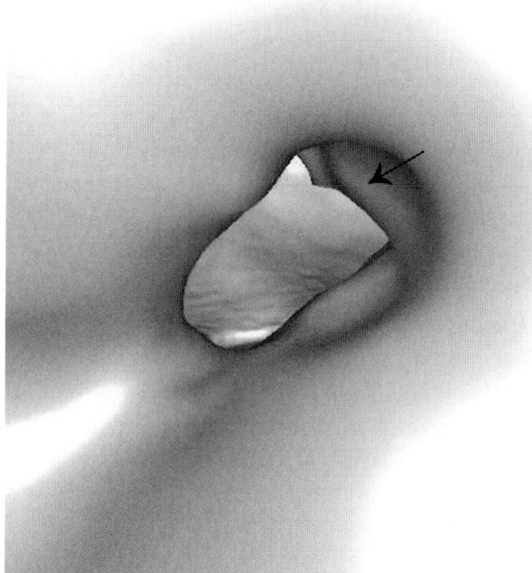

a b

Fig. 9.7a, b. View from the lateral ventricle into the foramen of Monro. The fornix forms the superomedial and frontal borders of the foramen. **a** True endoscopic image. Note the thalamostriate vein and the vein of septum pellucidum. *Arrow*, thalamostriate vein; *open arrow*, vein of septum pellucidum (Reproduced by courtesy of Dr. Kehler, Department of Neurosurgery, Medical University of Lübeck, Germany)**b** Virtual endoscopic image. Identical projection. There is no visualization of the thalamostriate vein or the vein of septum pellucidum. *Arrow*, fornix

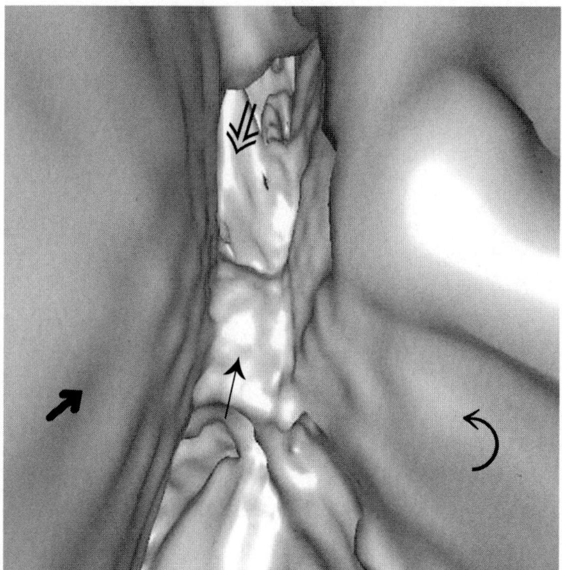

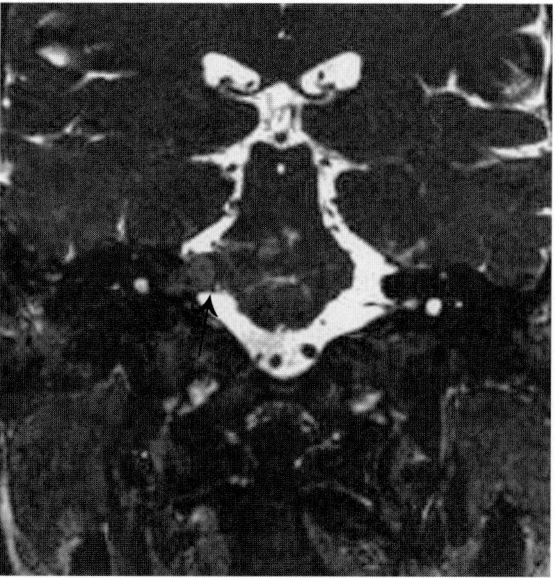

a b

Fig. 9.8a, b. Large extra- and intrameatal acoustic neurinoma. **a** Virtual endoscopic image. **b** Coronal scan acquired with a CISS sequence. *Arrow*, acoustic neurinoma; *open arrow*, trigeminal nerve; *thick arrow*, petrosal bone; *curved arrow*, brainstem

9.4 Virtual Endoscopy of the Intracranial Vessels

9.4.1 Imaging Protocols

Protocols for data acquisition for the endoscopic reconstruction of the intracranial vessels are available for two traditionally competing imaging modalities – CT angiography and MR angiography.

CT angiography is performed on a helical CT scanner. When scanning a volume with a width of no more than about 5–6 cm, which is sufficient for the depiction of the basal cranial arteries, a protocol with a table feed of 1 mm, a collimation of 1 mm, and reconstruction at a slice thickness of 1 mm or 0.5 mm can be used. A contrast administration regimen with infusion of a bolus of 70–100 ml of a nonionic contrast agent at a flow of about 2 ml/s and a scan delay of about 20 s has proved effective; slight deviations from this regimen are also in use. When a primary image matrix of 512×512 pixels is used with a field of view (FOV) of about 200–220 mm, a voxel size of less than 0.5 mm can be attained. Endoscopic rendering is done by segmentation of the contrast material column in the vessel. Where vessels border on bone, e.g., the head of the basilar artery on the dorsum sella, the similarity of the density values does not allow automated segmentation and requires manual editing. It is well established that CT angiography has technical limitations in depicting changes in small vessels, in particular small aneurysms (Ng et al. 1997; Young et al. 1999).

The alternative to CT is MR angiography using the time-of-flight (TOF) technique (Laub 1995). This technique is well established and is regarded as the most important MR angiographic technique in neuroradiology, in particular for depiction of the cerebral arteries. Drawbacks of this modality are the signal inhomogeneities resulting from nonlaminar flow or changes in flow velocity. These inhomogeneities impair the classification for rendering the virtual image. Administration of a superparamagnetic contrast agent can partly reduce these problems; in such cases shortening of TR may be helpful. The minimum slice thickness is about 0.6 mm. With a FOV of around 200 mm and a 256 matrix, it is likewise no problem to measure voxels less than 1 mm in size.

Both CT angiography and MR angiography are sensitive modalities for the assessment of stenoses (Shier et al. 1997), but MR angiography may overestimate their severity (Magarelli et al. 1998). Both modalities have a sensitivity of up to 95% in detecting intracranial aneurysms as small as 3–5 mm (Ross et al. 1990; Puskar et al. 1995; Vieco et al. 1995; Ogawa et al. 1996; Keogh and Vhora 1998) and can therefore be used for virtual endoscopy of well-defined vascular pathologies.

9.4.2 Clinical Applications in Neurosurgery and Neuroradiology

While angioscopic techniques have been described for extracranial arteries (White 1992; Yamakawa et al. 1992; Kuroda et al. 1993), true angioscopy is not available for the examination of intracranial vessels. Thus, the generation of virtual endoscopic images of the intracranial vessels is primarily a theoretical approach that does not simulate an already established technique, but rather aims at offering an alternative to angioscopy, which is too risky to perform in the brain.

Figure 9.9 shows a virtual angioscopic image from within the internal carotid artery looking into the origin of the anterior cerebral artery and medial ce-

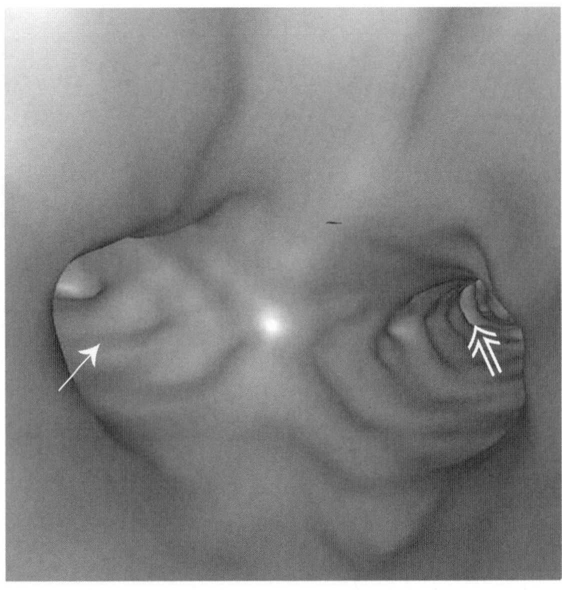

Fig. 9.9. Virtual angioscopic image of the internal carotid artery looking into the origin of the middle cerebral artery and anterior cerebral artery. The image, generated from an MR angiogram, may be affected by signal inhomogeneities due to nonlaminar flow. The irregular borders do not give an accurate representation of the status of the vessel wall._ *Thin arrow*, middle cerebral artery; *open arrow*, anterior cerebral artery

rebral artery. The image was generated from an MR angiogram and neither the rendered display nor the original image yields definite information on the status of the vessel wall. However, this figure should demonstrate that, in principle, depiction of the lumina of the large arteries and the origin of their branches is possible.

Advantages of reconstructed images of arterial vessels might be expected from the superior visualization of complicated anatomic structures. Thus, the most important application of virtual endoscopy is the depiction of aneurysms. Proper evaluation of an aneurysm comprises information on its location and spatial orientation, its size and shape, particularly the shape of the neck, the presence of thrombosis, and the relationship between adjacent vessel branches and those bearing the aneurysm.

Digital subtraction angiography (DSA) is the gold standard for the diagnostic assessment of intracranial aneurysms, and additional information regarding their location and shape can be obtained by rotational angiography (Hoff et al. 1994; Anxionnat et al. 1998). Computed tomography and magnetic resonance imaging can likewise be used to yield further information on size, the presence of thrombosis, and the spatial relationship to adjacent structures. CT angiography is also employed to determine the size of an aneurysm before embolization is performed (Jansen et al. 1998).

Several authors have explored the contribution of reconstructed virtual endoscopic images to an accurate determination of aneurysmal anatomy. Marro et al. (1997) reported the depiction of a 3-mm aneurysm of the basilar artery by shaded surface display generated from CT angiography. The rendering clearly showed that the aneurysm had no neck and that it involved the origin of the anterior superior cerebellar artery. Embolization of the aneurysm was not possible and the patient underwent surgery. Using data sets acquired by MR angiography for rendering, Shigematsu et al. (1998b) demonstrated that virtual endoscopy depicted the lumina of the large basal cerebral arteries, i.e., of the internal carotid artery, the basilar artery, and the middle cerebral artery. The anterior and posterior cerebral arteries as well as the posterior communicating artery were likewise visible if they were strong enough (Fig. 9.10). Although the authors showed, for instance, that it was possible to generate a view into the openings of the posterior cerebral artery from within a basilar artery aneurysm, they did not explain whether the virtual endoscopic view yielded any additional information compared with other diagnostic modalities.

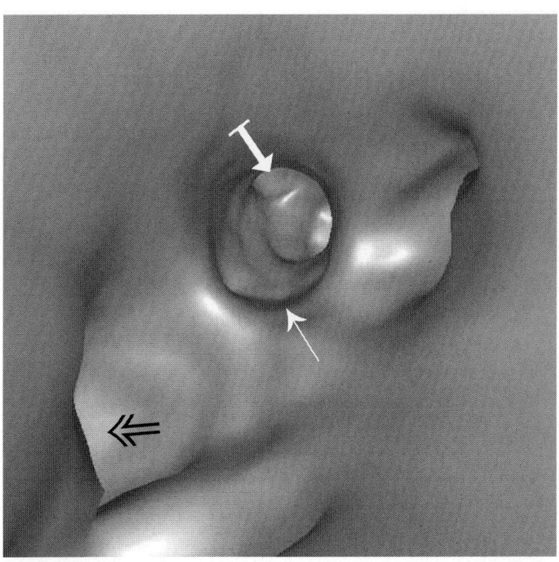

Fig. 9.10. Virtual angioscopic image of the basilar artery looking into the origin of the anterior superior cerebellar artery and posterior cerebral artery, reconstructed from a contrast enhanced MR angiography data set. *Thin arrow*, basilar artery; *open arrow*, left anterior superior cerebellar artery; *thick arrow*, left posterior cerebral artery

Kato et al. (1996) reported three aneurysms examined by CT angiography. The three-dimensional endoscopic image of a left-sided vertebral union aneurysm in combination with splitting of the basilar artery showed that the left part of the basilar artery formed part of the wall of the aneurysm and could not be separated from its dome. In a case of an aneurysm of the middle cerebral artery it was shown that the aneurysm had a wide neck and that the M2 segment originated from this neck. In a third case, virtual endoscopy accurately visualized the relationship of the neck of a vertebral union aneurysm, again combined with splitting of the basilar artery, to the fenestrated segments and to the origins of the anterior inferior cerebral artery. All three aneurysms were treated by surgery. The virtual topographic information complemented the findings of DSA and was considered to be useful for planning surgery (Kato et al. 1996).

Tomandl et al. (1997) presented a rendering algorithm based on CT angiography that creates an extraluminal view rather than an angioscopic one. The transparent display of the vessel walls enabled visualization of an aneurysm of the anterior communicating artery and depiction of the A1 and A2 segments without overlying structures (Fig. 9.11). This kind of display is useful for planning both neuroradiologic and surgical interventions.

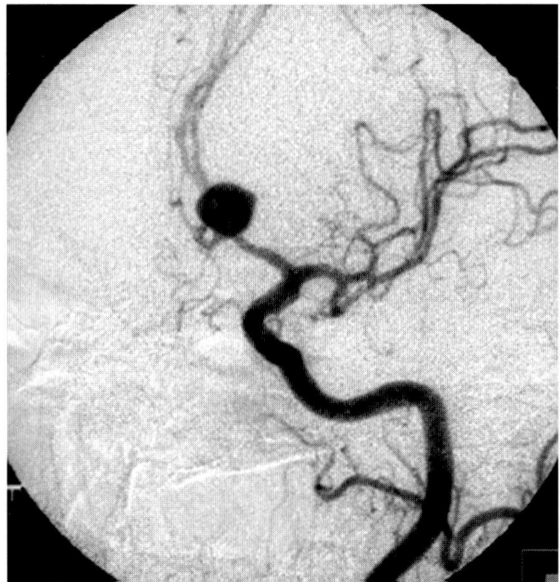

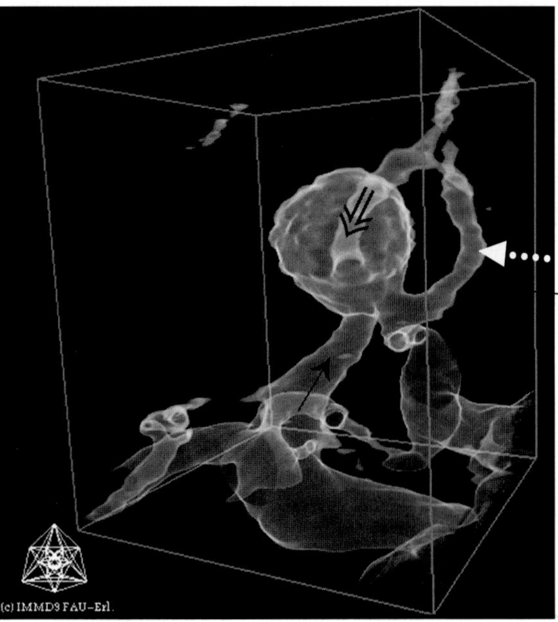

Fig. 9.11a, b. Aneurysm of the communicating cerebral artery. **a** Digital subtraction angiography. **b** Reconstruction from a CT angiography data set with transparent display of the vessel walls. Note that the aneurysm involves the right A1 and A2 segments of the anterior cerebral artery. *Heavy-pointed arrow*, left anterior cerebral artery (A2 segment); *plain arrow*, right anterior cerebral artery (A1 segment; *open arrow* right anterior cerebral artery (A2 segment). (Reproduced by courtesy of Dr. Tomandl, Department of Neuroradiology, University of Erlangen-Nürnberg, Germany)

Boor et al. (1998) and Fellner et al. (1998) also reported visualization techniques for creating extraluminal views of vessels. The virtual endoscopic displays of the basal cisterns in these studies were generated from angiography and from the data acquired with a CISS sequence. The authors investigated aneurysms, tumors of the posterior cranial fossa, and neurovascular compression syndromes. Despite the failure to visualize details such as small arteries and veins and cisternal membranes and the fact that only information which is already depicted on the original images is provided, the renderings were nevertheless described as being highly instructive because the surgeon could simply select endoscopic displays from various viewing angles depending on the individual case rather than having to mentally create such endoscopic views from looking at the individual scans.

9.5 Limitations of Virtual Endoscopy

Virtual endoscopy is a reconstruction technique aimed at providing complementary anatomic information rather than being used as the primary modality for making a diagnosis. The quality of the renderings depends on the quality of the original three-dimensional data sets. However, even with optimal image quality, fully homogeneous visualization of the subarachnoid space with adequate contrast relative to all anatomic structures within the space will not be achieved. A problem associated with the CISS sequence are variations in signal intensity induced by pulsation. MR angiography is limited by the occurrence of signal inhomogeneities in regions of turbulent flow. In CT angiography the difficulty lies in differentiating the luminal column of contrast material from thrombi or adjacent osseous structures. Information that is not available on the original angiographic images will not become available on the reconstructed images: a missed aneurysm will also be missed on the three-dimensional displays. The generation of endoscopic images is an operator-dependent rendering technique because it is based on a threshold which is subjectively selected by the operator. Through the selection of this threshold, the operator can make structures visible or obscure them. Selection of a wrong threshold value may lead to the enlargement of a structure, thereby giving the impression of a pathologic condition, or the connection to a vessel may be overestimated or eliminated.

It is not generally possible to visualize small vessels, despite the fact that they serve as anatomic landmarks in surgery. This drawback limits the potential use of three-dimensional displays as anatomic teaching aids. Thin membranes such as the walls of arachnoid cysts are likewise not depicted accurately: membrane defects cannot be differentiated from very delicate membranes (AUER and AUER 1998).

With these technical limitations kept in mind, virtual endoscopy nevertheless provides fascinating images that offer important complementary information on anatomy, from which both interventional neuroradiology and minimally invasive neurosurgery may benefit in the future.

References

Anxionnat R, Bracard S, Macho J, Da Costa E, Vaillant R, Launay L, Trousset Y, Romeas R, Picard L (1998) 3D angiography. Clinical interest. First applications in interventional neuroradiology. J Neuroradiol 25:251–62

Auer LM, Auer DP (1998) Virtual endoscopy for planning and simulation of minimally invasive neurosurgery. Neurosurgery 43:529–37

Benoudiba F, Iffenecker C, Fuerxer F, Huang J, Hadj-Rabia M, Francke JP, Doyon D (1998) Imaging cranial nerves with inframillimetric T2-weighted MRI. J Radiol 79:21–5

Blezek DJ, Robb RA (1997) Evaluating virtual endoscopy for clinical use. J Digit Imaging 10:51–55

Boor S, Resch KM, Perneczky A, Stoeter P (1998) Virtual endoscopy (VE) of the basal cisterns: its value in planning the neurosurgical approach. Minim Invasive Neurosurg 41:177–82

Fellner F, Blank M, Fellner C, Bohm-Jurkovic H, Bautz W, Kalender WA (1998) Virtual cisternoscopy of intracranial vessels: a novel visualization technique using virtual reality. Magn Reson Imaging 16:1013–22

Fenlon HM, McAneny DB, Nunes DP, Clarke PD, Ferrucci JT (1999) Occlusive colon carcinoma: virtual colonoscopy in the preoperative evaluation of the proximal colon. Radiology 210:423–8

Fries G, Perneczky A (1998) Endoscope-assisted brain surgery: part 2–analysis of 380 procedures. Neurosurgery 42:226–31

Gaab MR, Schroeder HWS (1997) Neuroendoscopy and endoscopic neurosurgery. Nervenarzt 68:459–465

Gangemi M, Maiuri F, Donati P, Sigona L, Iaconetta G, De Divitiis E (1998) Neuroendoscopy. Personal experience, indications and limits. J Neurosurg Sci 42:1–10

Grunert P, Perneczky A, Resch K (1994) Endoscopic procedures through the foramen interventriculare of Monro under stereotactical conditions. Minim Invasive Neurosurg 37:2–8

Harris LW (1994) Endoscopic techniques in neurosurgery. Microsurgery 15:541–46

Held P, Fellner C, Fellner F, Seitz J, Strutz J (1997) MRI of inner ear anatomy using 3D MP-RAGE and 3D CISS sequences. Br J Radiol 70:465–72

Hoff DJ, Wallace MC, terBrugge KG, Gentili F (1994) Rotational angiography assessment of cerebral aneurysms. Am J Neuroradiol 15:1945–48

Jansen O, Braks E, Hahnel S, Schramm T, Sartor K (1998) CT angiography to determine the size of intracranial aneurysms before GDC therapy. Rofo Fortschr Geb Rontgenstr Neuen Bildgeb Verfahr 169:175–81

Kato Y, Sano H, Katada K, Ogura Y, Kanaoka N, Yokoyama T, Kanno T (1996) Clinical usefulness of 3-D CT endoscopic imaging of cerebral aneurysms. Neurol Res 18:98–102

Keogh AJ, Vhora S (1998) The usefulness of magnetic resonance angiography in surgery for intracranial aneurysms that have bled. Surg Neurol 50:122–27

Kuroda S, Kamiyama H, Takahashi A, Houkin K, Abe H, Saitoh H (1993) Clinical application of angioscopy during carotid endarterectomy for patients with internal carotid artery stenosis. Neurol Med Chir (Tokyo) 33:815–19

Laub GA (1995) Time-of-flight method of MR angiography. Magn Reson Imaging Clin N Am 3:391–98

Magarelli N, Scarabino T, Simeone AL, Florio F, Carriero A, Salvolini U, Bonomo L (1998) Carotid stenosis: a comparison between MR and spiral CT angiography. Neuroradiology 40:367–73

Magnusson M, Lenz R, Danielsson PE (1991) Evaluation of methods for shaded surface display of CT volumes. Comput Med Imaging Graph 15:247–256

Marro B, Galanaud D, Valery CA, Zouaoui A, Biondi A, Casasco A, Sahel M, Marsault C (1997) Intracranial aneurysm: inner view and neck identification with CT angiography virtual endoscopy. J Comput Assist Tomogr 21:587–79

McAdams HP, Goodman PC, Kussin P (1998) Virtual bronchoscopy for directing transbronchial needle aspiration of hilar and mediastinal lymph nodes: a pilot study. Am J Roentgenol 170:1361–64

Ng SH, Wong HF, Ko SF, Lee CM, Yen PS, Wai YY, Wan YL (1997) CT angiography of intracranial aneurysms: advantages and pitfalls. Eur J Radiol 25:14–19

Ogawa T, Okudera T, Noguchi K, Sasaki N, Inugami A, Uemura K, Yasui N (1996) Cerebral aneurysms: evaluation with three-dimensional CT angiography. Am J Neuroradiol 17:447–54

Perneczky A, Fries G (1998) Endoscope-assisted brain surgery: part 1–evolution, basic concept, and current technique. Neurosurgery 42:219–24

Puskar G, Ruggieri PM (1995) Intracranial aneurysms. Magn Reson Imaging Clin N Am 3:467–83

Resch KD, Perneczky A, Tschabitscher M, Kindel S (1994) Endoscopic anatomy of the ventricles. Acta Neurochir Suppl (Wien) 61:57–61

Rogalla P, Nischwitz A, Gottschalk S, Huitema A, Kaschke O, Hamm B (1998) Virtual endoscopy of the nose and paranasal sinuses. Eur Radiol 8:946–50

Ross JS, Masaryk TJ, Modic MT, Ruggieri PM, Haacke EM, Selman WR (1990) Intracranial aneurysms: evaluation by MR angiography. Am J Neuroradiol 11:449–55

Rubin GD, Beaulieu CF, Argiro V, Ringl H, Norbash AM, Feller JF, Dake MD, Jeffrey RB, Napel S (1996) Perspective volume rendering of CT and MR images: applications for endoscopic imaging. Radiology 199:321–30

Shigematsu Y, Korogi Y, Hirai T, Okuda T, Ikushima I, Sugahara T, Liang L, Ge Y, Takahashi M (1998a) Virtual MRI endoscopy of the intracranial cerebrospinal fluid spaces. Neuroradiology 40:644–50

Shigematsu Y, Korogi Y, Hirai T, Okuda T, Sugahara T, Liang L, Ge Y, Takahashi M (1998b) New developments: 2. Virtual MR endoscopy in the central nervous system. J Magn Reson Imaging 8:289–96

Shrier DA, Tanaka H, Numaguchi Y, Konno S, Patel U, Shibata D (1997) CT angiography in the evaluation of acute stroke. Am J Neuroradiol 18:1011–20

Stehling MK, Nitz W, Holzknecht N (1995) Fast and ultra-fast magnetic resonance tomography. Basic principles, pulse sequences and special properties. Radiologe 35:879–93

Tomandl BF, Eberhardt KEW, Tröscher-Weber R, Huk WJ, Hastreiter P, Ertl T (1997) Virtual endoscopic CT angiography (VECTA) in patients with intracranial aneurysms. Klin Neuroradiol 7:212–15

Vieco PT, Shuman WP, Alsofrom GF, Gross CE (1995) Detection of circle of Willis aneurysms in patients with acute subarachnoid hemorrhage: a comparison of CT angiography and digital subtraction angiography. Am J Roentgenol 165:425–30

White GH (1992) Angioscopy. Surg Clin North Am 72:791–821

Wirtz CR, Bonsanto MM, Knauth M, Tronnier VM, Albert FK, Staubert A, Kunze S (1997) Intraoperative magnetic resonance imaging to update interactive navigation in neurosurgery: method and preliminary experience. Comput Aided Surg 2:172–79

Yamakawa K, Kondo T, Yoshioka M, Takakura K (1992) Application of superfine fiberscope for endovasculoscopy, ventriculoscopy, and myeloscopy. Acta Neurochir Suppl (Wien) 54:47–52

Young N, Dorsch NW, Kingston RJ (1999) Pitfalls in the use of spiral CT for identification of intracranial aneurysms. Neuroradiology 41:93–99

10 Virtual Otoscopy

R. Klingebiel

CONTENTS

10.1 Introduction

Complex anatomy and pathology are encountered in the middle and inner ear, representing a challenge to radiological assessment. High-resolution (HR) cross-sectional imaging (CSI) has become accepted for evaluation of the petrosal bone and its compartments (Valvassori et al. 1995). Postprocessing of CSI data permits three-dimensional (3D) visualization and endoscopic views, eliminating the need for mental translation of two-dimensional (2D) images into the real 3D subject.

Virtual endoscopy (VE) and its manifold applications are the subject of this book. As a tool for three-dimensional visualization of intraluminal surfaces, this non-invasive procedure represents a potential competitor for the established "real" endoscopy. Any organ permitting access via a natural orifice may be suitable for endoscopic evaluation, whether for diagnostic or therapeutic purposes. The middle and inner ear, however, do not have easily accessible natural orifices, meaning that in order to conduct a true endoscopic examination, a defect usually has to be created in the tympanic membrane. Iatrogenic dissection of the tympanic membrane for a transtympanic approach carries the risk of incomplete healing at suture sites. The resultant permanent access for pollutants and microbes to the middle ear cavity elevates the risk of infection in patients undergoing this procedure. Patient sedation is required, and the risk of damaging the middle ear structures by endoscopic manoeuvres has to be taken into account, especially if performed exclusively for diagnostic purposes. In endoscopic surgery, aberrant anatomic structures may not be recognised until preparation of the very structure concerned.

Several recent reports on virtual otoscopy (VO) and related 3D techniques (Frankenthaler et al. 1998; Hans et al. 1999; Pozzi-Muvelli et al. 1997; Seemann et al. 1998) indicate that this method may be a useful complementary imaging procedure. VO consists of a computer-generated three-dimensional view of the patient's ear anatomy based on CT or MR cross-sectional images. The computer rendering provides a continuous intraluminal view within which one can navigate along the inner surfaces, similar to other virtual and traditional endoscopy techniques.

In this chapter we report on our experiences with VE and related 3D techniques (VO/3D) using the volume rendering technique (VRT) for the elucidation of middle and inner ear structures and pathology as well as those of the internal acoustic meatus (IAM) and external acoustic meatus (EAM). All figures are derived from data acquired throughout routine diagnostic procedures, i.e. no time-consuming academic protocols without practical relevance were used. None of the images presented here required

R. Klingebiel, MD
Division of Neuroradiology, Department of Radiology, Charité Hospital, Humboldt-Universität zu Berlin, Schumannstrasse 20/21, 10117 Berlin, Germany

specific preparation of the patient, nor was any increase in radiation exposure or examination time necessary.

10.2 Material and Methods

Primary HR imaging was performed on patients transferred from the Department of Otolaryngology, Charité, Berlin, predominantly for assessment of sensorineural hearing impairment. Other common indications were pre- and postoperative imaging in patients with a cholesteatoma and preoperative evaluation for cochlear implantation procedures.

All routine CT or MR imaging techniques that provide HR CSI can be postprocessed to obtain 3D reconstructions (Fig. 10.1a-d).

CT scanning for assessment of bony structures can be performed either using a continuously rotating helical CT system or by incremental CT scanning, with only minor differences in imaging quality. Slice thickness should not exceed 1.5 mm. Overlapping of 1-mm-thick slices may further increase resolution. When performing incremental CT scanning (Somatom, Siemens, Germany), which is slightly superior to helical CT, the following parameters were applied: 120 kV, 85 mAs, 2 s. Further voltage reduction without significant loss of image quality can be achieved. Emphasis should be put on excluding the lenses from the scan area, as especially younger patients may repeatedly be subject to CT evaluation. If one temporal bone is of interest, magnification should be achieved using the raw data, thus preventing an increase in pixel size without any benefit in resolution as encountered by using zoom options available in most workstation software programs. High-resolution (sometimes also called ultra-high) data-processing algorithms are obligatory.

MRI is the method of choice for elucidation of soft tissue and fluid compartments such as the labyrinth and the IAM content. If clinical findings suggest neoplastic retrocochlear lesions, thin-slice (2–3 mm) T1-weighted (T1w) spin-echo images pre-/postcontrast, preferably in the coronary plane, should be obtained. The following parameters were applied: TR 525 ms, TE 14 ms, slice thickness (SL) 2 mm, FOV 160×160, matrix 256×256, number of acquisitions (AC) 2, time of acquisition (TA) 5.53 min.

Precontrast T1w images are indispensable because any ambiguous hyperintensity postcontrast

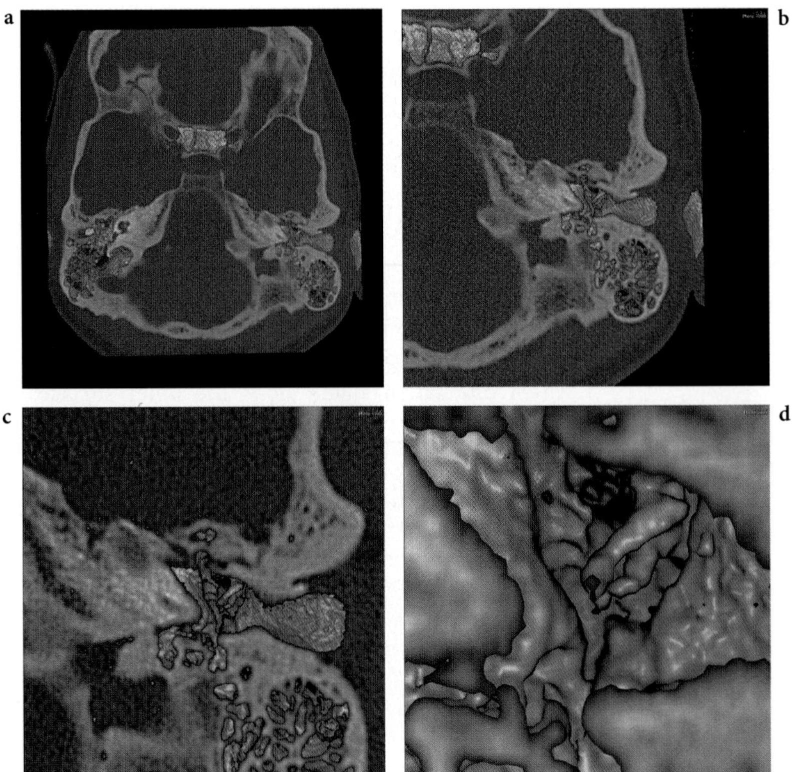

Fig. 10.1a–d. Volume rendering of an axial HRCT slice at the level of the mesotympanum

immediately raises the question of whether it was present precontrast; lipoma and bleeding are rare but important differential diagnoses to intrameatal neurinoma. If more detailed information is necessary or VO is intended, high-resolution 3D MR imaging is advantageous. Heavily T2-weighted gradient echo sequences are commonly applied. We used a 3D CISS sequence (constructive interference in steady state) rendering high contrast and resolution with the following parameters: TR 12,3 ms, TE 5,9 ms, SL 0,5 mm, flip angle 70°, AC 1, TA 10.04 min. We used a 1.5-T MR high-field scanner (Magnetom Vision), manufactured by Siemens, Erlangen, Germany.

The CT/MR images were transferred from the scanner workstations, using internal network connections, to a Spark Ultra 60 computer (Sun Microcomputers, USA) equipped with 3D processing software (Easy Vision 4.3, Philips Medical Systems, The Netherlands).

The data underwent volume rendering and/or segmentation using upper and lower threshold values in order to outline and/or isolate the anatomic structures of interest. Surface shaded views (SSV) were applied. Anatomic structures assessed by VO/3D were the tympanic cavity, the auditory tube, the oval and round windows, the labyrinth and the IAM. Depending on the clinical indication for the procedure, 3D intra- and extraluminal views were used as well as threshold segmentation, focusing on bony and/or soft tissue structures. Interactive endoscopic manoeuvres on the screen were performed in a standard resolution mode in order to reduce operation time, because moving in the *z*-axis especially turned out to be a time-consuming procedure using higher resolution algorithms. For documentation and demonstration purposes, a high-resolution mode or a 512 matrix was applied. The VO radiographs mostly feature a 1024 matrix that is impractical in daily clinical routine because image reconstruction takes so long. Colour-enhanced surface shading generally facilitated orientation but is unlikely to be available for demonstration purposes as most laser printers deliver black and white printouts. Depth cueing permitted selective foreground rendering to the structures of interest.

In order to provide easy access to the virtual endoscopic procedure as documented on film we reviewed and standardised the procedure, defining specific endoscopic viewpoints in accordance with our ENT physicians as seen in Fig. 10.2a-j, thus avoiding "spectacular" radiographic sights of little clinical interest. Our standard procedure comprised the following views: (1–3) 3D SSV of the petrosal bone while approaching the introitus of the external acoustic meatus with the virtual endoscope; (4–5) intraluminal views from a lateral viewpoint into the tympanic cavity; (6) a view from the mesotympanum looking towards the epitympanum; (7) a view from the epitympanum looking towards the meso- and hypotympanum with the articulation of the malleus and incus in the foreground; (8) a view into the auditory tube from the mesotympanum; (9) a view facing the oval and round window. Although the first three images may seem superfluous, they were included to enhance acceptance of VO, since untrained readers have been documented on film as saying that this makes it easier to follow the approach to the ear. Special indications such as detailed assessment of radical cavities after cholesteatoma operation profited from cooperative, interactive VO together with the ENT physician.

General technical information on hardware and software configuration for virtual endoscopy is given elsewhere in this book.

10.3 Anatomy

Applying virtual endoscopic techniques, we were able to visualise all middle ear structures of clinical interest with good correlation to the original 2D CT cross-sectional data in 3D. Especially the ossicles (Fig. 10.2f), the physiological orifices (Fig. 10.2j), the auditory tube (Fig. 10.2i) and the epitympanic recess (Fig. 10.2 g) were routinely assessed throughout VO evaluation. Suitable thresholding permitted imaging of soft tissue structures such as the tensor tympani muscle. Incomplete imaging of the stapes suprastructure was encountered due to partial volume effects of the tiny anterior and posterior crus.

For elucidation of the IAM we used HR CSI data and were able to image cranial nerves VII and VIII from an intraluminal viewpoint as well as their respective contours, tailoring the shape of the IAM as seen from an external anterior viewpoint (Fig. 10.3a-d). The superior and inferior vestibular, cochlear and facial nerves were able to be assessed by using the original CISS 3D images and their reconstructions as well as by VO. If the integrity of the bony walls of the IAM had to be demonstrated, evaluation of cross-sectional CT data was necessary with optional 3D imaging.

For 3D imaging of the labyrinth, CT and/or MRI data were used depending on the clinical indication. If

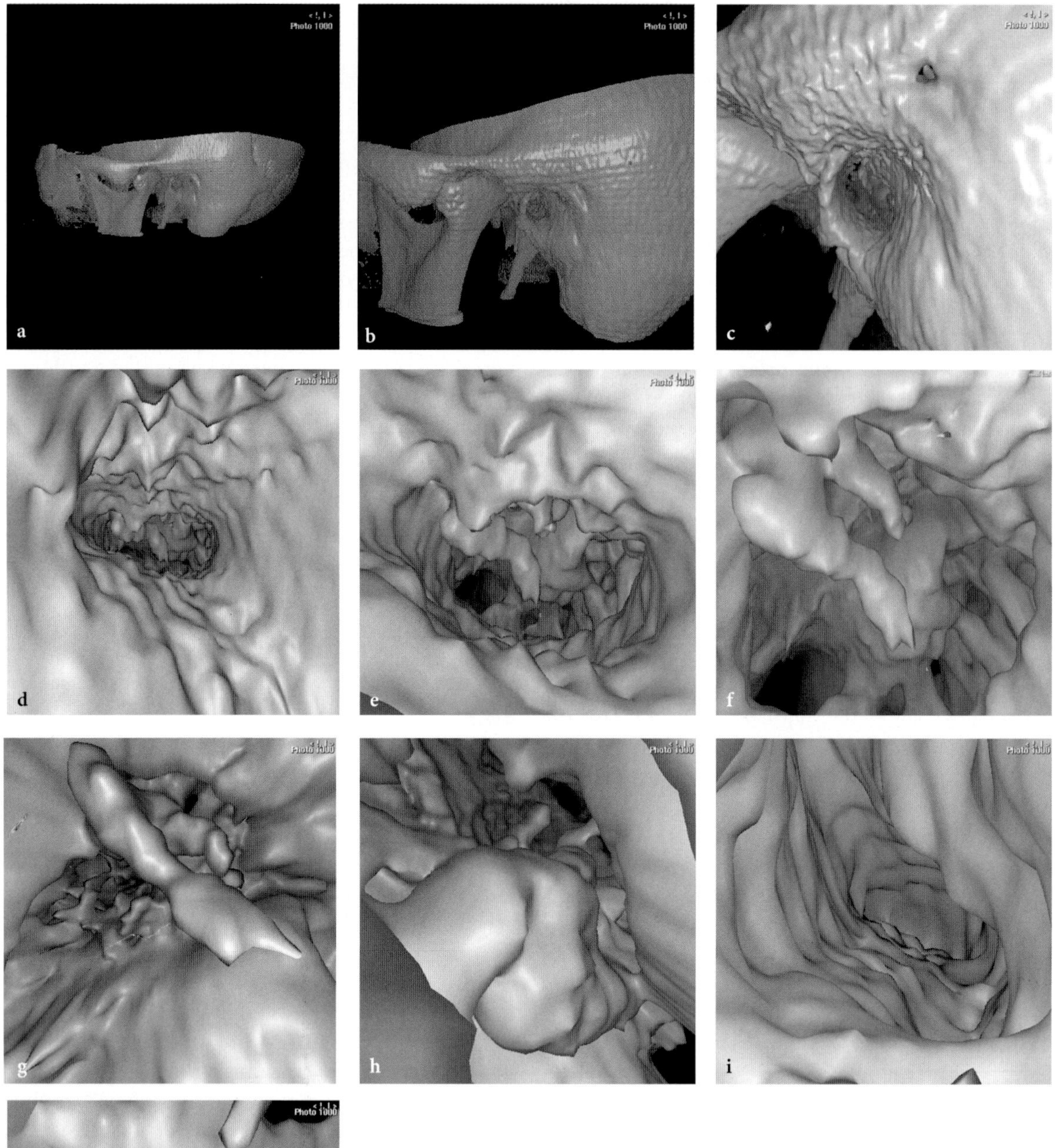

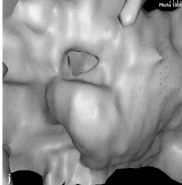

Fig. 10.2a–j. Virtual otoscopy. **a–c** The virtual otoscope (VOE) approaches the introitus of the left external acoustic meatus. **d** Intraluminal view of the EAM from the introitus. **e, f** The VOE approaches the entrance of the tympanic cavity, incus and malleus in the foreground. **g–i** Different endoscopic views: **g** up to the epitympanum, **h** down into the mesotympanum, **i** into the auditory tube. **j** Endoscopic view facing the oval window and promontory

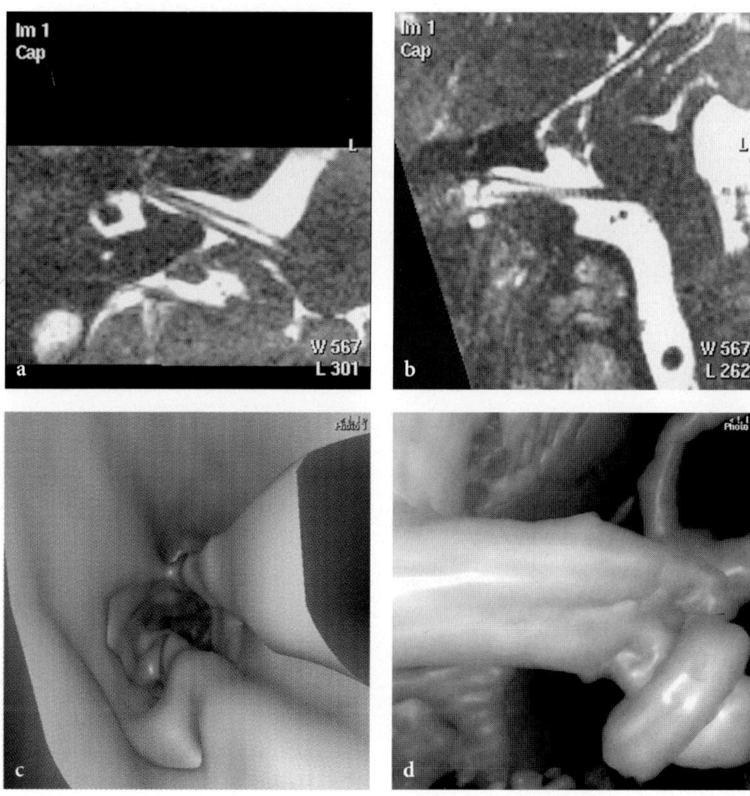

Fig. 10.3a–d. Visualisation of cranial nerves VII and VIII. **a, b** MPRs of HR T2w MRI data (CISS sequence), showing cranial nerves VII and VIII along their course from the brainstem into the IAM. **c** Endoluminal view of cranial nerves VII + VIII. **d** 3D SSV facing the internal acoustic meatus and the cochlea

bony obliteration of the cochlea is suspected, MRI for 3D imaging is not obligatory as subtracting the petrosal bone by segmentation leaves the operator with a soft-tissue-generated view of the cochlea (Fig. 10.4). In the case of preoperative assessment before placement of a cochlear implant, fibrous obliteration of the cochlea has to be excluded as well, creating a need for MRI work-up. In this case the VRT renders extraluminal 3D views of the labyrinth (Fig. 10.5a-c) as well as navigation through the cochlea and semicircular ducts (Fig. 10.6a,b) as an endoluminal approach.

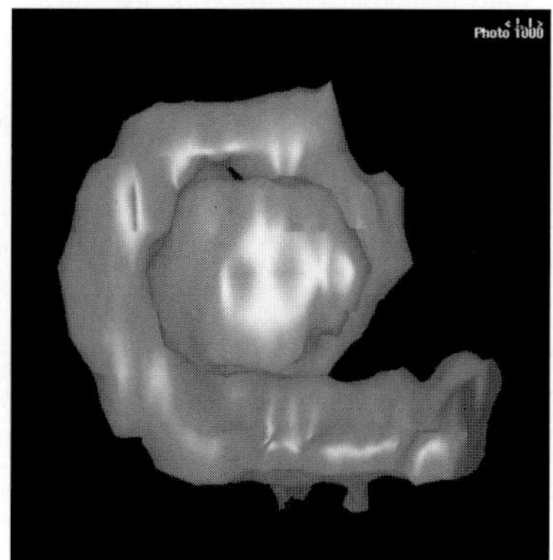

Fig. 10.4. SSV of the cochlea, derived from HRCT data

10.4 Pathology

10.4.1 Dysplasia/Malformation

Malformations of the middle ear may be expressed as slight ossicular dysplasia as well as almost complete agenesis. Associated abnormalities of the external auditory canal and the auricula such as microtia may also occur (Valvassori et al. 1995). Aberrance of the facial canal (Fig. 10.7a,b) or agenesis of the bony canal represents important information for the ENT surgeon before starting middle ear surgery.

Malformations of the ossicular chain are recognisable on HRCT images, but nevertheless 3D SSV/VO may be helpful to illustrate complex morphologic alterations (Fig. 10.8a–d).

Dysplasia of the inner ear such as a Mondini malformation can be assessed with MRI and HRCT as well (Fig. 10.9a–c). Dysplasia and agenesis of the semicircular ducts may be another indication for HRCT (Fig. 10.10a–d) and MRI. The bilateral enlargement of the endolymphatic duct and sac in Fig. 10.11a–c are depicted without additional 3D imaging, whereas the associated dysplasia of the semicir-

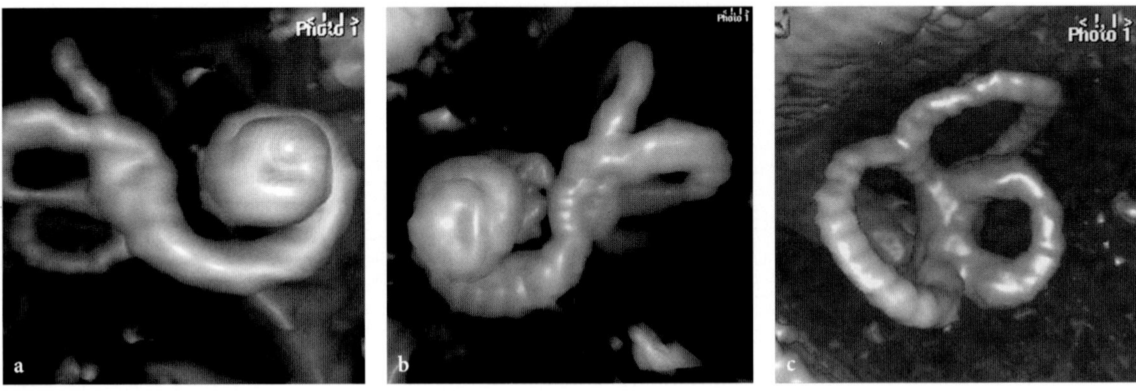

Fig. 10.5a–c. SSVs of the cochlea and vestibulum (**a**), the inner ear from anterior (**b**) and the semicircular ducts (SCDs) from craniolateral (**c**)

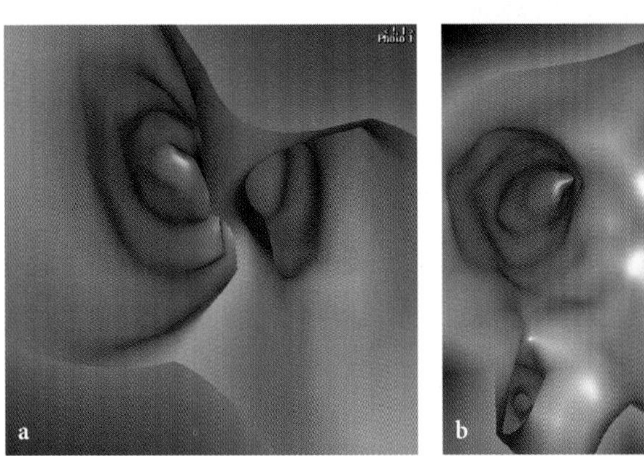

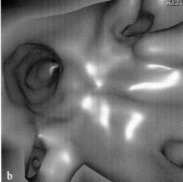

Fig. 10.6a,b. Endoluminal views of the labyrinth. **a** Endoluminal view of the basal turn of the cochlea, showing the interosseous spiral membrane as well as the vestibular and tympanic canal. **b** Endoluminal view of the vestibulum, facing the introitus of the SCDs

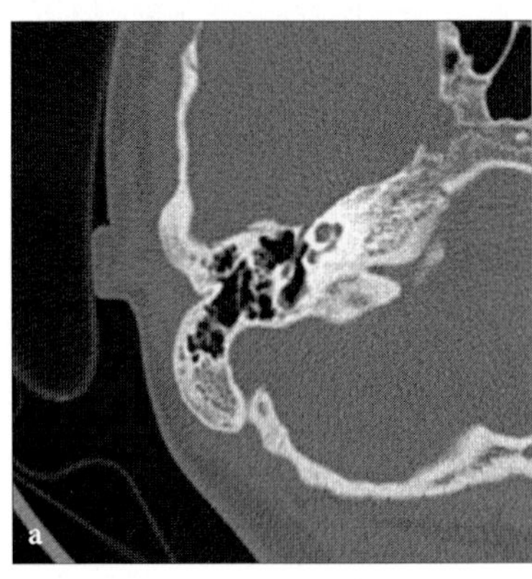

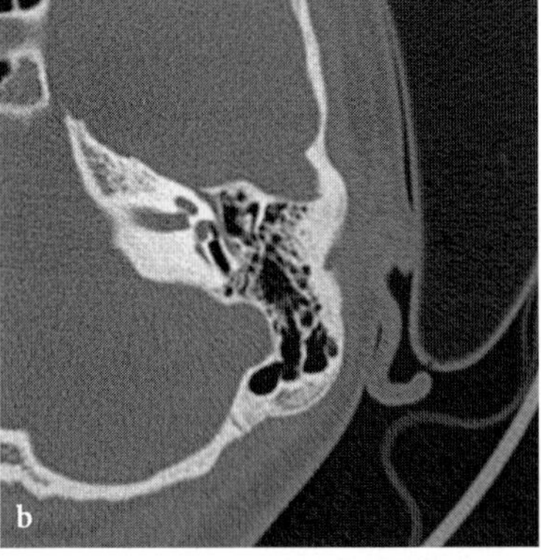

Fig. 10.7a,b. Laterally displaced right facial canal. **a** Axial HRCT slice; the facial canal is displaced towards the mesotympanum. **b** Contralateral axial HRCT slice; normal course of the facial canal

cular ducts is appreciated more comprehensively in the 3D SSV reconstruction.

10.4.2 Otodystrophy

Otodystrophy comprises a group of diseases which may affect the middle and inner ear, often characterised by pathologic ossifications and/or alterations of the bony micro- and macroarchitecture and by irregular intraluminal calcifications. HRCT is an excellent technique for imaging intra- and extraluminal bone pathology and can additionally detect bony enlargement and structural alterations (Paget's disease, fibrous dysplasia, osteopetrosis) as well as otosclerotic plaques in the tympanic cavity and labyrinth. Figure 10.12a–e shows reformatted HRCT images and VE

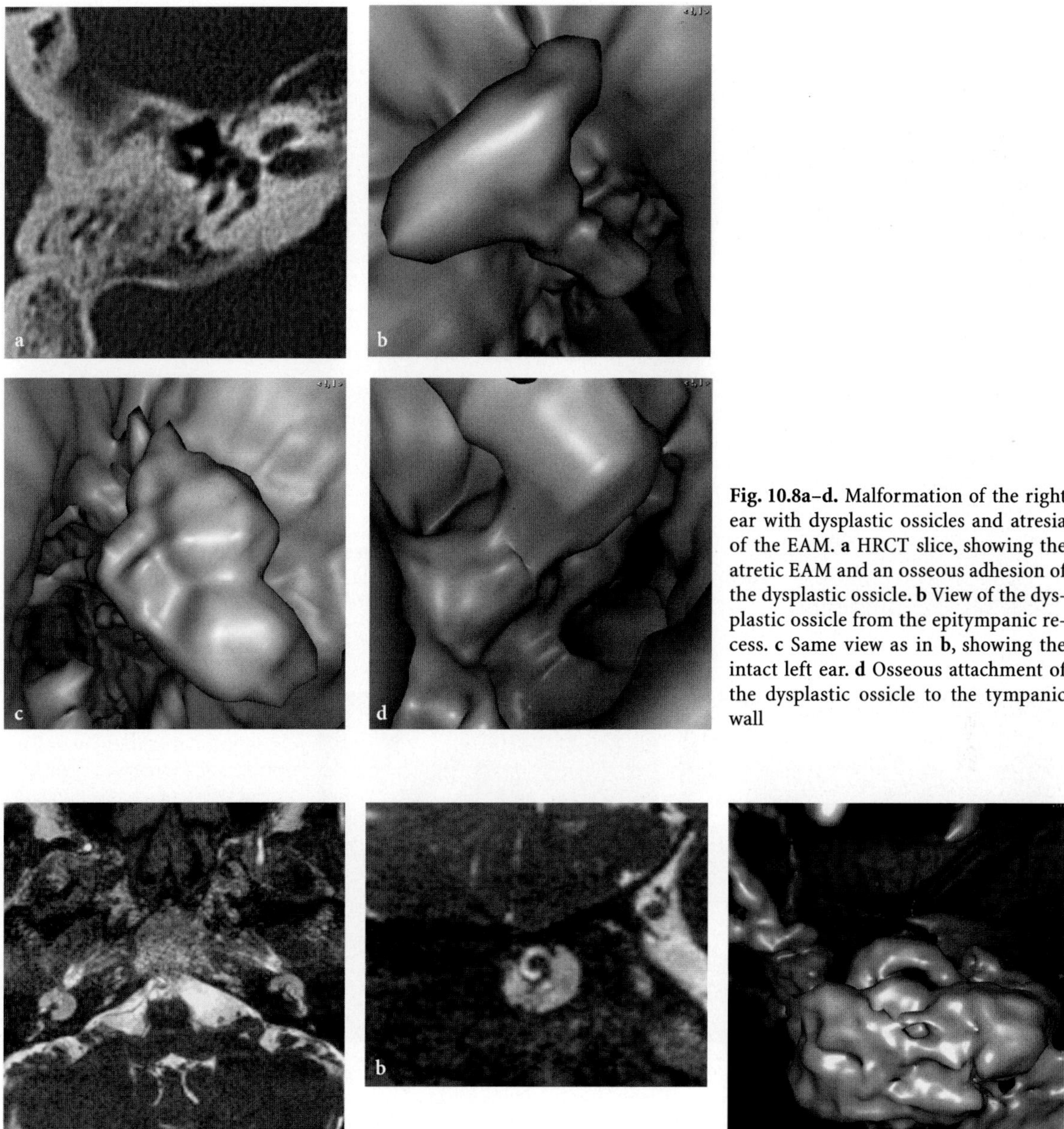

Fig. 10.8a–d. Malformation of the right ear with dysplastic ossicles and atresia of the EAM. **a** HRCT slice, showing the atretic EAM and an osseous adhesion of the dysplastic ossicle. **b** View of the dysplastic ossicle from the epitympanic recess. **c** Same view as in **b**, showing the intact left ear. **d** Osseous attachment of the dysplastic ossicle to the tympanic wall

Fig. 10.9a–c. Bilateral Mondini malformation. **a** Axial HR MRI slice (CISS sequence), showing bilateral enlargement of the basal cochlear turn. **b** Paracoronal MPR of the right cochlea. **c** SSV of the cochlea, showing an enlarged fluid-filled cavity at the site of the basal turn

images of a young boy being assessed for osteopetrosis. Focal petrosal bone sclerosis was demonstrated. Unfortunately, bilateral high-grade stenosis of the optic canal was present due to sphenoid bone hyperplasia aggravated by a bony septum in the left optic canal (virtual endoscopic view).

Exostosis may be another reason for bony obliteration, as in the patient in Fig. 10.13a–d, who suffered from bilateral high-grade narrowing of the EAM.

Enhancement of otosclerotic lesions has been described using dedicated T1w imaging (Casselmann 1996; Casselmann and Bensimon 1994; Casselmann et al. 1994) and should be performed especially if labyrinth involvement is suspected. VO/3D images may show endoluminal obliteration due to sclerotic plaques directly using CT data, or indirectly, by absence of fluid signal in CISS 3D MR images.

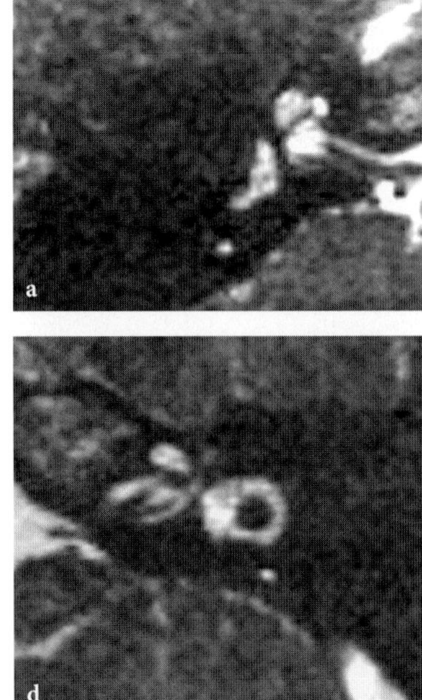
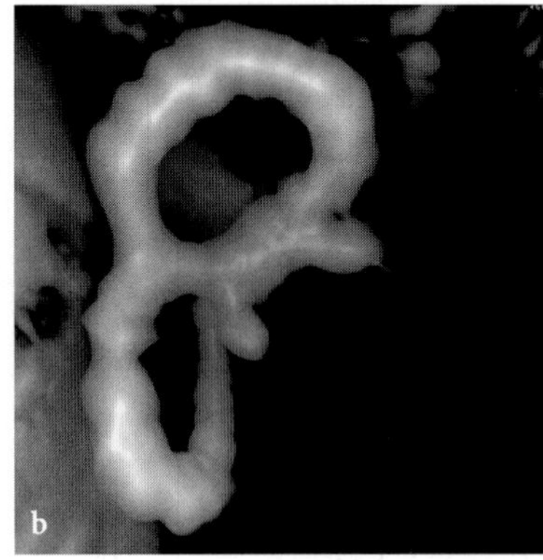
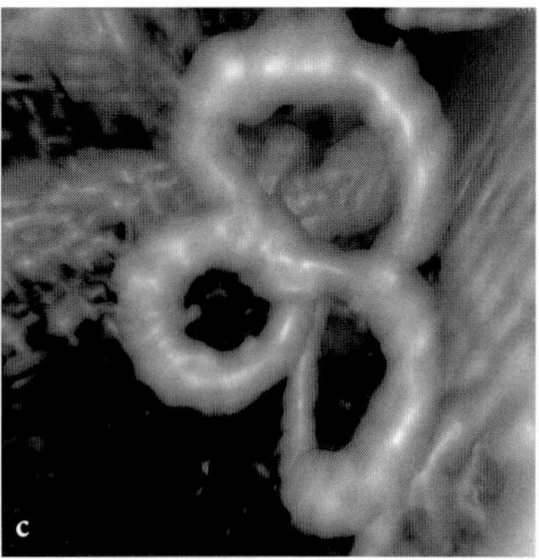

Fig. 10.10a–d. Dysplasia of the right lateral SCD. **a** Axial HR MRI slice (CISS sequence), showing the hypoplastic right lateral SCD. **b** 3D SSV corresponding to Fig. 9b. **c, d** Views of the left lateral SCD corresponding to Fig. 9a, b

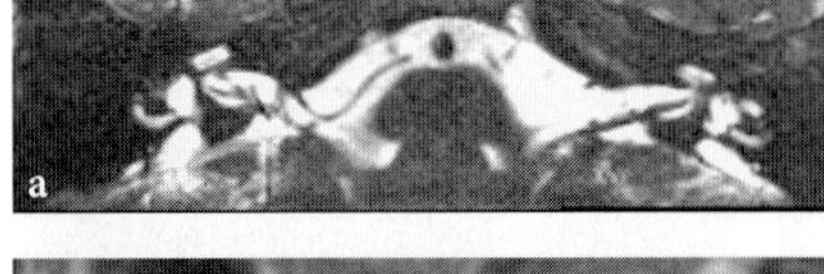
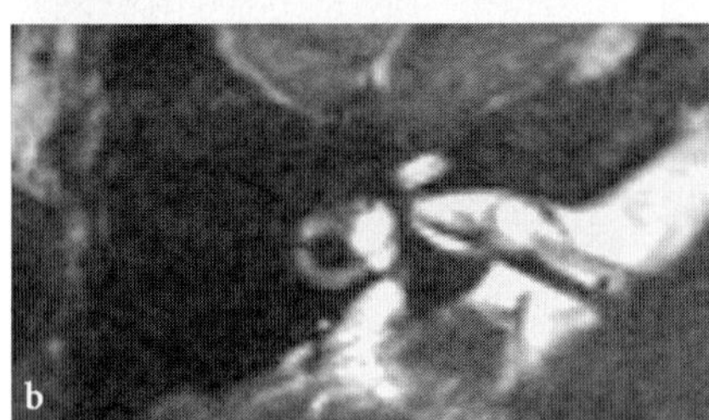
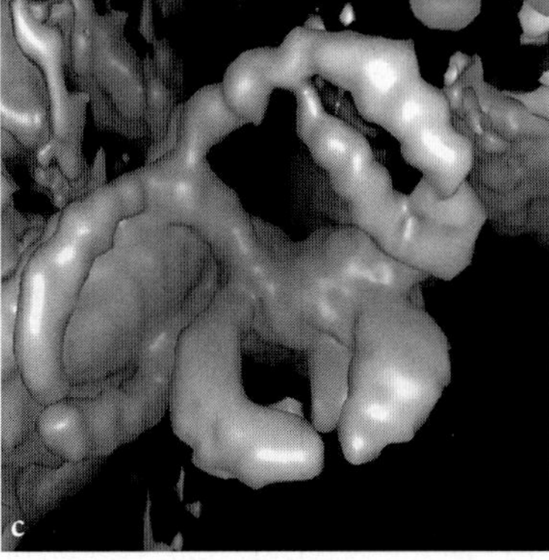

Fig. 10.11a–c. Bilaterally enlarged endolymphatic duct and sac. **a** Axial HR MRI slice, showing the enlarged endolymphatic duct and sac. **b** Axial HR MRI slice of the right side; the enlarged endolymphatic duct and a partial obliteration of the lateral SCD can be seen. **c** SSV of the right SCD; a complex dysplasia of all SCD is present

10.4.3 Trauma

If, following trauma, clinical neurological examination indicates the presence of a central neurological deficit, emergency CT to rule out intracranial haemorrhage is obligatory, using the soft tissue (brain) accompanied by the bone window. If there is any indication that temporal bone may have been fractured (otorrhoea, haematotympanum, peripheral paresis of the facial nerve), dedicated thin-slice CT (1–2 mm) will provide further information. Thus superior quality MPRs are available along with optional VO to elucidate ossicle trauma and involvement of the tympanic walls, especially when liquorrhoea suggests the presence of a dural fistula. Impairment of sound conduction is a common complication of longitudinal fractures of the petrosal bone, whereas a transverse fracture should raise suspicion of inner ear involvement. Fractures of the long axis of the temporal bone are more common and account for up to 80% of all petrosal fractures. The patient in Fig. 10.14a–f (original data not acquired in HR mode) has suffered from a transverse fracture of the petrosal bone; dislocation of the ossicles, as well as their bony adherence to the tympanic walls, are demonstrated.

Another possible complication of petrosal trauma may be intralabyrinthine haemorrhage, as can be detected with thin-slice T1w imaging. Post-traumatic alterations of the labyrinth, such as fibrous obliteration subsequent to a transverse fracture, are illustrated on

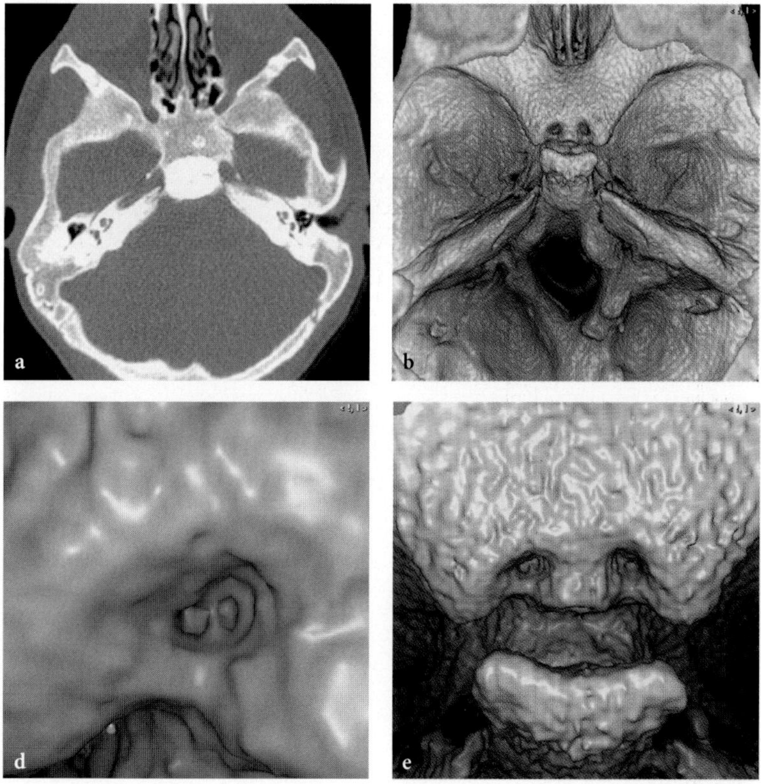

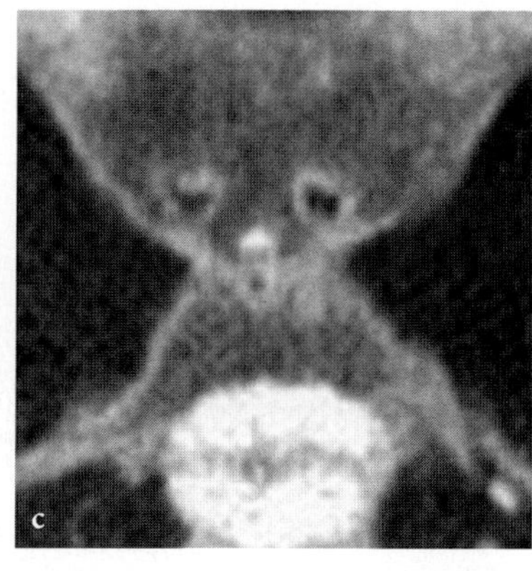

Fig. 10.12a–e. Osteopetrosis in a 17-year-old male. **a** Axial HRCT slice, showing bilateral osteosclerotic lesions in the petrosal bone. **b** SSV into the middle cranial fossa, showing a hypertrophied dorsum sellae. **c** Paraaxial HRCT MPR of the optic canal, showing high-grade bilateral narrowing and a small bony septum in the left canal. **d, e** SSV of the bilaterally stenosed optic canal, on the left side subdivided by a bony septum

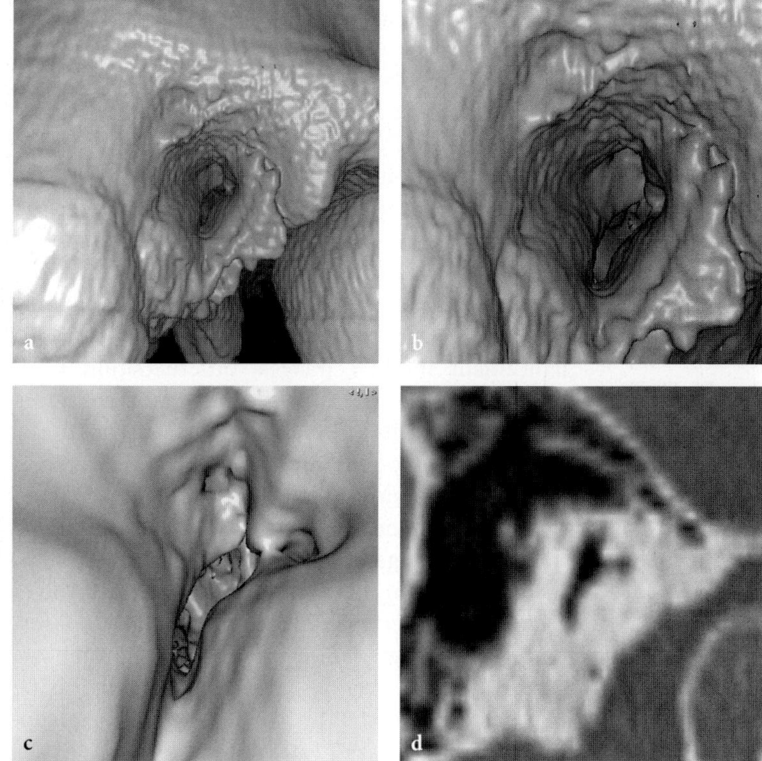

Fig. 10.13a–d. High-grade stenosis of the left EAM by exostosis. **a, b** External view into the left EAM; the bony stenosis can already be seen. **c** Endoluminal view of the left EAM, showing the small residual lumen that restricts the view into the tympanum. **d** Parasagittal MPR corresponding to **b, c**

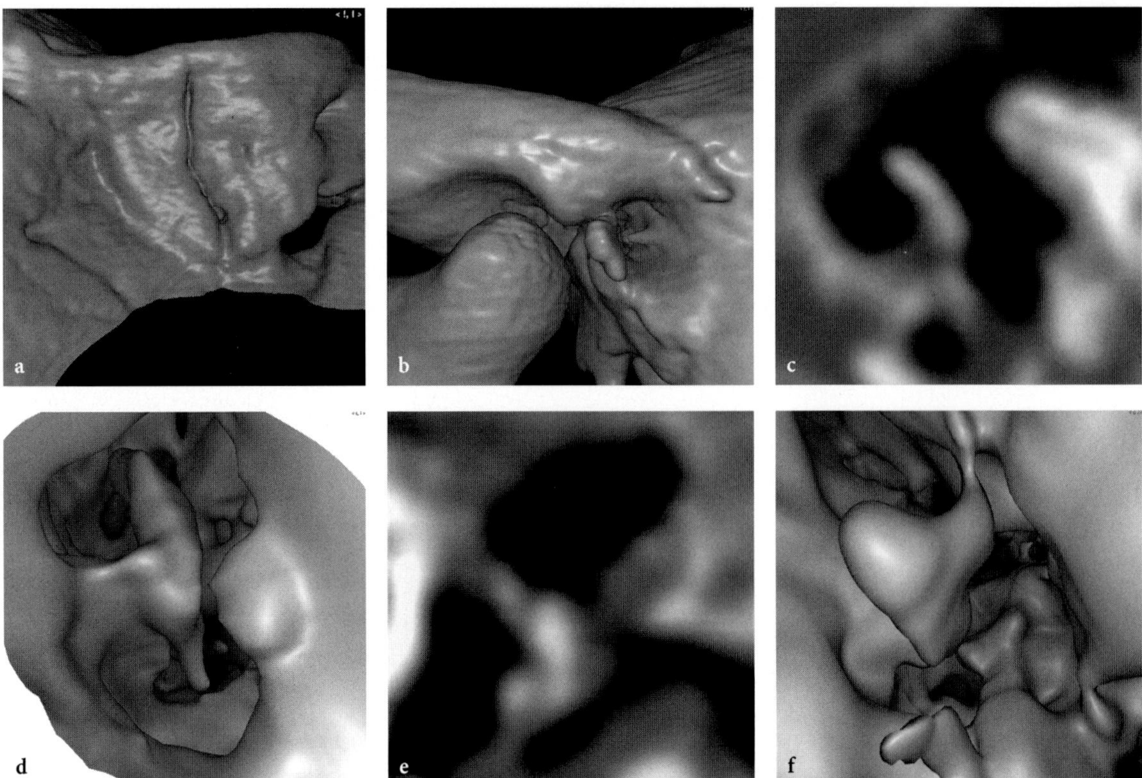

Fig. 10.14a–f. A 20-year-old female patient who had suffered a severe cranial trauma with transverse fracture of the left petrosal bone a year earlier; data were not acquired in a high-resolution mode. **a** SSV of the left temporal bone from posterior; the incomplete ossified fracture is well visualised. **b** View from lateral to the introitus of the EAM; a bony spur of the posterior wall is recognisable. **c** Parasagittal MPR of the tympanum; post-traumatic ossicle dysplasia with adhesion to the tympanic walls is visualised. **d** Endoluminal view corresponding to **c**. **e** Paracoronal MPR of the tympanum, showing further adhesive fixation of the ossicle. **f** Epitympanic endoluminal view onto the ossicle and its fibrous adhesion to the anterior tympanic wall

CISS 3D images. Subtle alterations of the labyrinthine fluid signal should prompt 3D reconstruction if 2D MIP reconstructions are inconclusive.

A traumatic perilabyrinthine fistula has been described as detectable on T1w images postcontrast due to the accompanying reactive inflammation (Karhuketo et al. 1997).

10.4.4 Inflammation

10.4.4.1 Acute Inflammation

Acute inflammatory diseases of the tympanic cavity are primarily subject to clinical rather than radiological investigation. Complications of acute otitis media, especially extension into the temporal bone, may be visualised by HRCT, showing opacification of the mastoid cells as well as destruction of their trabecular architecture. Mastoiditis is indicated by signal elevation in any MR sequence; however, increased signal intensity in the petrosal bone is also a common incidental finding. ENT physicians prefer the term "retained secretions" rather than "mastoiditis", in order to avoid unnecessary escalation of diagnostic and therapeutic procedures. As mastoid inflammation may lead to strong but inhomogeneous enhancement in T1w images, differentiation from non-inflammatory lesions such as glomus tumours requires HRCT to assess the trabecular structures.

Inflammatory penetration into the middle cranial fossa must be suspected if erosion of the tegmen tympani is evident in coronal and/or sagittal reformations. Once again, VO is not necessary but is helpful in visualising the bony defects. Dural involvement is indicated by enhancement in T1w images, and clinical signs of sigmoid sinus thrombosis should prompt venous MR angiography using phase-contrast or 2D time-of-flight (TOF) sequences. Also indicated are T2w turbo spin-echo (TSE)and gradient-echo (GE) sequences (dark fluid sequence/TIRM) to rule out encephalitis and intraparenchymal evidence of sinus venous thrombosis such as oedema and haemorrhage.

Acute labyrinthitis, as may occur following upper respiratory tract infections, can lead to a breakdown of the blood–labyrinth barrier, resulting in labyrinthine enhancement on T1w images.

Neuritis of the facial nerve may cause enhancement in the IAM in T1w thin-slice images pre- and postcontrast.

10.4.4.2 Chronic Inflammation

Inflammatory involvement of the auricula and the EAM is usually subject to clinical assessment. VE may assist in showing the extent of bony erosion beyond the overlying soft tissue, as in Fig. 10.15a–e. In this patient, the physician noticed ulcerations at the bottom of the EAM.

Chronic middle ear inflammation is characterised by an increase in size of the trabecular septa of the mastoid cells, followed by cell obliteration and a decrease in mastoid pneumatisation – a condition that can be nicely demonstrated by cross-sectional HRCT. Common complications are ossicle erosions, particularly concerning the long crus of the incus and the manubrium of the malleus (Czerny et al. 1997). Although the erosions may be depicted on axial HRCT images, they are much easier to demonstrate with VO views.

Common sequelae of labyrinthitis are obliterations, whether fibrous or calcified. Fibrous obliteration leads to an interruption of the labyrinthine fluid signals (Casselmann et al. 1994), as can be seen on CISS 3D images or, even better, on 3D SSV of the semicircular ducts. MRI alone does not permit differentiation between fibrous and osseous obliteration, so HRCT scans may be indicated.

10.4.5 Cholesteatoma

Cholesteatomas are subdivided into acquired and primary cholesteatomas, the latter also known as epidermoids. Primary cholesteatomas are often located in the petrosal apex and typically present with a hypointense signal in T1w and a hyperintense signal in T2w sequences. CT may show a soft tissue mass of low density.

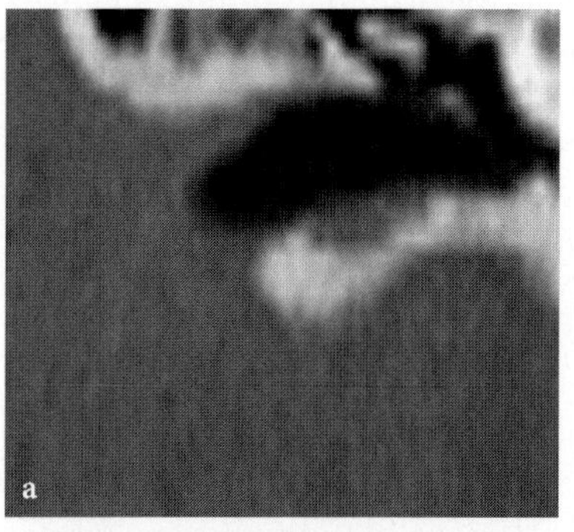

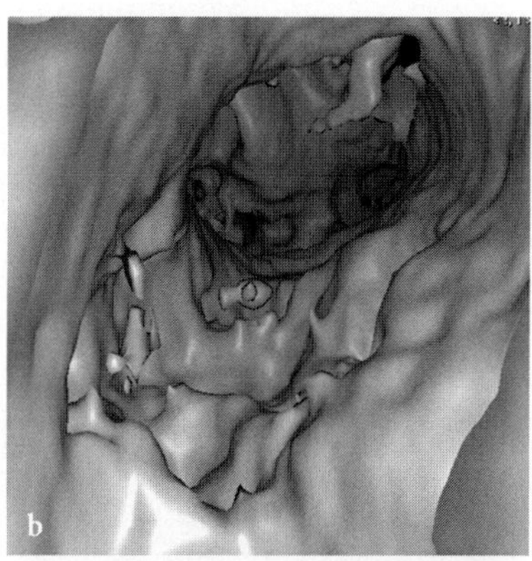

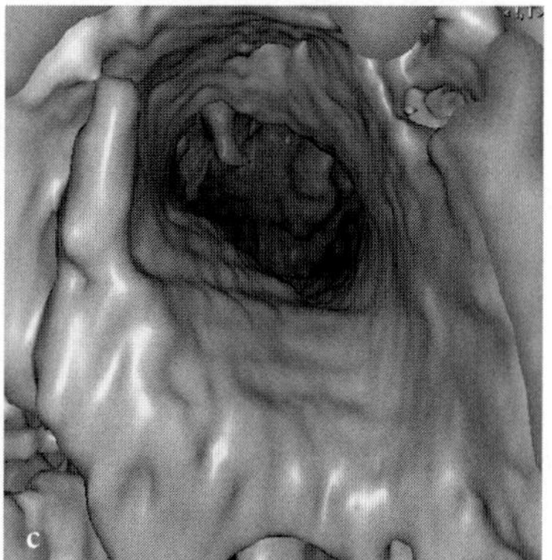

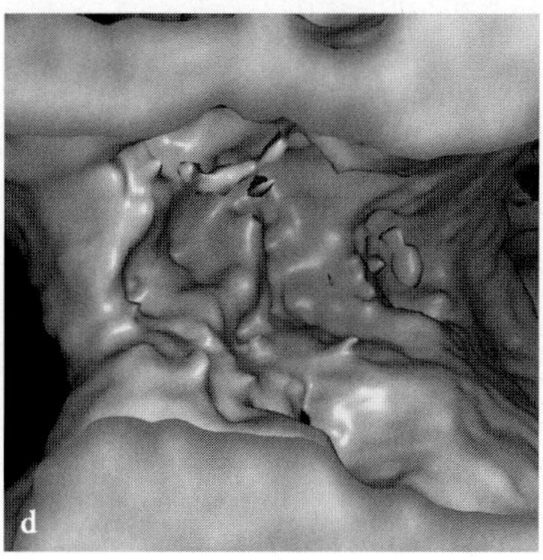

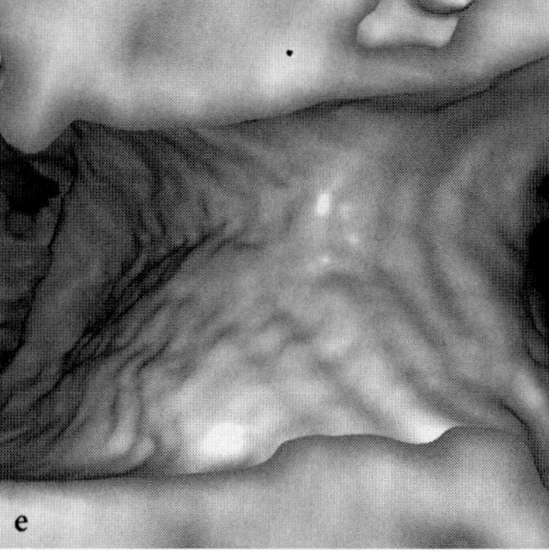

Fig. 10.15a–e. Ulcerations at the bottom of the right external acoustic meatus. **a** Coronal MPR, showing soft tissue eroding the EAM floor. **b, c** Endoluminal views (bone thresholding) of the right (**b**) and left (**c**) EAM. **d, e** Endoluminal views down to the bottom of the right (**d**) and left (**e**) EAM

Acquired cholesteatomas may arise from the pars flaccida or the pars tensa of the tympanic membrane, thus expanding differently within the tympanic cavity. Pars flaccida cholesteatomas should raise suspicion of bony epitympanic erosions including the caput mallei, whereas those derived from the pars tensa preferentially extend to the tympanic recess and may dislocate the ossicles and erode the malleus and incus. A cholesteatoma recurrence was suspected in the patient in Fig. 10.16a–c because of erosive irregularities of the epitympanum; the diagnosis was intraoperatively confirmed. For both types of cholesteatomas, HRCT provides all clinically important information. Nevertheless, orientation within the affected tympanic cavity, assessment of morphology and positioning of the ossicles is easier using VO. Both kinds of cholesteatoma may erode the bony wall of the lateral semicircular duct, inducing a labyrinthine fistula. Again, HRCT depicts the bony destruction whereas MRI assesses the replacement of discharged fluid by fibrous tissue.

3D visualization may again be advantageous in demonstrating bony destruction and should be employed for comprehensive assessment of the labyrinth.

The MRI signal intensities of cholesteatomas are rather unspecific, sometimes showing peripheral enhancement due to granulation tissue.

10.4.6 Tumours

10.4.6.1 Benign Tumours

The most common benign tumour in the middle ear is a tympanic glomus tumour, located near the promontory and showing strong enhancement in T1w images. It may be differentiated from high-riding jugular glomus tumours by assessing the edges of the promontory and the size of the jugular foramen/fossa, the latter being enlarged in jugular glomus tumours. Facial nerve Schwannomas (Fig. 10.17a-d), adenomas and cholesterol granulomas, amongst other benign lesions of the middle ear and mastoid, are assessed by cross-sectional imaging. MR imaging pre- and postcontrast is necessary as a supplementary diagnostic procedure to primary CT scanning. VO is performed in the same way as for cholesteatomas.

The labyrinth may be affected by intraluminal tumours such as Schwannomas which are accessible to T1w MR imaging pre-/postcontrast. Schwannomas may be differentiated from intraluminal postinflammatory fibrosis by their slightly hyperintense signal in precontrast T1w images. For other rare tumour entities, the reader is referred to specialist ENT textbooks. Involvement of the labyrinth may also occur by continuous expansion of glomus tumours, cholesterol granulomas, cholesteatomas and other tumours.

The destructive process in the petrosal apex of the patient in Fig. 10.18a,b was diagnosed as a chondroma; in this case, the extent of bony destruction is well

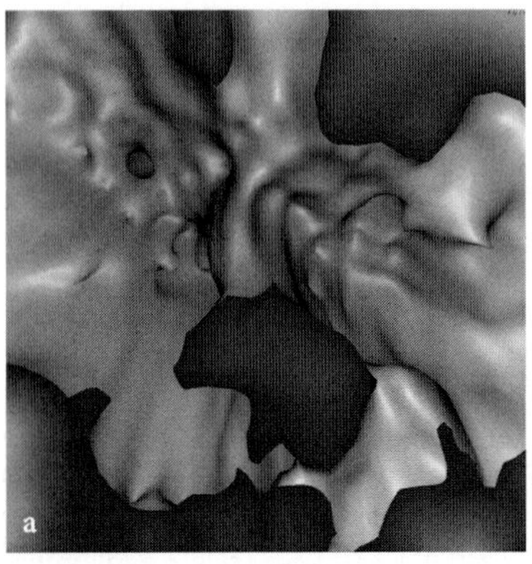

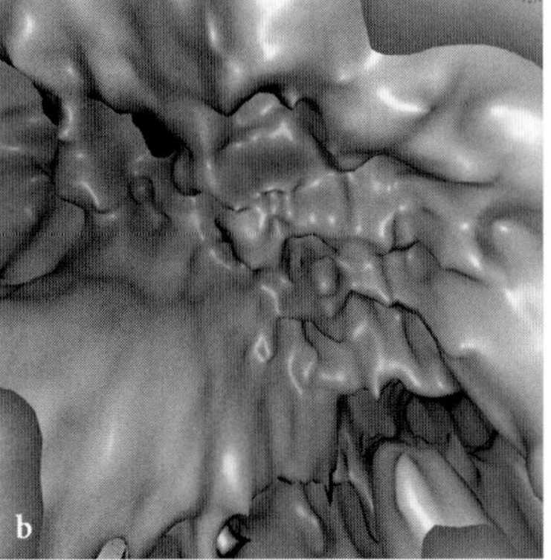

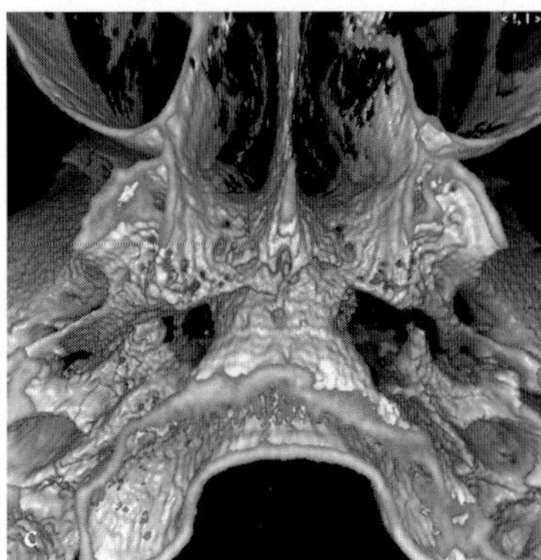

Fig. 10.16a–c. Cholesteatoma recurrence. **a** Coronal MPR, showing erosive irregularities of the tegmen tympani. **b** Endoluminal view to the tegmen tympani; data PP by the use of a bone thresholding protocol. **c** Same view as in **b**, using a soft tissue thresholding protocol. The difference between the real endoscopic view and pathologic findings beyond this view is well depicted

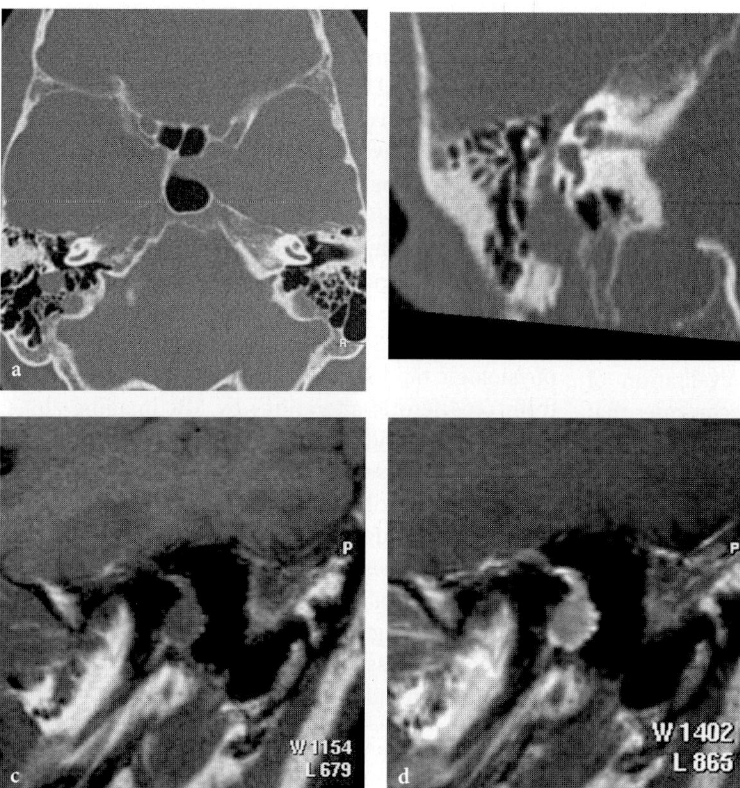

Fig. 10.17a–d. Schwannoma of the facial nerve. **a** Axial HRCT slice showing the mastoid segment of the facial canal. **b** MPR of the facial canal; enlarged mastoid segment. **c, d** T1w parasagittal slices pre-/postcontrast; the enhancing Schwannoma is well delineated

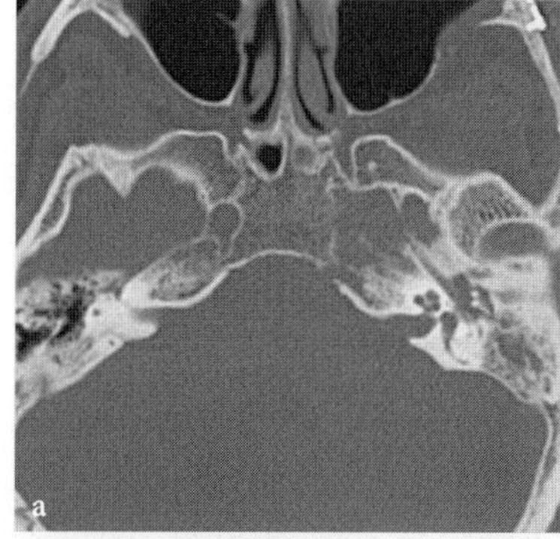

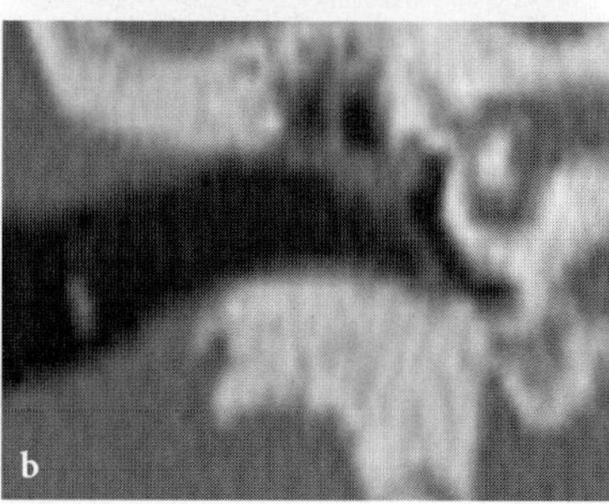

Fig. 10.18a,b. Chondroma of the left petrosal bone apex. **a** Axial HRCT slice; the irregularities of the petrosal apex are well recognisable. **b** 3D SSV corresponding to **a**

depicted by HRCT; 3D SSVs do not add substantially new information. In order to differentiate Schwannomas, bleeding, or rare lipomas from other lesions, pre- and postcontrast T1w imaging is indispensable. CISS 3D sequences and their MIP reformations are helpful for an appreciation of the labyrinthine invasion; VO/3D imaging serves as a supplement to the CISS protocol.

10.4.6.2
Malignant Tumors

Malignant neoplasms of the middle ear are a rather rare finding and demand extensive imaging preoperatively using pre- and postcontrast CT/MRI protocols. Tumours such as squamous cell carcinomas, adenocarcinomas, metastatic lesions and sarcomas may be mentioned here. If the tumour is accessible by "real" endoscopy, optional biopsy may be indicated. CT again shows the extension of bony destruction, whereas MRI may contribute to the specification of the neoplastic lesion and help identify intracranial dural or parenchymal invasion. As radical surgery is usually necessary, VO may not be of any additional benefit.

These tumours may secondarily affect the labyrinth, and the degree of labyrinth invasion can be visualised by CISS sequences, showing aborted fluid signal. VO may be considered if the case does not involve dealing with a mass lesion right away.

10.4.7 Preoperative Assessment

High-resolution cross-sectional imaging plays an important role in the preoperative evaluation of middle and inner ear pathology. The techniques that may be employed have been mentioned earlier and need to be adapted to the clinical findings.

A sigmoid sinus dislocation, an aberrant course of the facial nerve (Fig. 10.7a–b) or agenesis of its bony canal and a high-riding bulb of jugular vein are, amongst other findings, important information for the ENT surgeon. For special purposes, such as soft tissue obliterated radical cavities, documentation of the same endoscopic view in bone as well as soft tissue segmentation may be helpful. The extent of bony destruction behind the overlying soft tissue can thus be demonstrated (Fig. 10.19a–f).

If a (partial) ossicle resection has been performed and postoperative results have to be checked, VO views of the operation site are complementary to HRCT CSI (Fig. 10.20a,b).

If cochlear implantation is intended in a patient with sensorineural hearing loss, both CT and MRI are essential. Fibrous obliteration of the labyrinth can be detected by CISS sequences due to abortion of the physiologic fluid signal but may not be differentiated from otosclerotic alterations by MR imaging alone. Consequently both techniques, MRI as well as CT, are necessary because a fibrous obliteration restricted to only one canal still may permit CI whereas a labyrinthitis ossificans does not. In the case of purely fibrous obliteration, VO assessment of the patency of the vestibular and tympanic canals may be of special interest, although investigations into this procedure are currently in progress and therefore little information is available about its accuracy.

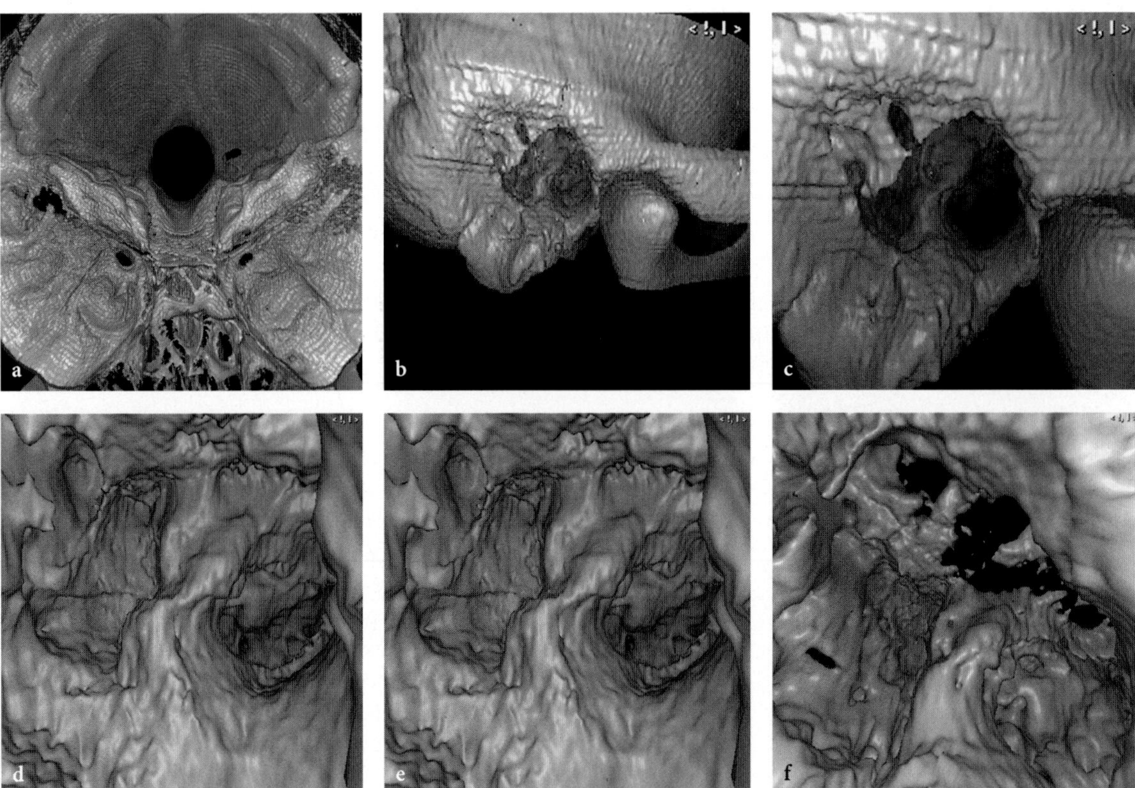

Fig. 10.19a–f. Postoperative radical cavity (cholesteatoma). **a** SSV from anterocranial onto the middle cranial fossa shows the defect of the right tegmen tympani. **b, c** The VO approaches the radical cavity. **d** Soft tissue thresholded view of the radical cavity. **e** Same view as in **d**. **f** Endoluminal view of the tegmen tympani; the bony defects of the tegmen tympani and the posterior cavity wall at the level of the sigmoid sinus are demonstrated

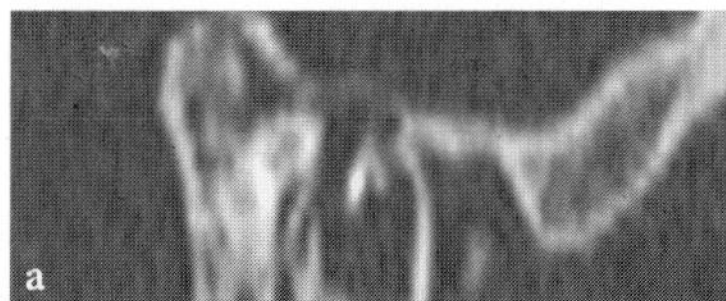

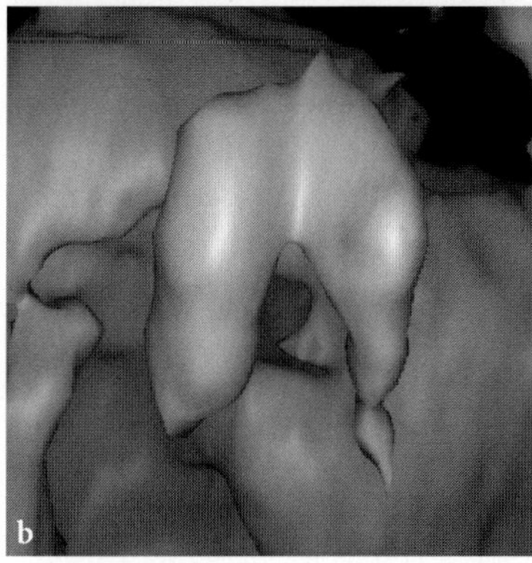

Fig. 10.20a,b. After tympanoplastic operation with partial ossicle resection. **a** Paracoronal MPR of the residual ossicles. **b** Endoluminal view corresponding to **a**

10.4.8 Postoperative Assessment

Postoperative management including CSI may be necessary for follow-up of tumour patients, assessment of the positioning of implant material and/or evaluation of postoperative complications such as infection, unexpected functional impairment, etc. Once again, the imaging technique must be closely related to the clinical information and standardised imaging protocols may be inadequate.

The enhancement encountered on CT/MR images postcontrast may simply represent granulation tissue, and hyperintensities on postcontrast T1w images may represent blood substrates rather than inflammatory enhancement. Imaging results should be discussed with the ENT surgeon concerned before releasing the final report, since the surgeon is best informed as to what may be a physiological postoperative finding.

In cochlear implant patients, electrode positioning sometimes cannot be performed in the normal way. Assessment of dislocation or malpositioning of the tip of the electrode can be achieved by CSI, whereas 3D SSV/VO may assist in illustrating the findings, as seen in Fig. 10.21a–e. The tip is located right in front of the round window; introduction into the basal cochlear turn has not been achieved. Other findings include fibrous adhesion of the malleus to the electrode (Fig. 10.21d,e). Endoscopy of the cochlea itself for evaluation of patency of areas scheduled for electrode implementation and preoperative simulation purposes is also possible, but this is still experimental work in our department. Another patient whose preoperative work-up suggested no especial problems, yet in whom there were difficulties with correct intraoperative placement of the electrode is shown in Fig. 10.22a,b. In this case the electrode is located in the basal cochlear turn, as introduction further in was not achieved.

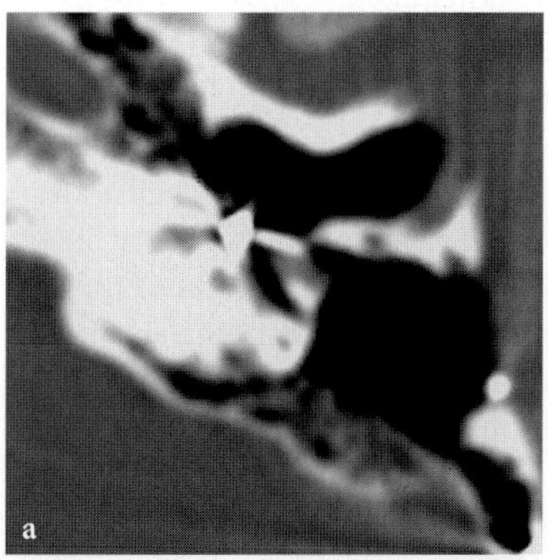

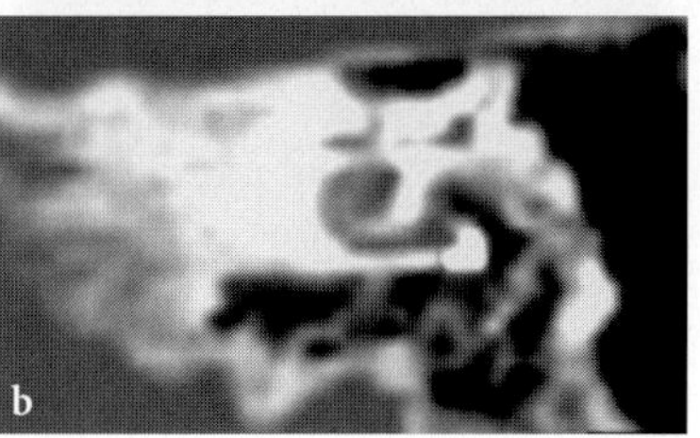

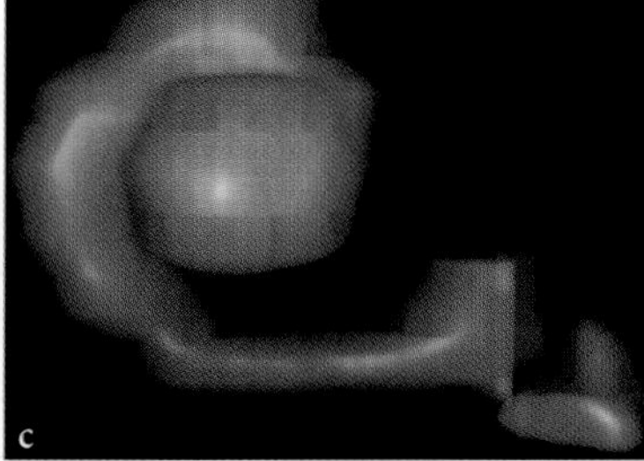

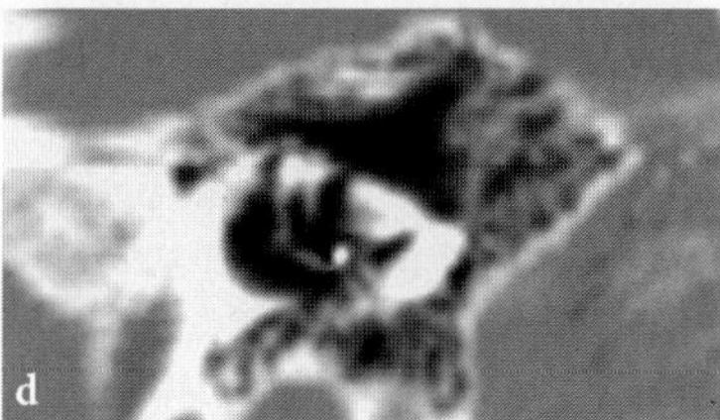

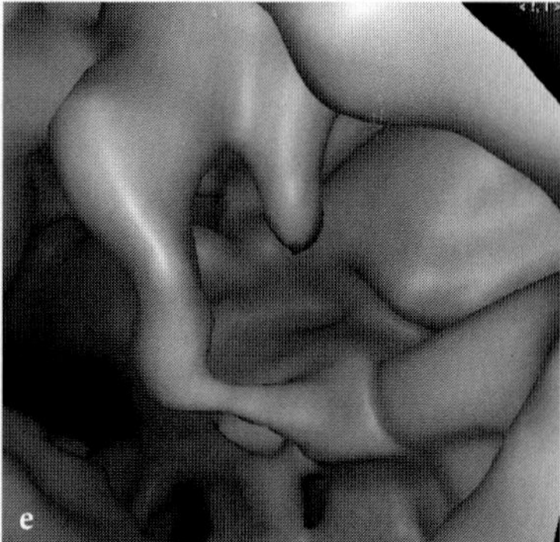

Fig. 10.21a–e. Malpositioning of the electrode of the cochlear implant at the round window. **a** Paraaxial MPR of the tympanum with the tip of the cochlear implant electrode at the round window. **b** Parasagittal MPR; introduction of the electrode into the basal cochlear turn has not been achieved. **c** 3D SSV of the cochlea and electrode tip, generated from HRCT data. **d** Axial HRCT, showing a tiny fibrous adhesion of the ossicle to the electrode. **e** Endoluminal view; the subtle finding of **d** is well recognisable by VO

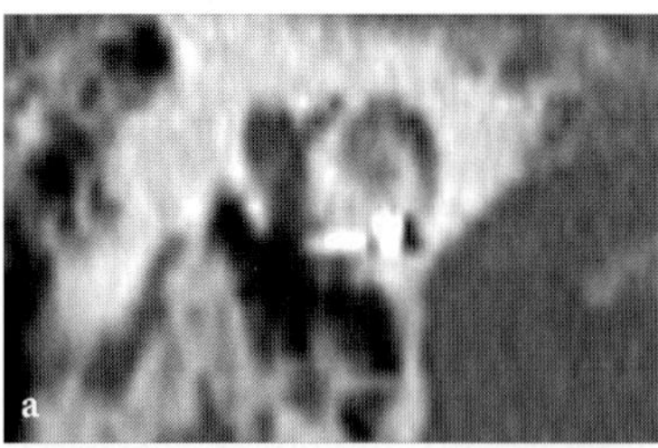

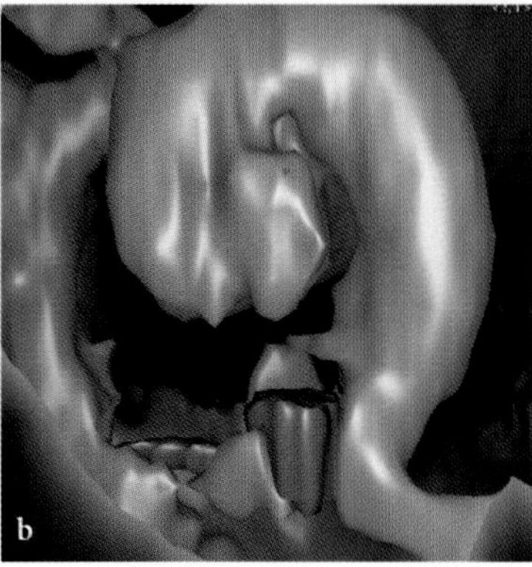

Fig. 10.22a,b. a, b Malpositioning of the cochlear implant electrode. **a** Parasagittal MPR; introduction of the electrode into the cochlea is incomplete. **b** 3D SSV generated from HRCT data, corresponding to **a**

10.5 Discussion

High-resolution cross-sectional data acquisition is required for middle and inner ear imaging. CT provides excellent visualisation of bony structures with insufficient resolution of soft tissue layers, and MR imaging provides excellent soft tissue characterisation with bony structures delivering low signal intensity, except bone marrow fat and marrow pathology. A first step in the process of working up 2D data may be multiplanar reformatting (MPR), generating 2D images along any chosen plane. This procedure is especially useful in imaging anatomic structures with longitudinal extension that cannot be captured in one orthogonal plane, such as cranial nerves VII and VIII. Assessing the integrity of physiological or iatrogenic cavities may be another reason for performing MPR. Defining a path along the facial canal in all three orthogonal planes permits complete 2D imaging of the facial canal in one picture, including the pars tympanica and pars petrosa. Maximum intensity projection (MIP) is helpful for imaging the labyrinth, but resolution of detail is limited.

Some reports about VO and related 3D techniques have been published recently (Frankenthaler et al. 1998; Hans et al. 1999; Pozzi-Muvelli et al. 1997; Seemann et al. 1998). A common finding is that VO/3D using volume rendering technique permits extensive access to middle and inner ear structures, overcoming the limitations associated with real otoscopy (Karhuketo et al. 1997) and standard postprocessing procedures.

Frankenthaler et al. commented on the start-up requirements for virtual otoscopy and listed a computer workstation, a software engineer and a research fellow. While the technical prerequisites may be affordable for a hospital with a busy ENT department, hiring a software engineer will most probably exceed budget limitations.

Hans et al. recently demonstrated that 3D labyrinth imaging superior to MIP imaging quality is achievable using VRT, although the small number of patients assessed in this study (n=13) may not permit general conclusions to be drawn regarding the routine use of this technique (Hans et al. 1999). In an ongoing study evaluating labyrinth imaging using VRT comparable to the procedure described by Hans et al., comprehensive labyrinth imaging was achieved in 19 of 21 patients. In one patient we encountered extensive fluid retention in adjacent mastoid cells, and in one patient incomplete labyrinth imaging was due to insufficient primary data acquisition.

In this chapter we have tried to outline relative indications for VO/3D as well as absolute ones. If up-to-date CSI does not reveal any abnormality or raise any suspicion whatsoever, usually there is no need to proceed with additional 3D imaging. If pathology is difficult to appreciate in the axial slices then we highly recommend considering additional imaging. The next step would be acquisition of MPR and/or MIP reconstructions. If this still is not satisfactory, VO/3D imaging should be performed. For some purposes it may be useful to consider VO right away, such as in cases of dysplasia of the ossicular chain and suspected malformation/obliteration of the labyrinth. In such cases, VO may increase the sensitivity of detecting a subtle pathological alteration and make it much easier to demonstrate such findings to the clinicians. In our experience, differences of opinion about morphologically subtle but clinically important pathology occur more rarely, since findings demonstrated by a 3D technique are often better accepted in the first place.

Virtual imaging may create virtual pathology by unintentionally eliminating structures of interest. Thus, profound knowledge of the secondary imaging techniques is indispensable for the investigator in order to identify possible artefacts and pitfalls at any point during the work-up process. If a suspicious finding cannot be retrospectively detected in both techniques, 2D as well as 3D, that "finding" probably originated somewhere in the working-up procedure.

VO/3D techniques, as secondary imaging procedures, do not deliver any information not provided by primary CSI. Nevertheless, appreciation especially of complex pathoanatomical alterations is much easier and faster with VO/3D SSV.

With the upcoming multislice detector scanners, the partial volume effects that still limit the visualisation of tiny osseous structures will be decreased further. In MRI, new imaging techniques such as 3D fast spin echo (FASE) have been reported to improve the signal-to-noise ratio and decrease the scanning time (NAGANAWA et al. 1998).

VO/3D does not require special preparation, nor are scanning time or the patient's radiation exposure increased. Compared to real endoscopic manoeuvres, emergency evaluation may not be possible as postprocessing takes time and the option of endoscopic microsurgery, of course, does not exist. On the other hand, healing defects at the membrane incision or accidental damage to middle ear structures do not occur. Other approaches, such as endoscopy via the auditory tube (EDELSTEIN et al. 1994), are still not widespread due to the requirement for special microfibreoptic equipment and to its limited intraluminal flexibility. Overall, no endoscopic technique provides more comprehensive access to the middle and inner ear than do virtual otoscopy and related 3D techniques.

10.6 Summary and Conclusion

Virtual otoscopy and related 3D techniques using VRT permit extensive access to the middle and inner ear. Complex anatomy and pathology can be displayed in an easily appreciable fashion, improving communication with the referring physician and the patient and eliminating the need for further and more invasive diagnostic procedures in some cases. Using VO/3D in the work-up may increase sensitivity in detection of slight abnormalities which are difficult to assess in cross-sectional imaging. The effectiveness of sophisticated and expensive therapeutic procedures such as cochlear implantation may benefit from the use of VO in the preoperative assessment and the postoperative follow-up. Although 3D imaging is not obligatory, it is a valuable supplementary imaging procedure.

Advances in computer and software technology may overcome the time and cost restrictions that presently prevent the widespread use of VO/3D.

It is up to the radiologist to ensure clinical acceptance of this promising new technique by carefully evaluating and correlating the 3D pathology with the original 2D data.

References

1. Casselmann JW (1996) Temporal boneimaging. Neuroimaging Clin North Am 6:265–289
2. Casselmann JW, Bensimon J-L (1994) Imaging of the inner ear. Radiologe 37:954–63
3. Casselmann JW, Majoor MHJM, Albers FW et al (1994) MR of the inner ear in patients with Cogan syndrome. Am J Neuroradiol 15: 131–138
4. Czerny C, Turetschek K, Duman M (1997) CT and MRI of the middle ear. Radiologe 37:945–53
5. Edelstein DR, Magnan, J, Parisier SC et al (1994) Microfiberoptic evaluation of the middle ear cavity. Am J Otol 15:50–53
6. Frankenthaler R, Moharir V, Kikinis R et al (1998) Virtual otoscopy. Otolaryngol Clin North Am 31:383–92
7. Hans P, Grant AJ, Laitt RD et al (1999) Comparison of three-dimensional visualization techniques for depicting the scala vestibuli and scala tympani of the cochlea by using high-resolution MR imaging. Am J Neuroradiol 20:1197–1206
8. Karhuketo TS; Puhakka HJ; Laippala PJ (1997) Endoscopy of the middle ear structures. Acta Otolaryngol Suppl Stockh 529:34–9
9. Mark AS, Fitzgerald D (1993) Segmental enhancement of the cochlea on contrast-enhanced MR:correlation with the frequency of hearing loss and possible sign of perilymphatic fistula and autoimmune labyrinthitis. Am J Neuroradiol 14:991–996
10. Naganawa S, Ito F, Fukatsu, H et al (1998) Three-dimensional fast spin echo MR of the inner ear: ultra-long ETL and half-Fourier technique. Am J Neuroradiol 19:739–41
11. Pozzi-Mucelli R, Morra A, Calgaro A. et al (1997) Virtual endoscopy with computed tomography of the anatomical structures of the middle ear. Radiol Med Torino 94:440–6
12. Seemann MD, Seemann O, Englmeier KH et al (1998) Hybrid rendering and virtual endoscopy of the auditory and vestibular system. Eur J Med Res 3:515–22
13. Valvassori G, Mafee MF, Carter BL (1995) (eds) Imaging of the head and neck, 2nd edn. Thieme, Stuttgart

Subject Index

List of Contributors

A.J. Aschoff, MD
Abteilung für Diagnostische Radiologie
Universitätsklinikum Ulm
Steinhövelstrasse 9
89075 Ulm
Germany

Clive I. Bartram, FRCP, FRCR
Intestinal Imaging 4V
St. Mark's Hospital
Northwick Park
Harrow HA1 3UJ
UK

Thorsten R. Fleiter, MD
Department of Diagnostic Imaging
University of Ulm
Steinhövelstrasse 9
89075 Ulm
Germany

Stefan Gottschalk, MD
Department of Radiology
Charité Hospital
Humboldt-Universität zu Berlin
Schumannstrasse 20/21
10117 Berlin
Germany
Medizinische Universität Lübeck
Institut für Radiologie, Neuroradiologie
Ratzeburger Allee 160
23538 Lübeck
Germany

R. Klingebiel, MD
Division of Neuroradiology
Department of Radiology
Charité Hospital
Humboldt-Universität zu Berlin
Schumannstrasse 20/21
10117 Berlin
Germany

Noga Meiri, RD
Department of Radiology
Charité Hospital
Humboldt-Universität zu Berlin
Schumannstrasse 20/21
10117 Berlin
Germany

E.M. Merkle, MD
Department of Diagnostic Imaging
University of Ulm
Steinhövelstrasse 9
89075 Ulm
Germany

Patrik Rogalla, MD
Department of Radiology
Charité Hospital
Humboldt-Universität zu Berlin
Schumannstrasse 20/21
10117 Berlin
Germany

Jeroen Terwisscha van Scheltinga, MSc
Philips Medical Systems
EasyVision Modules
P.O. Box 10000
5680 DA Best
The Netherlands

Till Hubertus Wiese, MD
Department of Radiology
Charité Hospital
Humboldt-Universität zu Berlin
Schumannstrasse 20/21
10117 Berlin
Germany

C. Wisianowsky, MD
Department of Diagnostic Imaging
University of Ulm
Steinhövelstrasse 9
89075 Ulm
Germany

Medical Radiology
Diagnostic Imaging and Radiation Oncology

Titles in the series already published

Diagnostic Imaging

Innovations in Diagnostic Imaging
Edited by J.H. Anderson

Radiology of the Upper Urinary Tract
Edited by E.K. Lang

The Thymus - Diagnostic Imaging, Functions, and Pathologic Anatomy
Edited by E. Walter, E. Willich, and W.R. Webb

Interventional Neuroradiology
Edited by A. Valavanis

Radiology of the Pancreas
Edited by A.L. Baert, co-edited by G. Delorme

Radiology of the Lower Urinary Tract
Edited by E.K. Lang

Magnetic Resonance Angiography
Edited by I.P. Arlart, G.M. Bongartz, and G. Marchal

Contrast-Enhanced MRI of the Breast
S. Heywang-Köbrunner and R. Beck

Spiral CT of the Chest
Edited by M. Rémy-Jardin and J. Rémy

Radiological Diagnosis of Breast Diseases
Edited by M. Friedrich and E.A. Sickles

Radiology of the Trauma
Edited by M. Heller and A. Fink

Biliary Tract Radiology
Edited by P. Rossi

Radiological Imaging of Sports Injuries
Edited by C. Masciocchi

Modern Imaging of the Alimentary Tube
Edited by A. R. Margulis

Diagnosis and Therapy of Spinal Tumors
Edited by P. R. Algra, J. Valk, and J. J. Heimans

Interventional Magnetic Resonance Imaging
Edited by J. F. Debatin and G. Adam

Abdominal and Pelvic MRI
Edited by A. Heuck and M. Reiser

Orthopedic Imaging
Techniques and Applications
Edited by A.M. Davies and H. Pettersson

Radiology of the Female Pelvic Organs
Edited by E.K.Lang

Magnetic Resonance of the Heart and Great Vessels
Clinical Applications
Edited by J. Bogaert, A. J. Duerinckx, and F. E. Rademakers

Modern Head and Neck Imaging
Edited by S. K. Mukherji and J. A. Castelijns

Radiological Imaging of Endocrine Diseases
Edited by J. N. Bruneton in collaboration with B. Padovani and M.-Y. Mourou

Trends in Contrast Media
Edited by H. S. Thomsen, R. N. Muller, and R. F. Mattrey

Functional MRI
Edited by C. T. W. Moonen and P. A. Bandettini

Radiology of the Pancreas
2nd Revised Edition
Edited by A. L. Baert
Co-edited by G. Delorme and L. Van Hoe

Emergency Pediatric Radiology
Edited by H. Carty

Spiral CT of the Abdomen
Edited by F. Terrier, M. Grossholz, and C. D. Becker

Liver Malignancies
Diagnostic and Interventional Radiology
Edited by C. Bartolozzi and R. Lencioni

Medical Imaging of the Spleen
Edited by A. M. De Schepper and F. Vanhoenacker

Radiology of Peripheral Vascular Diseases
Edited by E. Zeitler

Diagnostic Nuclear Medicine
Edited by C. Schiepers

Radiology of Blunt Trauma of the Chest
P. Schnyder and M. Wintermark

Portal Hypertension
Diagnostic Imaging-Guided Therapy
Edited by P. Rossi
Co-edited by P. Ricci and L. Broglia

Virtual Endoscopy and Related 3D Techniques
Edited by P. Rogalla, J. Terwisscha Van Scheltinga, and B. Hamm

Recent Advances in Diagnostic Neuroradiology
Edited by Ph. Demaerel

Transfontanellar Doppler Imaging in Neonates
A. Couture and C. Veyrac

Springer

MEDICAL RADIOLOGY
Diagnostic Imaging and Radiation Oncology

Titles in the series already published

RADIATION ONCOLOGY

Lung Cancer
Edited by C.W. Scarantino

Innovations in Radiation Oncology
Edited by H.R. Withers and L.J. Peters

Radiation Therapy of Head and Neck Cancer
Edited by G.E. Laramore

Gastrointestinal Cancer – Radiation Therapy
Edited by R.R. Dobelbower, Jr.

Radiation Exposure and Occupational Risks
Edited by E. Scherer, C. Streffer, and K.-R. Trott

Radiation Therapy of Benign Diseases - A Clinical Guide
S.E. Order and S.S. Donaldson

Interventional Radiation Therapy Techniques - Brachytherapy
Edited by R. Sauer

Radiopathology of Organs and Tissues
Edited by E. Scherer, C. Streffer, and K.-R. Trott

Concomitant Continuous Infusion Chemotherapy and Radiation
Edited by M. Rotman and C.J. Rosenthal

Intraoperative Radiotherapy – Clinical Experiences and Results
Edited by F.A. Calvo, M. Santos, and L.W. Brady

Radiotherapy of Intraocular and Orbital Tumors
Edited by W.E. Alberti and R.H. Sagerman

Interstitial and Intracavitary Thermoradiotherapy
Edited by M.H. Seegenschmiedt and R. Sauer

Non-Disseminated Breast Cancer
Controversial Issues in Management
Edited by G.H. Fletcher and S.H. Levitt

Current Topics in Clinical Radiobiology of Tumors
Edited by H.-P. Beck-Bornholdt

Practical Approaches to Cancer Invasion and Metastases
A Compendium of Radiation Oncologists' Responses to 40 Histories
Edited by A.R. Kagan with the Assistance of R.J. Steckel

Radiation Therapy in Pediatric Oncology
Edited by J.R. Cassady

Radiation Therapy Physics
Edited by A.R. Smith

Late Sequelae in Oncology
Edited by J. Dunst and R. Sauer

Mediastinal Tumors. Update 1995
Edited by D.E. Wood and C.R. Thomas, Jr.

Thermoradiotherapy and Thermochemotherapy

Volume 1:
Biology, Physiology, and Physics

Volume 2:
Clinical Applications
Edited by M.H. Seegenschmiedt, P. Fessenden, and C.C. Vernon

Carcinoma of the Prostate
Innovations in Management
Edited by Z. Petrovich, L. Baert, and L.W. Brady

Radiation Oncology of Gynecological Cancers
Edited by H.W. Vahrson

Carcinoma of the Bladder
Innovations in Management
Edited by Z. Petrovich, L. Baert, and L.W. Brady

Blood Perfusion and Microenvironment of Human Tumors
Implications for Clinical Radiooncology
Edited by M. Molls and P. Vaupel

Radiation Therapy of Benign Diseases. A Clinical Guide
2nd Revised Edition
S.E. Order and S.S. Donaldson

Carcinoma of the Kidney and Testis, and Rare Urologic Malignancies
Innovations in Management
Edited by Z. Petrovich, L. Baert, and L.W. Brady

Progress and Perspectives in the Treatment of Lung Cancer
Edited by P. Van Houtte, J. Klastersky, and P. Rocmans

Combined Modality Therapy of Central Nervous System Tumors
Edited by Z. Petrovich, L. W. Brady, M. L. Apuzzo, and M. Bamberg

Age-Related Macular Degeneration
Current Treatment Concepts
Edited by W. A. Alberti, G. Richard, and R. H. Sagerman

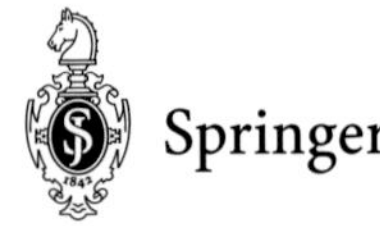

Springer